D1366645

THE POCKET

calorie counter

the complete, discreet, and portable guide for managing your health

SUZANNE BEILENSON

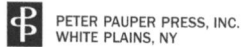

PETER PAUPER PRESS, INC.
WHITE PLAINS, NY

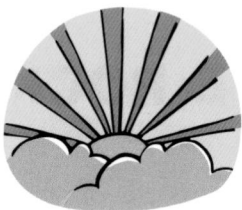

Designed by Heather Zschock
Illustrations copyright © 2010 Kerren Barbas Steckler

Copyright © 2010
Peter Pauper Press, Inc.
202 Mamaroneck Avenue
White Plains, NY 10601
All rights reserved
ISBN 978-1-59359-648-4
Printed in Hong Kong
7 6 5 4 3

Visit us at www.peterpauper.com

The content contained within this book is for general information purposes only, and is not meant to substitute for the advice provided by a medical practitioner. Consult your physician before initiating any dietary or exercise program. Peter Pauper Press, Inc., makes no claims or guarantees whatsoever regarding the accuracy, interpretation, or utilization of any information provided in this book. The nutrient values for prepared foods are subject to change and may differ from the listings contained in this book, which are based on the USDA guidelines. The information presented in this book does not constitute a recommendation or endorsement of any company or product. The author and publisher disclaim any liability arising directly or indirectly from the use of this book.

THE POCKET

calorie counter

the complete, discreet, and portable guide for managing your health

contents

introduction

It's all about choice. Every day, we have to choose what foods we are going to put into our bodies. And those decisions really matter because they affect our weight, our health, and our longevity.

It can be daunting to choose well when we have so many options. Not only are our kitchens full of different foods, but we have a huge variety of restaurant and take-out foods available. Did you know that supermarkets on average carry 45,000 items? (It's estimated that in 1949 supermarkets carried only 3,750 items.) The choices are overwhelming, and it's no wonder we have trouble making the right decisions.

That's where *The Pocket Calorie Counter* can help you simplify your life, lose weight, and become healthier. We've compiled information on the **calories**, **total fat**, **saturated fat**, **sodium**, **carbohydrates**, **fiber**, and **protein** for thousands and thousands of foods. Not only will you find this information on the foods that we buy and cook ourselves based on data provided by the United States Department of Agriculture (www.usda.gov), but you'll also find nutritional information from many popular **chain restaurants** and **fast-food outlets**. As you consider which foods to eat, simply look them up and find out which ones have fewer calories, less fat and sodium, and more fiber and protein.

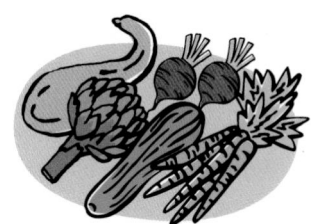

Bring *The Pocket Calorie Counter* with you wherever you go. It can help you make better choices. (And its discreet design lets you make those choices privately!)

understanding nutrition

As the saying goes, we are what we eat. But what exactly are we eating? A French fry may just be a fried potato (and a yummy one at that!), but at a chemical level, it's a combination of fat, carbohydrates, protein, sodium, and more.

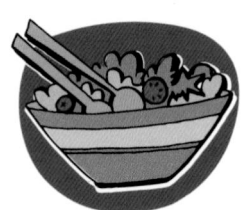

We can compare different foods by looking at the energy and nutrients they provide. Understanding the nutritional content of food is vital to ensure we provide our bodies with what they need to function properly. Since there's no one perfect food, we must eat a variety of foods to capture all the nutrients we need to stay healthy. It can be complicated, however, to follow a diet that's nutrient-rich, but not overloaded with calories.

energy and weight loss
CALORIES

Calories are the measure of energy contained in a food. Calories are not bad—in fact, they are essential. Our bodies need them to function properly, from taking a breath to running a marathon. Without calories, our bodies would come to a grinding halt.

Your body converts calories into physical energy. Any extra calories you consume that aren't used are stored as fat. If you consume fewer calories than your body needs, your body will start burning stored fat to get the energy it requires.

WEIGHT LOSS

For all the hype and fad diets that abound, weight loss really comes down to a simple equation. *Calories consumed minus calories used* determines whether you gain or lose weight. If you consume more calories than your body burns, you gain weight. If you burn more calories than you consume, you lose weight.

Every pound of fat on your body is equivalent to 3,500 calories that did not get used. So to lose a pound a week, divide 3,500 calories by 7 days, and reduce your intake by 500 calories per day or burn an extra 500 calories a day—or some combination of the two.

The bottom line? To lose weight, you have to eat less, burn more, or do both.

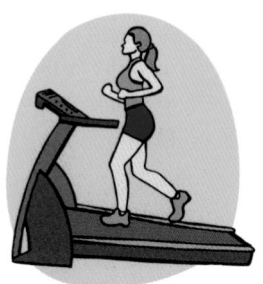

But note: Consuming too *few* calories will not necessarily get you to your goal faster! If you're not eating enough, your body will lower your BMR (Basal Metabolic Rate, *see page 12*) in order to conserve its fat stores. A lower BMR means that instead of needing perhaps 1,500 calories a day, you may only require 1,000. So, if you're consuming 1,200 that may be 200 too many, and you may actually gain weight! See what a tricky business this can be?

It's also important to lose *no more than two pounds* per week. When you lose weight faster than that, you actually lose muscle, not fat. You definitely want to avoid doing that. Losing muscle tissue slows down your metabolism, making you work even harder to burn the same calories!

On the other hand, the more muscle you have, the more calories you burn and the easier it is to burn them. That's because the body uses up more calories to simply sustain muscle tissue. What a great reason to get to the gym!

Our best tips to tip the scale in the right direction:

- Get moving. The more you move, the more calories you burn. So, while it's terrific if you're working out at the gym, don't forget that you can add more activity to your day without "exercising." How? Take the stairs instead of the elevator. Walk the kids to school instead of driving them. Carry a basket while you shop for food instead of using a cart. (You'll buy less too!) Any movement you can build into your daily routine can quickly add up to a surprising number of calories burned.

- Break up your exercise. Many people don't feel like they have an hour or more to spend exercising. So, take a 20-minute walk after every meal. It doesn't matter to your body whether you exercise all at once or if you split it up.

- Take ownership of your food. If you're a fast food junkie or always buying pre-made, pre-packaged food, consider a cooking class. A cooking class, and I'm trying to lose weight? Yup. Because when you cook for yourself, you are fully conscious of what's going into the food you eat, from the amount of salt you add to the type of oil you use. You can often prepare the same dish that you might have bought, but with fewer calories and more wholesome ingredients. And when you've gone to the trouble to cook, enjoy the fruits of your labor . . . which brings us to the next weight loss tip.

- Slow down. Don't be a turkey and gobble your food. Enjoy it. Savor it. Chew it thoroughly. Put your fork down between bites. It takes 15 minutes or more for your brain to get the message that you're full. Eating slower means you'll have consumed less by the time your brain realizes you're satisfied.

- Ditch the "grab" habit. A handful of chips here, a spoonful of ice cream there. When you grab a little food, it may seem like it doesn't count . . . but the calories do. Be aware that whether you eat at the table, in the car, or on the go, it all counts.

- Write it down. Keep a daily food diary, recording everything you eat *before* you eat it. Not only will writing down *everything* you eat help you say "no" to that handful of chips, it can also reveal your eating patterns and triggers. Are you eating the leftovers off your kids' plates because you hate waste? Has your late-morning coffee break turned into a coffee and muffin break? Are you eating after you had a fight with your mother? Being aware of when and why you eat is the first step to making real changes in your diet.

- Snack! The reason we often "grab" food is because we're hungry. If you want to make good eating choices and lose weight, you can't be hungry! That's when the pangs in your stomach overpower your good intentions. So snack, but plan your snacks in advance and be sure to include some protein, which will leave you feeling fuller for longer. So, cut up extra celery sticks to have with low-fat peanut butter. Or have low-fat string cheese and a piece of fresh fruit. A couple of well-timed snacks each day will help keep you on track.

- Quit drinking up calories! Just because you're not chewing doesn't mean you're not swallowing. If you currently drink a can of regular soda or a glass of wine a day, and you replace it with water, you'll lose 10 pounds in a year.

- Use a plate! When you eat directly out of a bag of chips or a container of ice cream, it's difficult to know how much you're actually consuming. Put your food on a plate or in a bowl so that you can control your portion size.

- Now use a smaller plate—because the "eyes" have it. It's important that what you see looks satisfying. It's natural to want to fill up that plate. Just use smaller ones. The same portion of food that looked skimpy on a large dinner plate will seem far more generous on a smaller lunch plate. A similar strategy can work for dessert too. Fill half your bowl with fresh fruit before adding ice cream or frozen yogurt. You'll reduce the amount of high-calorie food, but it will be visually filling!

- Weigh yourself regularly. Get on the scale at least once a week. If you've had a small weight gain, it's easier to get back on track. If you've lost weight, it's a big motivator to keep up the good work!

basal metabolic rate

Welcome to your Basal Metabolic Rate! Your BMR indicates the calories your body needs per day to survive without moving. First, calculate your BMR using the formula below. Now, multiply that number by 1.2—the result is the number of calories you need to maintain weight. If you don't ingest enough calories for the day, you'll do more harm than good. Cutting too many calories will lower your BMR. In general, if you're trying to lose weight, aim for a loss of 1 to 2 pounds a week, no more.

Here's the formula:

Women: BMR = 655 + (4.35 x weight in pounds) + (4.7 x height in inches) - (4.7 x age in years)

Men: BMR = 66 + (6.23 x weight in pounds) + (12.7 x height in inches) - (6.8 x age in years)

daily recommended caloric intake

According to American College of Sports Medicine (ACSM), calories consumed should be no less than 1,200 for women, and 1,800 for men.

If you reduce net calories (by eating 500 fewer calories a day and/or exercising), you'll be able to lose 1 pound a week. You need 3,500 fewer calories than required by your BMR to burn off one pound (500 x 7 days = 3,500 calories).

body mass index

The dreaded Body Mass Index! A good indicator of body fatness, your BMI should stay below 25. The formula below tells how to find yours. Height is measured without shoes and weight without clothes.

BMI = Weight in pounds divided by height in inches squared. Multiply result by 703. End product is your BMI.

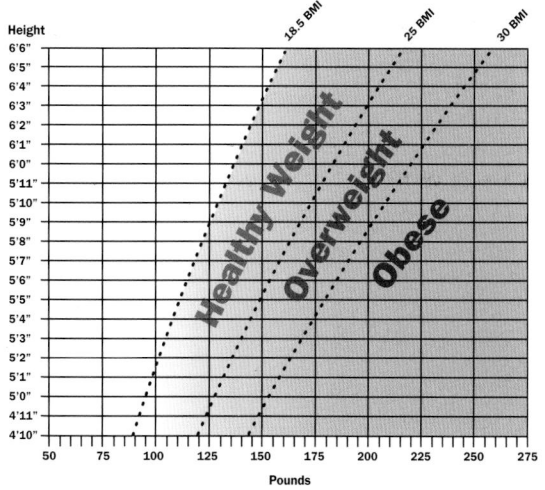

Here are guidelines for healthy body fat percentages, by age and gender. You can ascertain your body fat with a specialized scale or with help from a personal trainer.*

AGE	WOMEN	MEN
20-39	21% to 32%	8% to 19%
40-59	23% to 33%	11% to 21%
60 and up	24% to 35%	13% to 24%

*In addition, BMI should be between 18.5 and 24.9

portion control

American food industry portions are out of control. Ask someone from another country what they think of an individual restaurant portion here and you'll likely hear it would feed their entire family!

Here are some USDA guidelines that may help you visualize proper portion sizes:

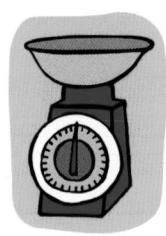

Protein/meat	3 oz (size of your palm or a deck of cards)
Carbs/pasta/rice	1/2 cup (size of a tennis ball or baseball cut in half)
Fruits	1 cup (size of a tennis ball or baseball)
Cheese	1 oz (size of 4 dice or your thumb)
Bagel	Average serving: hockey puck size
Potato	Medium serving: size of a computer mouse
Peanut butter/butter	1 tsp (the tip of your thumb)
Bread	1 slice
Pancake	1 (size of a CD/DVD)
Vegetables	1/2 cup cooked (size of a tennis ball or baseball cut in half)
Lettuce	1 cup (4 leaves)
Milk/yogurt	1 cup (size of a tennis ball or baseball)
Nuts	8 (handful)

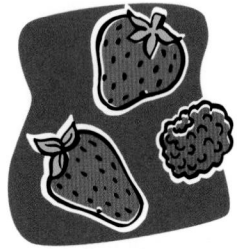

If you're having a hard time judging sizes, consider investing in a food scale. That way you can weigh and portion out food in advance. Do it when you get home from the grocery store. Try putting meats, veggies, and especially snacks in individual storage bags.

food groups

When it comes to supplying the calories our bodies need for fuel, there are three energy- and nutrient-loaded food groups: **fat**, **carbohydrates** (which include **fiber**), and **protein**. Fat provides nine calories per gram, while carbohydrates and protein provide four calories per gram. Fat, carbohydrates, and protein are sometimes called **macronutrients** because we require large quantities of them. Other substances like vitamins and minerals are considered micronutrients because, while necessary, we need far less of them in our diet.

FAT

You need fat. You really do. It's an important nutrient that ensures your body functions properly, from providing you with energy to helping you make estrogen, testosterone, and even Vitamin D. **In fact, it's recommended that 25% to 30% of your calories come from fat!**

So what's the problem? First, fat is a high-calorie nutrient. It doesn't take much fat to hit your recommended intake. Second, the foods found in nature contain two types of fat—saturated and unsaturated—and they're not created equal. Saturated fat is linked to a whole host of health problems, particularly coronary heart disease. What's more, your body can produce all of the saturated fat it requires, so there's no health benefit to eating it.

Luckily, *unsaturated* fats have great health benefits. These fats can improve cholesterol levels, reduce inflammation, and help your heart. Better yet, most people don't get enough unsaturated fats. So make it a habit to consume unsaturated fats while watching your overall calorie intake.

Tips for getting the right fats into your diet:

- Eat foods that are good sources of unsaturated fats. These include nuts, avocados, pumpkin and sesame seeds, flax seeds, and fish and vegetable oils (canola, peanut, olive, sunflower, corn, and soybean).

- Reduce saturated fat by avoiding these foods: butter, whole-fat milk, ice cream, palm and coconut oils, high-fat cheeses, and high-fat cuts of meat.

- Swap out solid fats like butter or stick margarine with liquid oils. Try dipping bread in olive oil rather than spreading on the butter.

- Check the label on pre-packaged food to avoid palm and coconut oils which are often used in commercial bakeries.

- Replace whole milk with low-fat or skim milk.

- Ditch the skin on poultry. Don't eat the skin or leave it on when you cook.

- Eat more fish and less meat, and when you do go for red meat, opt for a leaner cut like sirloin.

CARBOHYDRATES

Carbohydrates come in all shapes, sizes, and colors, from red raspberries to milk, from orange sweet potatoes to wild rice. Of all the nutrients we need, carbs offer the greatest choice and provide our main source of energy, along with vitamins, minerals, and fiber. Talk about multitasking!

But different carbs are digested at different rates. Some are slowly processed into blood sugar, while others, such as potatoes, are quickly converted into blood sugar and give us quick bursts of energy. Diabetes, heart disease, and other conditions have been linked to diets high in these types of "fast" carbs.

About 50% of the calories you consume should come from carbohydrates, and complex, "slow" carbs should dominate your

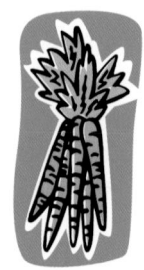

diet. "Slow" carbs keep you feeling fuller, and may improve your blood pressure and cholesterol. You can find these carbs (and not a lot of added calories!) in fruits, vegetables, beans, and whole-grain foods. See the next page for information about incorporating fiber—that carb essential for digestive health—into your diet.

Some good ideas to get good carbs:

- Make your diet colorful. Choose foods that are richly colored, from fuchsia beets and dark green broccoli to blueberries and peachy peaches.

- Skip the added sugar. Packaged foods often come with added sugar, not to mention added calories and fewer nutrients.

- Switch out potatoes with grains such as barley, quinoa, and millet.

- Less processing is better. The more processing a food has undergone before you eat it, the faster your body will convert it to blood sugar. So, skip the fruit juice and eat whole fruits instead. Also, stay away from "milled," "refined," or "finely ground" grains.

- Expand your horizons. Try whole-wheat pasta!

- Give beans a whirl. They'll keep you satisfied longer since your body digests them slowly.

FIBER

Fiber is the freebie of the carbohydrate world. The body can't digest fiber, so it passes through us, grabbing fatty substances as it goes, thus helping to reduce cholesterol levels. Fiber also gets things moving in the intestinal track—say goodbye to constipation! And if that weren't enough, fiber keeps food in your stomach longer, thereby keeping you feeling fuller longer. Now that's a nutrient everyone can love. **Recommended amounts of fiber: 25–40 grams daily.**

How can you get recommended daily amounts of fiber?

- Eat "slow" carbs; fruits, vegetables, beans, and whole grains are good sources of fiber.

- Swap out those potato chips for popcorn!

- Make legumes the main course. Try black bean soup or chili made with beans for a high-fiber entrée.

- Throw a handful of rinsed chickpeas into your salad.

- Choose breads with a fiber content of more than 3 grams per slice.

PROTEIN

Protein is the one nutrient of which most people get enough. Eating a varied diet generally takes care of our protein needs. That's good news because proteins are found in every cell of our bodies.

So what exactly is protein? Proteins are strings of molecules known as amino acids. Our bodies can actually produce some of those amino acids. The others have to come from the foods we eat. Sometimes you'll hear a food called a "complete protein," which means that it contains all of the essential amino acids we need. Complete proteins are often found in animal-based foods like meat, chicken, fish, and dairy. Vegetarians have to be extra careful to get enough complete proteins. Many foods are high only in certain amino acids, but can provide a complete package when combined with other foods. For example, rice and beans is a power pair, as is peanut butter on whole wheat bread!

Protein is your friend. Eating protein keeps you feeling fuller longer than eating carbohydrates. The extra bonus? Your body burns more calories digesting protein than it does carbs! **Protein should make up 25%–35% of your daily caloric intake**. On a 1,500 calories a day plan, that would be 375–525 calories (or 94–132 grams/3.5 to 4 oz).

Take your pick of these excellent protein choices:

- Leaner cuts of meat
- Skinless chicken and turkey
- Low-fat or fat-free dairy products like milk, yogurt, or cheese
- Nuts, seeds, and legumes such as beans, lentils, or chickpeas
- Tofu, soybeans, or other soy-based foods

about sodium

When it comes to sodium, a little goes a long way. Sodium helps balance the amount of water in your cells, but too much sodium leads to excess fluid in your blood. Excess fluid makes your heart work harder, and that in turn, can lead to hypertension, kidney disease, and even diabetes.

How much sodium do you need? **The experts recommend a diet that has between 1,500 and 2,400 milligrams per day**. If you think that sounds like a lot, think again. One teaspoon of table salt contains over 2,300 milligrams of sodium!

For most people, though, overusing the salt shaker is not the problem. More than 70% of our sodium intake comes from processed and prepared food. When you're at the store, it's crucial to read the ingredient list! Also, many foods are packed *with* sodium even if they don't contain salt. Look out for any ingredient that contains the word *sodium* or *soda*, such as "monosodium glutamate," "baking soda," and "sodium nitrate."

Keep your sodium intake in check with these strategies:

- Condiments, salad dressings, and sauces are often high in sodium. Limit how much ketchup, mustard, and relish you use at your next barbecue.

- Wave bye-bye to breakfast meat. That bacon, sausage, or ham you're having with your omelet is shooting your sodium levels sky-high.

- Spice up your diet. Add flavor with herbs and spices, rather than salt.

- Be fresh. Fresh meats, fruits, and vegetables generally have lower sodium levels than their processed counterparts.

- Wash it. When you rinse canned food, you wash away some of the sodium.

- De-salt your fat! Substitute canola or olive oil for butter or margarine.

nutrition label tips

Nutrition labels contain a wealth of information. Here are things to note:

- Watch the serving size!

- 5% is low and 20% is high for all nutrients.

- 40 calories is low, 100 is moderate, and 400 is high.

- Keep saturated fats, sodium, and sugar LOW.

- Keep protein and fiber HIGH.

- Keep in mind Nutrition Facts are based on a 2,000 calorie/day diet—adjust accordingly.

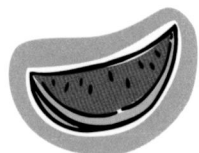

using *the pocket calorie counter*

For every food in *The Pocket Calorie Counter*, we've given the calorie and nutrient information for a designated portion size. However, you may want to use a different measure. The table below will help you easily convert one portion size to another.

Equivalents

Teaspoon	Tablespoon	Cup	Fluid Ounce	Pints+
1 tsp	1/3 tbsp			
3 tsp	1 tbsp			
	2 tbsp	1/8 cup	1 fl oz	
	4 tbsp	1/4 cup	2 fl oz	
	8 tbsp	1/2 cup	4 fl oz	
	12 tbsp	3/4 cup	6 fl oz	
	16 tbsp	1 cup	8 fl oz	1/2 pint
		2 cups	16 fl oz	1 pint
		4 cups	32 fl oz	1 quart
		16 cups	128 fl oz	1 gallon

setting goals: where we want to be

It's time to set some goals. Want to drop 20 pounds by summer? Want to firm up and lower your blood pressure? Find out where you need to be, then set small goals. Sometimes larger goals throw us off track because they seem so, well, big. Small steps help us get there without despair.

WEIGHT

Check out the accompanying government chart of healthy, overweight, and obese weights. Remember, these are only guidelines. Not everyone is made the same. Some people will be healthy at a higher weight than this suggests. Some may need to weigh less. Each of us is unique. Our cultural background can predetermine our body composition through DNA. Strive to be healthy, not thin.

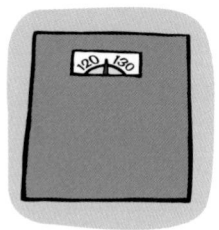

BMI	19	20	21	22	23	24	25	26	27	28	29	30	31	32	33	34	35
Height								Weight in pounds									
4'10"	91	96	100	105	110	115	119	124	129	134	138	143	148	153	158	162	167
4'11"	94	99	104	109	114	119	124	128	133	138	143	148	153	158	163	168	173
5'	97	102	107	112	118	123	128	133	138	143	148	153	158	163	168	174	179
5'1"	100	106	111	116	122	127	132	137	143	148	153	158	164	169	174	180	185
5'2"	104	109	115	120	126	131	136	142	147	153	158	164	169	175	180	186	191
5'3"	107	113	118	124	130	135	141	146	152	158	163	169	175	180	186	191	197
5'4"	110	116	122	128	134	140	145	151	157	163	169	174	180	186	192	197	204
5'5"	114	120	126	132	138	144	150	156	162	168	174	180	186	192	198	204	210
5'6"	118	124	130	136	142	148	155	161	167	173	179	186	192	198	204	210	216
5'7"	121	127	134	140	146	153	159	166	172	178	185	191	198	204	211	217	223
5'8"	125	131	138	144	151	158	164	171	177	184	190	197	203	210	216	223	230
5'9"	128	135	142	149	155	162	169	176	182	189	196	203	209	216	223	230	236
5'10"	132	139	146	153	160	167	174	181	188	195	202	209	216	222	229	236	243
5'11"	136	143	150	157	165	172	179	186	193	200	208	215	222	229	236	243	250
6'	140	147	154	162	169	177	184	191	199	206	213	221	228	235	242	250	258
6'1"	144	151	159	166	174	182	189	197	204	212	219	227	235	242	250	257	265
6'2"	148	155	163	171	179	186	194	202	210	218	225	233	241	249	256	264	272
6'3"	152	160	168	176	184	192	200	208	216	224	232	240	248	256	264	272	279
	Healthy						Overweight						Obese				

BLOOD PRESSURE

Your blood pressure should be below 120/80.

RESTING HEART RATE (RHR)

You should be aiming for a RHR between 60 and 80 beats per minute. In order to determine your RHR, first take your pulse, best done when you get up in the morning. Place your forefinger and middle finger on your wrist pulse point. Have a clock or watch with a second hand (or a digital version) nearby. Count the number of pulses in a given time period (i.e., count for 10 seconds, and multiply that number by 6 to get your beats per minute. Or count for 30 seconds and multiply by 2). That's your

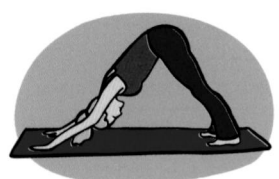

RHR. It should be between 50 and 100. Most people have a RHR around 70. The more active you are, the lower your RHR will get. The lower your RHR, the better your cardiovascular health.

You want to get your heart rate up during activity to burn more calories. Your Maximum Heart Rate is 220 minus your age. If you're 33, that would be 187 beats per minute (220 – 33 = 187 MHR). For optimum fat-burning benefits during exercise, keep that heart rate between 60% and 85% of your MHR. Do the math, multiplying your MHR by .6 or .85, to figure out where your heart rate should be for the best fat burn.

Now, while the "fat-burning zone" will burn a higher percentage of fat, the cardio zone will burn more calories and a higher *amount* of fat. Thus, if you can keep it up in the cardio zone, you'll see better results. The faster your heart beats, the speedier your metabolism.

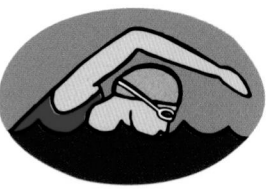

(That's why most "diet" pills have caffeine in them.)

WAIST TO HIP RATIO

This is actually said to be one of the best indicators of overall health, as body fat stored around your midsection is a risk factor for heart disease. Work to get and keep this ratio low. To determine Waist to Hip Ratio, you'll need a tape measure. Measure your hips around the widest part of your buttocks. Then measure your waist where it's smallest, above the belly button. Divide the waist measurement by the hip measurement. Cardiovascular risk is higher for women with ratios higher than 0.85, and for men with ratios above 0.90.

getting started

First, take some time to check the nutritional information on the foods you eat on a regular basis. You may find some foods are more caloric than you realize or that your protein intake is too low. Armed with that knowledge, you can begin to make modifications to your diet that will get you healthier and more energetic. Most important, make changes that you can live

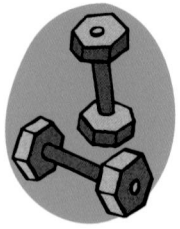

with over the long haul. Because it's not just about losing weight, adding fiber, or eating good fats in the short term. It's about being able to maintain a new style of eating for years to come.

You've already taken the first step. Now just turn the page and you'll be on your way to a more nutritious way of life!

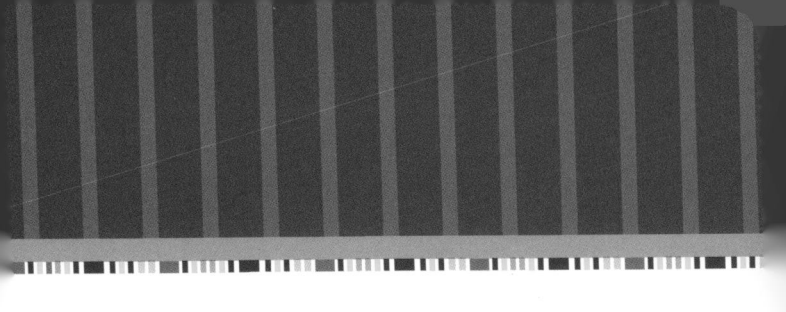

food

ITEM DESCRIPTION	Serving Size	Calories	Total Fat (g)	Saturated Fat (g)	Sodium (mg)	Carbohydrates (g)	Fiber (g)	Protein (g)
ABALONE (fried)	3 oz	161	6	1	502	9	0	17
ABIYUCH (fresh)	1/2 cup	79	0	0	23	20	6	2
ACEROLA (fresh)	1 fruit	2	0	0	0	0	0	0
ACEROLA JUICE (fresh)	1 cup	56	1	0	7	12	1	1
ACORN FLOUR	1 oz	142	9	1	0	15	0	2
ACORN SQUASH								
Baked, cubed	1 cup	115	0	0	8	30	9	2
Boiled, mashed	1 cup	83	0	0	7	22	6	2
Fresh, cubed	1 cup	56	0	0	4	15	2	1
ADOBO FRESCO	1 tbsp	49	4	1	3087	3	0	0
ADZUKI BEANS								
Canned, sweetened	1 cup	702	0	0	645	163	0	11
Dried, boiled	1 cup	294	0	0	18	57	17	17
Yokan	1 slice	36	0	0	12	9	0	0
ALFALFA SPROUTS (fresh)	1/4 cup	2	0	0	0	0	0	1
ALLSPICE (ground)	1 tbsp	16	1	0	5	4	1	0
ALMOND BUTTER								
Plain, w/o salt	1 tbsp	101	9	1	2	3	1	2
Plain, w/ salt	1 tbsp	101	9	1	72	3	1	2
ALMOND OIL	1 tbsp	120	14	1	0	0	0	0
ALMOND PASTE	1 oz	130	8	1	3	13	1	3
ALMONDS								
Blanched	1 oz	165	14	1	8	6	3	6
Dry roasted, w/o salt	1 oz	169	15	1	0	5	3	6
Dry roasted, w/ salt	1 oz	169	15	1	96	5	3	6
Honey roasted, unblanched	1 oz	168	14	1	37	8	4	5
Oil roasted, w/o salt	1 oz	172	16	1	0	5	3	6
Oil roasted, w/ salt	1 oz	172	16	1	96	5	3	6
Raw	10	69	6	0	0	3	2	3
Sugar coated	1 pc	17	1	0	0	2	0	0
AMARANTH								
Grain, cooked	1 cup	251	4	0	15	46	5	9
Leaves, boiled	1 cup	28	0	0	28	5	0	3
Leaves, fresh	1 cup	6	0	0	6	1	0	1

ITEM DESCRIPTION	Serving Size	Calories	Total Fat (g)	Saturated Fat (g)	Sodium (mg)	Carbohydrates (g)	Fiber (g)	Protein (g)
ANCHOVY								
European, canned in oil	1 oz	60	3	1	1040	0	0	8
European, fresh	3 oz	111	4	1	88	0	0	17
ANISE SEED (whole)	1 tbsp	23	1	0	1	3	1	1
APPLE BUTTER	1 tbsp	29	0	0	3	7	0	0
APPLE CRISP	1/2 cup	227	5	1	495	43	2	2
APPLE DRINKS								
Apple cider-flavored drink, low calorie	8 fl oz	2	0	0	34	1	0	0
Apple-grape juice	8 fl oz	125	0	0	18	31	0	0
Apple-grape-pear juice	8 fl oz	130	0	0	13	32	0	0
APPLE JUICE								
Canned or bottled, (unsweetened)	8 fl oz	114	0	0	10	28	0	0
Concentrate, unsweetened, diluted	8 fl oz	112	0	0	17	28	0	0
Concentrate, unsweetened, undiluted	6 fl oz	350	1	0	53	87	0	1
APPLE PIE FILLING (canned)	21 oz	595	1	0	280	155	6	1
APPLES								
Boiled, w/o skin, slices	1 cup	91	1	0	2	23	4	0
Canned, sweetened, slices	1 cup	137	1	0	6	34	4	0
Dried, stewed, w/ added sugar	1 cup	232	0	0	53	58	5	1
Dried, stewed, w/o added sugar	1 cup	145	0	0	51	39	5	1
Dried, uncooked	1 cup	209	0	0	75	57	7	1
Fresh, whole	1 med	72	0	0	1	19	3	0
Fresh, w/o skin, slices	1 cup	53	0	0	0	14	1	0
Fresh, w/ skin, slices	1 cup	57	0	0	1	15	3	0
Frozen, unsweetened, heated, slices	1 cup	97	1	0	6	25	4	1
Frozen, unsweetened, unheated, slices	1 cup	83	1	0	5	21	3	0
Microwaved, w/o skin, slices	1 cup	95	1	0	2	25	5	0
APPLESAUCE								
Sweetened, w/o salt	1 cup	167	0	0	5	43	3	0
Sweetened, w/ salt	1 cup	194	0	0	71	51	3	0
Unsweetened	1 cup	102	0	0	5	28	3	0

ITEM DESCRIPTION	Serving Size	Calories	Total Fat (g)	Saturated Fat (g)	Sodium (mg)	Carbohydrates (g)	Fiber (g)	Protein (g)
APPLE STRUDEL	1 pc	195	8	1	191	29	2	2
APPLE TURNOVERS (Pepperidge Farm, frozen)	1 serv	284	16	4	176	31	2	4
APRICOT NECTAR (canned)	1 cup	141	0	0	8	36	2	1
APRICOTS								
Canned in heavy syrup, halves, w/ skin	1 cup	214	0	0	10	55	4	1
Canned in juice, halves, w/ skin	1 cup	117	0	0	10	30	4	2
Canned in light syrup, halves, w/ skin	1 cup	159	0	0	10	42	4	1
Canned in water, halves, w/ skin	1 cup	66	0	0	7	16	4	2
Dehydrated, stewed	1 cup	314	1	0	12	81	0	5
Dehydrated, uncooked	1 cup	381	1	0	15	99	0	6
Dried, stewed, halves, w/o sugar	1 cup	212	0	0	10	55	7	3
Dried, stewed, halves, w/ sugar	1 cup	305	0	0	8	79	11	3
Dried, uncooked, halves	1 cup	313	1	0	13	81	9	4
Fresh, slices	1 cup	79	1	0	2	18	3	2
Fresh, whole	1 med	17	0	0	0	4	1	0
Frozen, sweetened	1 cup	237	0	0	10	61	5	2
ARROWHEAD (boiled)	1 corm	9	0	0	2	2	0	1
ARROWROOT (fresh, slices)	1 cup	78	0	0	31	16	2	5
ARROWROOT FLOUR	1 cup	457	0	0	3	113	4	0
ARTICHOKES								
Boiled	1 med	64	0	0	72	14	10	3
Canned or jarred, marinated	1/2 cup	58	3	0	244	7	2	2
Fresh, whole	1 med	60	0	0	120	13	7	4
Frozen, boiled	9 oz pkg	108	1	0	127	22	11	7
Jerusalem, fresh, slices	1 cup	110	0	0	6	26	2	3
ARUGULA (fresh)	1/2 cup	3	0	0	3	0	0	0
ASPARAGUS								
Boiled, cut	1/2 cup	20	0	0	13	4	2	2
Canned, drained	1/2 cup	23	0	0	347	3	1	3
Fresh, cut	1/2 cup	13	0	0	1	3	1	1
Frozen, boiled	10 oz pkg	53	1	0	9	6	5	9

ITEM DESCRIPTION	Serving Size	Calories	Total Fat (g)	Saturated Fat (g)	Sodium (mg)	Carbohydrates (g)	Fiber (g)	Protein (g)
AVOCADO								
California, fresh, whole	1 fruit	227	21	3	11	12	9	3
Common varieties, cubed	1 cup	240	22	3	10	13	10	3
Florida, fresh, whole	1 fruit	365	31	6	6	24	17	7
AVOCADO OIL	1 tbsp	124	14	2	0	0	0	0
BABASSU OIL	1 tbsp	120	14	11	0	0	0	0
BACON								
Baked	1 slice	44	4	1	178	0	0	3
Bits, meatless	1 tbsp	33	2	0	124	2	1	2
Broiled or roasted	1 slice	43	3	1	185	0	0	3
Broiled or roasted, reduced sodium	1 slice	43	3	1	82	0	0	3
Canadian style, grilled	1 slice (1 oz)	43	2	1	363	0	0	6
Grease	1 tsp	39	4	2	6	0	0	0
Hormel Canadian style	1 serv	68	3	1	569	1	0	9
Microwaved	1 slice	25	2	1	104	0	0	2
Pan fried	1 slice	42	3	1	192	0	0	3
BACON & BEEF STICKS	1 oz	145	12	4	398	0	0	8
BACON SUBSTITUTE								
Breakfast strips, pork, cooked	1 slice	52	4	1	238	0	0	3
Meatless, cooked	1 oz	50	5	1	234	1	0	2
Morningstar Farms Veggie Bacon Strips, frozen	2 strips	55	4	1	234	2	1	2
Worthington Stripples, frozen	2 strips	55	4	1	234	2	1	2
BAGELS								
Cinnamon-raisin (3" dia)	1 bagel	156	1	0	184	31	1	6
Egg (3" dia)	1 bagel	192	1	0	348	37	2	7
Oat bran (3" dia)	1 bagel	145	1	0	289	30	2	6
Onion (3" dia)	1 bagel	146	1	0	255	29	1	6
Plain (3" dia)	1 bagel	146	1	0	255	29	1	6
Poppy (3" dia)	1 bagel	146	1	0	255	29	1	6
Sesame (3" dia)	1 bagel	146	1	0	255	29	1	6
BAKED BEANS								
Campbell's, brown sugar & bacon	1 cup	320	5	1	941	60	16	10
Canned, w/ beef	1 cup	322	9	4	1264	45	0	17

ITEM DESCRIPTION	Serving Size	Calories	Total Fat (g)	Saturated Fat (g)	Sodium (mg)	Carbohydrates (g)	Fiber (g)	Protein (g)
Canned, w/ franks	1 cup	368	17	6	1114	40	18	17
Canned, w/o salt	1 cup	266	1	0	3	52	14	12
Canned, w/ pork	1 cup	268	4	2	1047	51	14	13
Canned, w/ pork & sweet sauce	1 cup	283	4	1	845	53	11	13
Canned, w/ pork & tomato sauce	1 cup	231	2	1	1075	46	10	13
Canned, w/ salt	1 cup	239	1	0	871	54	10	12
Homemade	1 cup	392	13	5	1068	55	14	14
Vegetarian	1 cup	339	3	0	441	65	15	15
BAKING CHOCOLATE								
Unsweetened, liquid	1 oz	134	14	7	3	10	5	3
Unsweetened, squares	1 sq	145	15	9	7	9	5	4
BAKING POWDER								
Sodium aluminum sulfate	1 tsp	2	0	0	488	1	0	0
Straight phosphate	1 tsp	2	0	0	363	1	0	0
Low sodium	1 tsp	5	0	0	4	2	0	0
BAKING SODA	1 tsp	0	0	0	1259	0	0	0
BALSAM PEAR								
Leafy tips, boiled	1 cup	20	0	0	8	4	1	2
Pods, boiled (1/2" pcs)	1 cup	24	0	0	7	5	3	1
BAMBOO SHOOTS								
Boiled (1/2" slices)	1 cup	14	0	0	5	2	1	2
Canned (1/8" slices)	1 cup	25	1	0	9	4	2	2
BANANA BREAD (Made w/margarine, homemade)	1 slice	196	6	1	181	33	1	3
BANANA CHIPS	1 oz	147	10	8	2	17	2	1
BANANA POWDER	1 tbsp	21	0	0	0	5	1	0
BANANAS								
Dehydrated	1 cup	346	2	1	3	88	10	4
Fresh, slices	1 cup	134	0	0	2	34	4	2
Fresh, whole	1 med	105	0	0	1	27	3	1
BARBEQUE SAUCE								
Low sodium	2 tbsp	52	0	0	46	13	0	0
Regular	2 tbsp	52	0	0	386	13	0	0
BARLEY (pearled, cooked)	1 cup	193	1	0	5	44	6	4

ITEM DESCRIPTION	Serving Size	Calories	Total Fat (g)	Saturated Fat (g)	Sodium (mg)	Carbohydrates (g)	Fiber (g)	Protein (g)
BARLEY FLOUR								
Or barley meal	1 cup	511	2	0	6	110	15	16
w/ malt	1 cup	585	3	1	18	127	12	17
BASIL								
Dried, leaves	1 tbsp	5	0	0	1	1	1	0
Fresh, chopped	2 tbsp	1	0	0	0	0	0	0
BASS								
Freshwater, cooked in dry heat	3 oz	124	4	1	76	0	0	21
Sea bass, cooked in dry heat	3 oz	105	2	1	74	0	0	20
BAY LEAF (crumbled)	1 tbsp	6	0	0	0	1	0	0
BEECHNUTS (dried)	1 oz	163	14	2	11	10	0	2
BEEF								
Bottom round, 0" fat, braised	3 oz	190	9	3	36	0	0	28
Bottom round, 0" fat, roasted	3 oz	190	8	3	30	0	0	23
Bottom round, 1/8" fat, braised	3 oz	210	11	4	36	0	0	28
Bottom round, 1/8" fat, roasted	3 oz	190	11	4	29	0	0	22
Bottom sirloin, tri-tip roast, 0" fat, all grades, roasted	3 oz	175	9	3	45	0	0	22
Bottom sirloin, tri-tip steak, 0" fat, all grades, roasted	3 oz	231	11	4	62	0	0	26
Brisket, flat half, 0" fat, all grades, braised	3 oz	175	7	3	46	0	0	28
Brisket, flat half, 1/8" fat, all grades, braised	3 oz	246	16	6	41	0	0	25
Brisket, point half, 0" fat, all grades, braised	3 oz	304	24	10	58	0	0	20
Brisket, point half, 1/8" fat, all grades, braised	3 oz	297	23	9	59	0	0	21
Brisket, whole, 0" fat, all grades, braised	3 oz	247	17	6	55	0	0	23
Brisket, whole, 1/8" fat, all grades, braised	3 oz	281	21	8	54	0	0	22
Chuck, arm pot roast, 0" fat, all grades, braised	3 oz	252	16	6	40	0	0	25
Chuck, arm pot roast, 1/8" fat, all grades, braised	3 oz	257	16	6	42	0	0	26

ITEM DESCRIPTION	Serving Size	Calories	Total Fat (g)	Saturated Fat (g)	Sodium (mg)	Carbohydrates (g)	Fiber (g)	Protein (g)
Chuck, blade roast, 0" fat, USDA Choice, braised	3 oz	296	22	9	55	0	0	23
Chuck, blade roast, 1/8" fat, all grades, braised	3 oz	290	21	9	55	0	0	23
Chuck, clod roast, 0" fat, all grades, roasted	3 oz	176	9	3	60	0	0	22
Chuck, clod steak, top & center, 0" fat, all grades, grilled	3 oz	155	7	2	51	0	0	22
Chuck, clod steak, top blade, 0" fat, all grades, grilled	3 oz	189	11	4	65	0	0	21
Chuck, mock tender steak, 0" fat, all grades, broiled	3 oz	136	5	2	60	0	0	22
Chuck, shoulder clod steak, top & center, 0" fat, USDA Choice, grilled	3 oz	155	7	2	51	0	0	22
Chuck, top blade, 0" fat, all grades, broiled	3 oz	184	10	3	57	0	0	22
Cured beef, corned beef brisket, cooked	3 oz	213	16	5	964	0	0	15
Cured beef, corned beef, canned	3 oz	213	13	5	856	0	0	23
Cured beef, dried	1 slice	4	0	0	78	0	0	1
Cured beef, luncheon meat, jellied	1 slice	31	1	0	375	0	0	5
Cured beef, pastrami	1 slice	41	2	1	248	0	0	6
Cured beef, sausage, smoked	3 oz	265	23	10	962	2	0	12
Cured beef, smoked, chopped beef	1 slice	37	1	1	352	1	0	6
Cured beef, thin slices	1 slice	4	0	0	30	0	0	1
Eye of round, 0" fat, all grades, roasted	3 oz	143	4	1	32	0	0	25
Eye of round, 1/8" fat, all grades, roasted	3 oz	177	8	3	31	0	0	24
Flank, 0" fat, all grades, broiled	3 oz	200	7	3	48	0	0	24
Full cut, 1/8" fat, USDA Choice, broiled	3 oz	230	11	4	53	0	0	23
Ground beef, 30% fat, crumbles, pan browned	3 oz	175	15	6	82	0	0	22
Ground beef, 30% fat, loaf, baked	3 oz	205	13	5	62	0	0	20
Ground beef, 30% fat, patty, broiled	3 oz	232	15	6	69	0	0	22

ITEM DESCRIPTION	Serving Size	Calories	Total Fat (g)	Saturated Fat (g)	Sodium (mg)	Carbohydrates (g)	Fiber (g)	Protein (g)
Ground beef, 30% fat, patty, pan browned	3 oz	202	13	5	78	0	0	19
Ground beef, 25% fat, crumbles, pan browned	3 oz	239	15	6	79	0	0	22
Ground beef, 25% fat, loaf, baked	3 oz	216	14	5	60	0	0	21
Ground beef, 25% fat, patty, broiled	3 oz	236	16	6	66	0	0	22
Ground beef, 25% fat, patty, pan broiled	3 oz	211	14	5	74	0	0	20
Ground beef, 20% fat, crumbles, pan browned	3 oz	231	15	6	77	0	0	23
Ground beef, 20% fat, loaf, baked	3 oz	216	14	5	57	0	0	21
Ground beef, 20% fat, patty, broiled	3 oz	230	15	6	64	0	0	22
Ground beef, 20% fat, patty, pan broiled	3 oz	209	14	5	71	0	0	20
Ground beef, 15% fat, crumbles, pan browned	3 oz	218	13	5	76	0	0	24
Ground beef, 15% fat, loaf, baked	3 oz	204	12	5	54	0	0	22
Ground beef, 15% fat, patty, pan broiled	3 oz	197	12	5	67	0	0	21
Ground beef, 10% fat, crumbles, pan browned	3 oz	196	10	4	74	0	0	24
Ground beef, 10% fat, loaf, baked	3 oz	182	9	4	52	0	0	23
Ground beef, 10% fat, patty, broiled	3 oz	184	10	4	58	0	0	22
Ground beef, 10% fat, patty, pan broiled	3 oz	173	9	4	64	0	0	21
Ground beef, 5% fat, crumbles, pan browned	3 oz	164	6	3	72	0	0	25
Ground beef, 5% fat, loaf, baked	3 oz	148	5	2	49	0	0	23
Ground beef, 5% fat, patty, broiled	3 oz	145	6	3	55	0	0	22
Ground beef, 5% fat, patty, pan broiled	3 oz	139	5	2	60	0	0	22
Loin, bottom sirloin butt, tri-tip, 0" fat, all grades, roasted	3 oz	155	7	3	47	0	0	23
Outside round, bottom round steak, 0" fat, all grades, grilled	3 oz	155	6	2	49	0	0	23

ITEM DESCRIPTION	Serving Size	Calories	Total Fat (g)	Saturated Fat (g)	Sodium (mg)	Carbohydrates (g)	Fiber (g)	Protein (g)
Rib eye, small end, 0" fat, all grades, broiled	1 steak	576	34	13	130	0	0	64
Ribs, large end, 0" fat, USDA Choice, roasted	3 oz	316	26	10	54	0	0	19
Ribs, large end, 1/8" fat, all grades, broiled	3 oz	287	23	9	54	0	0	18
Ribs, large end, 1/8" fat, all grades, roasted	3 oz	302	24	10	54	0	0	20
Ribs, large end, 1/8" fat, USDA Prime, broiled	3 oz	343	30	12	53	0	0	18
Ribs, large end, 1/8" fat, USDA Prime, roasted	3 oz	334	28	12	54	0	0	19
Ribs, short ribs, USDA Choice, braised	3 oz	400	36	15	43	0	0	18
Ribs, small end, 0" fat, all grades, broiled	3 oz	212	13	5	48	0	0	23
Ribs, small end, 1/8" fat, all grades, broiled	3 oz	247	17	7	45	0	0	22
Ribs, small end, 1/8" fat, all grades, roasted	3 oz	290	23	9	54	0	0	19
Ribs, small end, 1/8" fat, USDA Prime, broiled	3 oz	301	24	10	54	0	0	21
Ribs, small end, 1/8" fat, USDA Prime, roasted	3 oz	349	30	12	55	0	0	19
Ribs, whole, 1/8" fat, all grades, broiled	3 oz	286	23	9	54	0	0	19
Ribs, whole, 1/8" fat, all grades, roasted	3 oz	298	24	10	54	0	0	19
Ribs, whole, 1/8" fat, USDA Prime, broiled	3 oz	328	28	11	53	0	0	19
Ribs, whole, 1/8" fat, USDA Prime, roasted	3 oz	340	29	12	55	0	0	19
Roast beef spread	1/4 cup	127	9	4	413	2	0	9
Round, knuckle, tip center steak, 0" fat, all grades, grilled	1 steak	266	10	4	78	0	0	41
Round, knuckle, tip side steak, 0" fat, all grades, grilled	3 oz	143	4	2	46	0	0	25
Short loin, Porterhouse steak, 0" fat, all grades, broiled	3 oz	235	16	6	55	0	0	20

ITEM DESCRIPTION	Serving Size	Calories	Total Fat (g)	Saturated Fat (g)	Sodium (mg)	Carbohydrates (g)	Fiber (g)	Protein (g)
Short loin, Porterhouse steak, 1/8" fat, all grades, broiled	3 oz	252	19	7	54	0	0	20
Short loin, T-bone steak, 0" fat, all grades, broiled	3 oz	210	14	5	57	0	0	21
Short loin, T-bone steak, 1/8" fat, all grades, broiled	3 oz	238	17	6	56	0	0	21
Short loin, top loin, 0" fat, all grades, broiled	3 oz	164	7	3	50	0	0	25
Short loin, top loin, 1/8" fat, all grades, broiled	3 oz	224	14	6	46	0	0	22
Short loin, top loin, 1/8" fat, USDA Prime, broiled	3 oz	264	19	8	54	0	0	22
Sirloin, tri-tip steak, 0" fat, all grades, broiled	3 oz	225	13	5	61	0	0	25
Skirt steak, 0" fat, all grades, broiled	3 oz	187	10	4	64	0	0	22
Skirt steak, outside, 0" fat, all grades, broiled	3 oz	217	15	6	78	0	0	20
Tenderloin, 0" fat, all grades, broiled	3 oz	185	9	4	48	0	0	23
Tenderloin, 1/8" fat, all grades, broiled	3 oz	227	15	6	46	0	0	22
Tenderloin, 1/8" fat, all grades, roasted	3 oz	275	21	8	48	0	0	20
Tenderloin, 1/8" fat, USDA Prime, broiled	3 oz	262	19	8	50	0	0	21
Tenderloin, 1/8" fat, USDA Prime, roasted	3 oz	292	23	9	47	0	0	20
Tip round, 0" fat, all grades, roasted	3 oz	160	7	3	30	0	0	23
Tip round, 1/8" fat, all grades, roasted	3 oz	186	10	4	54	0	0	23
Top round, 0" fat, all grades, braised	3 oz	178	5	2	38	0	0	30
Top round, 0" fat, all grades, broiled	3 oz	175	5	2	35	0	0	27
Top round, 1/8" fat, all grades, braised	3 oz	202	9	3	38	0	0	29
Top round, 1/8" fat, all grades, broiled	3 oz	173	8	3	35	0	0	26
Top round, 1/8" fat, USDA Choice, pan fried	3 oz	226	12	4	58	0	0	28
Top sirloin, 0" fat, all grades, broiled	3 oz	180	7	2	55	2	0	29
Top sirloin, 1/8" fat, all grades, broiled	3 oz	207	12	5	48	0	0	23
Top sirloin, 1/8" fat, USDA Choice, pan fried	3 oz	266	18	7	60	0	0	24

ITEM DESCRIPTION	Serving Size	Calories	Total Fat (g)	Saturated Fat (g)	Sodium (mg)	Carbohydrates (g)	Fiber (g)	Protein (g)
BEEF BOUILLON								
(powder, prepared w/ water)	1 cube	9	0	0	611	1	0	1
BEEF BROTH								
Broth & tomato juice, canned	1 cup	90	0	0	320	21	0	1
Campbell's Red & White, condensed	1 cup	15	0	0	636	1	0	3
Canned, ready to serve	1 cup	17	1	0	782	0	0	3
Cubed, prepared w/ water	1 cube	6	0	0	864	1	0	1
BEEF JERKY	1 lg pc	82	5	2	443	2	0	7
BEEF STEW								
Canned	1 serv	220	12	5	947	16	4	11
Hormel Dinty Moore, canned	1 cup	222	13	6	984	16	3	11
BEEF STICKS	1 stick	110	10	4	296	1	0	4
BEEF STOCK (homemade)	1 cup	31	0	0	475	3	0	5
BEEF SUBSTITUTE, BRAND NAME								
Carl Buddig Smoked Slices, beef	2 oz	79	4	1	816	0	0	11
Loma Linda Dinner Cuts, canned	2 slices	96	1	0	456	4	2	18
Loma Linda Swiss Stake, w/ gravy, canned	1 pc	130	6	1	433	10	3	9
Lorna Linda Tender Bits, canned	6 pcs	115	4	1	521	7	4	13
Loma Linda Tender Rounds, w/ gravy, canned	6 pcs	116	5	1	354	6	3	13
Worthington Choplets, canned	2 slices	95	1	0	420	4	3	18
Worthington Prime Stakes, canned	1 pc	124	7	1	442	7	1	9
Worthington Stakelets, frozen	1 pc	150	7	1	462	7	2	14
Worthington Vegetable Steaks, canned	2 slices	81	1	0	300	4	2	15
BEER								
Bud Light	12 fl oz	110	0	12	11	7	0	1
Budweiser	12 fl oz	146	0	0	11	11	0	1
Budweiser Select	12 fl oz	99	0	0	11	3	0	1
Light, all	12 fl oz	103	0	0	14	6	0	1
Michelob Ultra Light	12 fl oz	96	0	0	11	3	0	1
Regular, all	12 fl oz	153	0	0	14	13	0	2

ITEM DESCRIPTION	Serving Size	Calories	Total Fat (g)	Saturated Fat (g)	Sodium (mg)	Carbohydrates (g)	Fiber (g)	Protein (g)
BEET GREENS								
Boiled (1" pcs)	1 cup	39	0	0	347	8	4	4
Fresh	1 cup	8	0	0	86	2	1	1
BEETS								
Boiled (2" dia)	1 beet	22	0	0	39	5	1	1
Canned, diced	1 cup	49	0	0	305	11	3	1
Canned, no salt	1 cup	69	0	0	52	16	3	2
Canned, reg	1 cup	74	0	0	352	18	3	2
Fresh (2" dia)	1 beet	35	0	0	64	8	2	1
Harvard, canned	1 cup	180	0	0	399	45	6	2
Pickled, canned	1 cup	148	0	0	599	37	6	2
BISCUITS								
Martha White Buttermilk Biscuit	1 serv	159	5	2	531	24	1	3
Mixed grain, refrigerated (2.5" dia)	1 biscuit	116	2	1	295	21	0	3
Pillsbury Buttermilk Biscuits, refrigerated	1 serv	150	2	0	570	29	1	4
Pillsbury Golden Layer Buttermilk Biscuits, refrigerated	1 serv	104	5	1	360	14	0	2
Pillsbury Grands Buttermilk Biscuits, refrigerated	1 serv	193	8	3	631	25	1	4
Plain or buttermilk, commercial (2.5" dia)	1 biscuit	128	6	1	368	17	0	2
Plain or buttermilk, dry mix, prepared	1 oz	95	3	1	271	14	1	2
Plain or buttermilk, homemade (2.5" dia)	1 biscuit	212	10	3	348	27	1	4
Plain or buttermilk, refrigerated (2.5" dia)	1 biscuit	95	4	1	292	13	0	2
Plain or buttermilk, refrigerated, lower fat (2.25" dia)	1 biscuit	63	1	0	305	12	0	2
BLACK BEANS (boiled)	1 cup	227	1	0	2	41	15	15
BLACKBERRIES								
Canned in heavy syrup	1 cup	236	0	0	8	59	9	3
Fresh	1 cup	62	1	0	1	14	8	2
Frozen, unsweetened	1 cup	97	1	0	2	24	8	2
Juice, canned	1 cup	95	2	0	3	20	0	1

ITEM DESCRIPTION	Serving Size	Calories	Total Fat (g)	Saturated Fat (g)	Sodium (mg)	Carbohydrates (g)	Fiber (g)	Protein (g)
BLUEBERRIES								
Canned in heavy syrup	1 cup	225	1	0	8	56	4	2
Canned in light syrup	1 cup	215	1	0	7	55	6	3
Fresh	1 cup	84	0	0	1	21	4	1
Frozen, sweetened	1 cup	186	0	0	2	50	5	1
Frozen, unsweetened	1 cup	79	1	0	2	19	4	1
Frozen, wild	1 cup	71	0	0	4	19	6	0
Pie filling, canned	1 cup	474	1	0	31	116	7	1
BLUEFISH (cooked in dry heat)	3 oz	135	5	1	65	0	0	22
BOLOGNA								
Beef	1 oz slice	87	8	3	302	1	0	3
Beef & pork	1 oz slice	87	7	3	206	2	0	4
Beef & pork, low fat	1 oz slice	64	5	2	310	1	0	3
Beef, low fat	1 oz slice	57	4	2	330	1	0	3
Beef, reduced sodium	1 oz slice	88	8	3	191	1	0	3
Chicken & pork	1 oz slice	94	9	3	347	1	0	3
Chicken, pork, beef	1 oz slice	76	6	2	314	2	0	3
Chicken, turkey, pork	1 oz slice	83	7	2	258	2	0	3
Oscar Mayer, beef	1 oz slice	88	8	4	330	1	0	3
Oscar Mayer, beef, light	1 oz slice	56	4	2	322	2	0	3
Oscar Mayer, chicken, pork & beef	1 oz slice	89	8	3	289	1	0	3
Oscar Mayer, fat free	1 oz slice	22	0	0	274	2	0	4
Oscar Mayer, light	1 oz slice	57	4	2	313	2	0	3
Pork	1 oz slice	69	6	2	332	0	0	4
Pork & turkey lite	1 oz slice	59	5	2	200	1	0	4
Pork, turkey & beef	1 oz slice	95	8	3	299	2	0	3
Turkey	1 oz slice	59	4	1	351	1	0	3
BOYSENBERRIES								
Canned, heavy syrup	1 cup	225	0	0	8	57	7	3
Frozen, unsweetened	1 cup	66	0	0	1	16	7	1
BRAN								
Corn, crude	1 cup	170	1	0	5	65	60	6
Wheat, crude	1 cup	125	2	0	1	37	25	9

ITEM DESCRIPTION	Serving Size	Calories	Total Fat (g)	Saturated Fat (g)	Sodium (mg)	Carbohydrates (g)	Fiber (g)	Protein (g)
BRAZIL NUTS								
(Dried, unblanched, whole)	1 cup	874	89	20	4	16	10	19
BREAD								
Boston brown	1 slice	88	1	0	284	19	2	2
Cracked wheat	1 slice	65	1	0	135	12	1	2
Egg	1 slice	113	2	1	197	19	1	4
French or Vienna (2" slice)	1 slice	92	1	0	208	18	1	4
Irish soda	1 oz	82	1	0	113	16	1	2
Italian	1 slice	54	1	0	117	10	1	2
Multi-grain	1 slice	69	1	0	109	11	2	3
Oat bran	1 slice	71	1	0	122	12	1	3
Oat bran, reduced calorie	1 slice	46	1	0	81	10	3	2
Oatmeal	1 slice	70	1	0	121	12	1	3
Oatmeal, reduced calorie	1 slice	48	1	0	89	10	1	2
Pepperidge Farm Crusty Italian Bread, garlic	1 serv	186	10	2	200	21	0	4
Pillsbury Crusty French Loaf, refrigerated	1 serv	149	2	1	358	29	1	5
Pita, white (4" dia)	1 pita	77	0	0	150	16	1	3
Pita, whole wheat (4" dia)	1 pita	74	1	0	149	15	2	3
Protein, including gluten	1 slice	47	0	0	104	8	1	2
Pumpernickel	1 slice	65	1	0	174	12	2	2
Raisin	1 slice	71	1	0	101	14	1	2
Rice bran	1 slice	66	1	0	119	12	1	2
Rye	1 slice	83	1	0	211	15	2	3
Rye, reduced calorie	1 slice	47	1	0	93	9	3	2
Sourdough (2" slice)	1 slice	92	1	0	208	18	1	4
Wheat	1 slice	66	1	0	130	12	1	3
Wheat bran	1 slice	89	1	0	175	17	1	3
Wheat, reduced calorie	1 slice	46	1	0	118	10	3	2
White, commercial	1 slice	66	1	0	170	13	1	2
White, commercial, low sodium	1 slice	67	1	0	7	13	0	2
White, homemade, w/ lowfat milk	1 slice	120	2	0	151	21	1	3

ITEM DESCRIPTION	Serving Size	Calories	Total Fat (g)	Saturated Fat (g)	Sodium (mg)	Carbohydrates (g)	Fiber (g)	Protein (g)
White, homemade, w/ nonfat dry milk	1 slice	121	1	0	148	24	1	3
White, reduced calorie	1 slice	48	1	0	104	10	2	2
Whole wheat, commercial	1 slice	69	1	0	132	12	2	4
Whole wheat, homemade	1 slice	128	2	0	159	24	3	4
BREAD CRUMBS								
Dry, grated, plain	1 cup	427	6	1	791	78	5	14
Dry, grated, seasoned	1 cup	460	7	2	2111	82	6	17
Kraft Shake 'n' Bake Original Recipe, coating for pork	1 serv	106	1	0	795	22	0	2
White, commercial	1 cup	120	1	0	306	23	1	3
White, commercial, low sodium	1 cup	120	2	0	12	22	1	4
BREADSTICKS plain (4.25")	1 stick	21	0	0	33	3	0	1
BREAD STUFFING								
Dry mix, prepared	1 oz	50	2	0	154	6	1	1
Cornbread, prepared	1 oz	51	2	0	129	6	1	1
BREAKFAST STRIPS (Cured beef, cooked)	1 slice	51	4	2	255	0	0	4
BROAD BEANS (boiled)	1 cup	187	1	0	8	33	9	13
BROCCOLI								
Boiled, chopped	1/2 cup	27	0	0	32	6	3	2
Fresh, chopped	1 cup	31	0	0	30	6	2	3
Fresh, flowers	1 cup	20	0	0	19	4	0	2
Frozen, boiled, chopped	1 cup	20	0	0	20	10	6	6
Frozen, boiled, spears	10 oz pkg	70	0	0	60	13	8	8
Green Giant Broccoli in Cheese Flavored Sauce, frozen	1 cup	113	4	1	806	15	0	4
Stalks, fresh	1 stalk	32	0	0	31	6	0	3
BROCCOLI RABE								
Cooked	1 cup	144	2	0	245	14	12	17
Fresh, chopped	1 cup	9	0	0	13	1	1	1
BROWNIES								
Commercial (2-3/4" sq)	1	227	9	2	175	36	1	3
Homemade (2" sq)	1	112	7	2	82	12	0	1

ITEM DESCRIPTION	Serving Size	Calories	Total Fat (g)	Saturated Fat (g)	Sodium (mg)	Carbohydrates (g)	Fiber (g)	Protein (g)
Martha White Chewy Fudge Brownies	1 serv	114	2	0	128	23	1	1
Pillsbury Traditional Fudge Brownies	1 serv	132	4	1	88	23	0	1
BRUSSELS SPROUTS								
Boiled	1/2 cup	28	0	0	16	6	2	2
Frozen, boiled	1/2 cup	33	0	0	12	6	3	3
BUCKWHEAT								
Flour, whole groat	1 cup	402	4	1	13	85	15	15
Groats, roasted, cooked	1 cup	155	1	0	7	34	5	6
Groats, roasted, dry	1 cup	567	4	1	18	123	17	19
BULGUR (cooked)	1 cup	151	0	0	9	34	8	6
BURBOT (cooked in dry heat)	3 oz	98	1	0	105	0	0	21
BURDOCK ROOT								
Boiled (1" pcs)	1 cup	110	0	0	5	26	2	3
Fresh (1" pcs)	1 cup	85	0	0	6	20	4	2
BURRITO								
Bean & cheese, microwavable	1	309	9	2	758	48	12	10
Beef & bean, frozen	1	332	13	4	816	43	6	10
BUTTER								
No salt	1 tbsp	102	12	7	2	0	0	0
Salted	1 tbsp	102	12	7	82	0	0	0
Whipped, w/ salt	1 tbsp	67	8	5	78	0	0	0
BUTTER BLEND								
Butter-margarine, stick, w/o salt	1 tbsp	101	11	4	4	0	0	0
Butter-vegetable oil, spread, reduced calorie, w/ salt	1 tbsp	63	7	2	85	0	0	0
Butter-vegetable oil, spread, w/ salt	1 tbsp	51	6	1	110	0	0	0
BUTTERBUR (canned, chopped)	1 cup	4	0	0	5	0	0	0
BUTTERFISH (cooked in dry heat)	3 oz	159	9	0	97	0	0	0
BUTTERMILK								
Low fat	1 cup	98	2	1	257	12	0	8
Reduced fat	1 cup	137	5	3	211	13	0	10
BUTTERMILK SQUASH (baked, cubed)	1 cup	82	0	0	8	22	0	2
BUTTERNUT SQUASH (frozen, boiled, mashed)	1 cup	94	0	0	5	24	0	3

ITEM DESCRIPTION	Serving Size	Calories	Total Fat (g)	Saturated Fat (g)	Sodium (mg)	Carbohydrates (g)	Fiber (g)	Protein (g)
BUTTER OIL	1 tbsp	112	13	8	0	0	0	0
BUTTERNUTS (dried)	1 cup	734	68	2	1	14	6	30
BUTTER REPLACEMENT (powder, no fat)	1 cup	298	1	0	960	71	0	2
BUTTERSCOTCH TOPPING	2 tbsp	103	0	0	143	27	0	1
CABBAGE								
Chinese (bok choy), boiled, shredded	1 cup	20	0	0	58	3	2	3
Chinese (bok choy), fresh, shredded	1 cup	9	0	0	46	2	1	1
Chinese (pe tsai), boiled, shredded	1 cup	17	0	0	11	3	2	2
Chinese (pe tsai), fresh, shredded	1 cup	12	0	0	7	2	1	1
Common, fresh, shredded	1 cup	17	0	0	13	4	2	1
Japanese style, fresh, pickled	1 cup	45	0	0	416	9	5	2
Mustard, boiled, shredded	1 cup	36	0	0	13	7	4	1
Napa, cooked	1 cup	13	0	0	12	2	0	1
Red, boiled, shredded	1 cup	44	0	0	42	10	4	2
Red, fresh, shredded	1 cup	22	0	0	19	5	1	1
Savoy, boiled, shredded	1 cup	35	0	0	35	8	4	3
Savoy, fresh, shredded	1 cup	19	0	0	20	4	2	1
CAKE								
Angelfood, commercial (12 oz cake)	1/12 cake	72	0	0	210	16	0	2
Angelfood, from mix (10" dia cake)	1/12 cake	129	0	0	255	29	0	3
Betty Crocker Super Moist Party Cake Swirl	1 serv	178	3	1	266	35	0	2
Betty Crocker Super Moist Yellow Cake	1 serv	178	3	1	289	35	0	2
Boston cream pie, commercial	1/6 pie	232	8	2	132	39	1	2
Cheesecake, commercial (17 oz cake)	1/6 cake	257	18	8	166	20	0	4
Cheesecake, from no-bake mix (9" dia)	1/12 cake	271	13	7	376	35	2	5
Cherry fudge, w/ chocolate frosting	1/8 cake	187	9	4	160	27	1	2

ITEM DESCRIPTION	Serving Size	Calories	Total Fat (g)	Saturated Fat (g)	Sodium (mg)	Carbohydrates (g)	Fiber (g)	Protein (g)
Chocolate, commercial, w/ chocolate frosting (18 oz cake)	1/8 cake	235	10	3	214	35	2	3
Chocolate, from pudding-type mix	1 oz	112	3	1	253	22	1	1
Chocolate, homemade w/o frosting (9" dia)	1/12 cake	352	14	5	299	51	2	5
Coffee cake, cheese (16 oz cake)	1/6 cake	258	12	4	258	34	1	5
Coffee cake, cinnamon w/ crumb topping, commercial (20 oz cake)	1/9 cake	263	15	4	221	29	1	4
Coffee cake, cinnamon w/crumb topping, from mix	1/8 cake (2 oz)	178	5	1	236	30	1	3
Coffee cake, crème filled, w/ chocolate frosting (19 oz cake)	1/6 cake	298	10	3	291	48	2	5
Coffee cake, fruit	1/8 cake	156	5	1	193	26	1	3
Fruitcake, commercial	1 pc	139	4	0	116	26	2	1
German chocolate, from pudding-type mix	1 oz	114	3	1	182	23	1	1
Gingerbread, homemade (8" sq cake)	1/9 cake	101	5	1	93	14	0	1
Pineapple upside-down, homemade (8" sq cake)	1/9 cake	367	14	3	367	58	1	4
Pound, commercial, fat free (12 oz cake)	1/12 cake	80	0	0	97	17	0	2
Pound, commercial, w/ butter (12 oz cake)	1/12 cake	109	6	3	111	14	0	2
Pound, commercial, w/o butter (12 oz cake)	1/12 cake	109	5	1	112	15	0	1
Shortcake, biscuit, homemade (12 oz cake)	1/12 cake	98	4	1	143	14	0	2
Snackwell's Fat Free Devil's Food Cookie Cakes	1 serv	49	0	0	28	12	0	1
Sponge, commercial (16 oz cake)	1/12 cake	110	1	0	93	23	0	2
Sponge, homemade (10" dia)	1/12 cake	187	3	1	144	36	0	5
White, homemade w/ coconut frosting (9" dia)	1/12 cake	399	12	4	318	71	1	5
White, homemade, w/o frosting (9" dia)	1/12 cake	264	9	2	242	42	1	4

ITEM DESCRIPTION	Serving Size	Calories	Total Fat (g)	Saturated Fat (g)	Sodium (mg)	Carbohydrates (g)	Fiber (g)	Protein (g)
Yellow, commercial, w/ chocolate frosting (18 oz cake)	1/8 cake	243	11	3	216	35	1	2
Yellow, commercial, w/ vanilla frosting (18 oz cake)	1/8 cake	239	9	2	220	38	0	2
Yellow, homemade w/o frosting (8" dia)	1/12 cake	245	10	3	233	36	0	4
CALABASH GOURD								
Boiled, cubed	1 cup	22	0	0	3	5	0	1
Fresh (1" pcs)	1 cup	16	0	0	2	4	0	1
CANDY								
Butterscotch	1 pc	21	0	0	21	5	0	0
Candy corn	1 oz	105	0	0	57	27	0	0
Caramels	1 pc	39	1	0	25	8	0	0
Caramels, chocolate-flavored roll	1 pc	26	0	0	3	6	0	0
Caramels, w/ nuts, chocolate covered	1 pc	66	3	1	3	8	1	1
Carob, unsweetened	3 oz bar	470	27	25	93	49	3	7
Coffee beans, dark chocolate coated	1 pc	8	0	0	0	1	0	0
Divinity, homemade	1 pc	40	0	0	4	10	0	0
Gumdrops, dietetic, w/ Sorbitol	1 pc	8	0	0	0	4	1	0
Gumdrops, starch jelly pieces	1 pc	14	0	0	2	4	0	0
Hard	1 pc	24	0	0	2	6	0	0
Hard, dietetic, w/ Sorbitol	1 pc	11	0	0	0	3	0	0
Jellybeans	1 sml	4	0	0	1	1	0	0
Milk chocolate, w/ almonds	1.45 oz bar	216	14	7	30	22	3	4
Milk chocolate, w/ rice cereal	1.45 oz bar	230	13	7	39	27	1	3
Nougat, w/ almonds	1 pc	56	0	0	5	13	0	0
Peanut bar	1.4 oz bar	209	13	2	62	19	2	6
Peanuts, milk chocolate coated	1 pc	21	1	1	2	2	0	1
Praline, homemade	1 pc	189	10	1	19	23	1	1
Raisins, milk chocolate coated	1 pc	4	0	0	0	1	0	0
Sesame crunch	1 pc	10	1	0	3	1	0	0
Taffy, homemade	1 pc	60	0	0	8	14	0	0
Toffee, homemade	1 pc	67	4	2	16	8	0	0
Truffles, homemade	1 pc	61	4	2	8	5	0	1

ITEM DESCRIPTION	Serving Size	Calories	Total Fat (g)	Saturated Fat (g)	Sodium (mg)	Carbohydrates (g)	Fiber (g)	Protein (g)
CANDY, BRAND NAME								
100 Grand Bar	1.5 oz bar	201	8	5	87	31	0	1
3 Musketeers Bar	2.13 oz bar	259	8	5	117	47	1	2
5th Avenue Candy Bar	2 oz bar	270	13	4	126	35	2	5
After Eight Thin Mints	5 mints	170	5	3	0	32	1	1
Almond Joy Bites	18 pcs	218	14	8	16	23	2	2
Almond Joy Candy Bar	1.76 oz pkg	235	13	9	70	29	2	2
Baby Ruth Bar	2.1 oz bar	273	13	7	137	39	1	3
Bit-O-Honey Candy Chews	6 pcs	150	3	2	118	32	0	1
Butterfinger Bar	2.1 oz bar	273	11	6	137	43	1	3
Caramello Candy Bar	1.25 oz bar	162	7	4	43	22	0	2
Chunky Bar	1.4 oz bar	190	11	5	15	24	1	3
Dove Dark Chocolate	1.3 oz bar	192	12	7	1	22	3	2
Dove Milk Chocolate	1.3 oz bar	201	12	7	23	22	1	2
Golden Almond Solitaires	13 pcs	234	15	6	21	19	2	5
Goobers Chocolate Covered Peanuts	1.375 oz pkg	200	13	5	14	21	4	4
Heath Bites	15 pcs	207	12	6	96	25	1	2
Hershey's Nuggets	17 pcs	215	14	7	29	20	1	4
Hershey's Skor Toffee Bar	1.4 oz bar	209	13	7	124	24	1	1
Hershey's Special Dark Chocolate Bar	1.45 oz bar	228	13	0	2	25	3	2
Hershey's Symphony Milk Chocolate Bar	1.5 oz bar	223	13	8	42	24	1	4
Kit Kat Bites	15 pcs	199	10	7	26	25	1	3
Kit Kat, big bar	1.94 oz bar	286	15	10	35	35	1	3
Kit Kat, wafer bar	1.5 oz bar	218	11	8	23	27	0	3
Krackel Chocolate Bar	1.45 oz bar	210	11	7	80	26	1	3
M&M's Almond Chocolate Candies	1.31 oz bar	189	10	4	17	22	2	3
M&M's Milk Chocolate Candies	1.48 oz box	207	9	5	26	30	1	2
M&M's Minis Milk Chocolate Candies	1 oz tube	151	7	4	20	21	1	1
M&M's Peanut Butter Chocolate Candies	1.63 oz bag	244	14	9	98	26	2	5

ITEM DESCRIPTION	Serving Size	Calories	Total Fat (g)	Saturated Fat (g)	Sodium (mg)	Carbohydrates (g)	Fiber (g)	Protein (g)
M&M's Peanut Chocolate Candies	1 bag	280	14	6	27	33	2	5
Mars Almond Bar	1.76 oz bar	234	12	4	85	31	1	4
Milky Way Bar	2.05 oz bar	263	10	7	97	41	1	2
Milky Way Minis, dark chocolate covered	5 pcs	202	9	6	108	30	1	2
Milky Way Minis, milk chocolate covered	5 pcs	204	8	6	120	30	0	2
Milky Way Midnight Bar	1.76 oz bar	221	9	6	84	36	1	2
Mounds Candy Bar, snack size	1 bar	92	5	4	28	11	1	1
Mr. Goodbar Chocolate Bar	1.75 oz bar	264	16	7	20	27	2	5
Nestle Crunch Bar & Dessert Topping	1.55 oz bar	220	11	7	66	29	1	2
Oh Henry! Bar	2 oz bar	263	13	5	110	37	1	4
Pop'ables 3 Musketeers Bite Size	15 pcs	182	6	4	71	31	1	1
Pop'ables Milky Way Brand Bite Size	13 pcs	177	7	3	57	28	0	1
Pop'ables Snickers Brand Bite Size	13 pcs	187	9	4	87	24	1	3
Raisinets Chocolate Covered Raisins	1.58 oz bag	189	8	5	15	32	1	2
Reese's Bites	16 pcs	203	12	7	70	22	1	4
Reese's Fast Break	1 bar	277	13	5	180	36	2	5
Reese's Fast Break, milk chocolate, peanut butter	2 oz bar	265	13	5	185	34	2	5
Reese's NutRageous	1.92 oz bar	281	17	5	77	29	2	6
Reese's Peanut Butter Cups	1 PB cup	88	5	2	53	9	1	2
Reese's Pieces	10 pcs	40	2	1	16	5	0	1
Reesesticks Crispy Wafers, peanut butter, milk chocolate	1.5 oz	219	13	6	111	23	1	4
Rolo Caramels, milk chocolate	7 pcs	199	9	6	79	29	0	2
Skittles Original Bite Size Candies	2.17 oz pk	249	3	3	9	56	0	0
Skittles Sours Original	1.8 oz bag	202	2	2	7	44	0	0
Skittles Tropical Bite Size Candies	2.1 oz bag	249	3	0	9	56	0	0
Skittles Wild Berry Bite Size	2.1 oz bag	249	3	3	9	56	0	0
Snickers Almond Bar	1.76 oz bar	236	11	4	78	32	1	3

ITEM DESCRIPTION	Serving Size	Calories	Total Fat (g)	Saturated Fat (g)	Sodium (mg)	Carbohydrates (g)	Fiber (g)	Protein (g)
Snickers Bar	2 oz bar	271	14	5	140	35	1	4
Snickers Cruncher	1.66 oz bar	230	11	6	89	30	1	3
Snickers Munch Bar	1.42 oz bar	216	15	4	144	18	2	6
Starburst Fruit Chews, original	8 chews	163	3	3	1	33	0	0
Starburst Fruit Chews, tropical	8 chews	164	3	3	1	33	0	0
Starburst Sour Fruit Chews	2.07 oz pck	235	5	4	52	47	0	0
Tootsie Roll, chocolate-flavored roll	6 pcs	155	1	0	18	35	0	1
Twix Caramel Cookie Bars	2 oz pkg	286	14	11	113	37	1	3
Twix Peanut Butter Cookie Bars	2 bars	289	18	9	122	29	2	5
Twizzlers Cherry Bites	18 pcs	135	1	0	104	32	0	1
Twizzlers Nibs Cherry Bits	27 pcs	139	1	0	78	32	0	1
Twizzlers Strawberry Twists Candy	4 pcs	133	1	0	109	30	0	1
Whatchamacallit Candy Bar	1.7 oz bar	237	11	8	144	30	1	4
York Bites	15 pcs	154	3	2	18	32	1	1
York Peppermint Pattie	1.5 oz patty	163	3	2	12	34	1	1
CANDY COATING								
Butterscotch	1 oz	153	8	7	25	19	0	1
Peanut butter	1 oz	153	8	4	71	13	1	5
Yogurt	1 oz	153	8	7	25	18	0	2
CANOLA OIL								
Canola oil	1 tbsp	124	14	1	0	0	0	0
Natreon	1 tbsp	124	14	1	0	0	0	0
CANTALOUPE (fresh, cubed)	1 cup	54	0	0	26	13	1	1
CAPERS (canned)	1 tbsp	2	0	0	255	0	0	0
CARAMBOLA (STARFRUIT) (fresh, cubed)	1 cup	41	0	0	3	9	4	1
CARAMEL CUSTARD FLAN (homemade)	1/2 cup	223	6	3	81	35	0	7
CARAMEL TOPPING	2 tbsp	103	0	0	143	27	0	1
CARDAMOM (ground)	1 tbsp	18	0	0	1	4	2	1
CARDOON (fresh, shredded)	1 cup	30	0	0	303	7	3	1
CAROB FLOUR	1 cup	229	1	0	36	92	41	5
CARP (cooked in dry heat)	3 oz	138	6	1	54	0	0	19
CARROT JUICE (canned)	1 cup	94	0	0	68	22	2	2

ITEM DESCRIPTION	Serving Size	Calories	Total Fat (g)	Saturated Fat (g)	Sodium (mg)	Carbohydrates (g)	Fiber (g)	Protein (g)
CARROTS								
Baby, fresh	1 med	4	0	0	8	1	0	0
Boiled, slices	1/2 cup	27	0	0	45	6	2	1
Canned, w/o salt	1/2 cup	18	0	0	31	4	1	0
Canned, w/ salt	1/2 cup	18	0	0	177	4	1	0
Dehydrated	1/2 cup	126	1	0	102	29	9	3
Fresh, whole	1 med	25	0	0	42	6	2	1
Frozen, boiled	1/2 cup	27	0	0	43	6	2	0
CASABA MELON (fresh, cubed)	1 cup	48	0	0	15	11	2	2
CASHEW BUTTER								
Plain, w/o salt	1 tbsp	94	8	2	2	4	0	3
Plain, w/ salt	1 tbsp	94	8	2	98	4	0	3
CASHEW NUTS								
Dry roasted, w/o salt, halves	1 cup	786	64	13	22	45	4	21
Dry roasted, w/ salt, halves	1 cup	786	64	13	877	45	4	21
Fresh	1 oz	157	12	2	3	9	1	5
Oil roasted, w/o salt, whole	1 cup	748	62	11	17	39	4	22
Oil roasted, w/ salt, whole	1 cup	750	62	11	397	39	4	22
CASSAVA (fresh)	1 cup	330	1	0	29	78	4	3
CATFISH								
Channel, breaded & fried	3 oz	195	11	3	238	7	1	15
Channel, farmed, cooked in dry heat	3 oz	129	7	2	68	0	0	16
Channel, wild, cooked in dry heat	3 oz	89	2	1	42	0	0	16
CATSUP								
Catsup	1 tbsp	15	0	0	167	4	0	0
Low sodium	1 tbsp	15	0	0	3	4	0	0
CAULIFLOWER								
Boiled (1" pcs)	1/2 cup	14	0	0	9	3	1	1
Fresh	1 cup	25	0	0	30	5	3	2
Frozen, boiled (1" pcs)	1/2 cup	17	0	0	16	3	2	1
CAULIFLOWER GREENS								
Cooked	1/5 head	29	0	0	21	6	3	3
Fresh	1 cup	20	0	0	15	4	2	2
CAVIAR (black & red, granular)	1 tbsp	40	3	1	240	1	0	4

ITEM DESCRIPTION	Serving Size	Calories	Total Fat (g)	Saturated Fat (g)	Sodium (mg)	Carbohydrates (g)	Fiber (g)	Protein (g)
CELERIAC								
Boiled	1 cup	42	0	0	95	9	2	1
Fresh	1 cup	66	0	0	156	14	3	2
CELERY								
Boiled, diced	1 cup	27	0	0	136	6	2	1
Fresh, chopped	1 cup	16	0	0	81	3	2	1
Seed	1 tbsp	25	2	0	10	3	1	1
CEREAL								
Bran flakes	3/4 cup	96	1	0	220	24	5	3
Bran, malted flour	1/3 cup	83	1	0	121	23	8	4
Chocolate flavored rings, presweetened	3/4 cup	112	2	0	128	22	2	1
Corn flakes, low sodium	1 cup	100	0	0	2	22	0	2
Corn flakes, plain	1 cup	101	0	0	266	24	1	2
Corn, rice, wheat, oat, presweetened, w/fruit & almonds	1-1/4 cup	211	2	0	266	43	2	4
Crispy brown rice	1 cup	124	1	0	4	28	2	2
Farina, cooked w/ water	1 cup	112	0	0	5	24	1	3
Muesli, dried fruit & nuts	1 cup	289	4	1	196	66	6	8
Oat cereal, frosted w/marshmallows	1 cup	109	1	0	158	24	1	2
Oat, corn & wheat squares, presweetened, maple flavored	1 cup	129	3	0	130	24	1	2
Oats, instant, cinnamon & spice, cooked w/ water	1 cup	257	3	1	362	52	4	6
Oats, instant, plain, cooked w/ water	1 cup	159	3	1	115	27	4	6
Oats, instant, raisins & spice, cooked w/ water	1 cup	240	3	0	362	49	4	5
Oats, reg & quick & instant, cooked w/ water	1 cup	166	4	1	9	28	4	6
Puffed corn, chocolate frosted	1 cup	122	1	0	201	26	1	1
Puffed oats, corn mixture, presweetened	1 cup	130	1	0	212	27	1	3
Puffed oats, corn, presweetened, w/marshmallows	1 cup	115	1	0	206	25	0	2
Puffed rice	1 cup	56	0	0	0	13	0	1

ITEM DESCRIPTION	Serving Size	Calories	Total Fat (g)	Saturated Fat (g)	Sodium (mg)	Carbohydrates (g)	Fiber (g)	Protein (g)
Puffed rice, presweetened, fruit flavored	3/4 cup	108	1	0	158	24	0	1
Puffed rice, presweetened, w/ cocoa	3/4 cup	115	1	1	157	25	1	1
Puffed wheat	1 cup	44	0	0	0	10	1	2
Puffed wheat, presweetened	3/4 cup	107	0	0	40	25	0	1
Shredded wheat bran, plain, salt & sugar free	1-1/4 cup	197	1	0	3	47	8	7
Shredded wheat, plain, salt & sugar free	2 biscuits	155	1	0	3	36	6	5
Shredded wheat, plain, salt & sugar free, spoon size	1 cup	167	1	0	3	41	6	5
Shredded wheat, presweetened	1 cup	183	1	0	10	44	5	4
Shredded whole wheat, presweetened	1 cup	200	2	0	11	42	4	5
Wheat & bran, presweetened, w/ nuts & fruit	1 cup	212	3	0	280	42	5	4
Wheat & malt barley flakes	3/4 cup	106	1	0	140	24	3	3
Wheat germ, toasted, plain	1 cup	432	12	2	5	56	17	33
Whole wheat & oats, presweetened, w/ nuts & fruit	2/3 cup	204	5	1	156	40	4	4
Whole wheat & oats, presweetened, w/ pecans	2/3 cup	216	6	1	214	38	4	5
Whole wheat & oats, presweetened, w/ walnuts & fruit	1 cup	249	6	1	253	44	4	5
Whole wheat, corn & oats, presweetened, w/ almonds	3/4 cup	126	3	0	187	24	1	2
Whole wheat, hot natural cereal, cooked w/ water	1 cup	150	1	0	0	33	4	5
Whole wheat, oats & rice, maple flavored, w/ pecans	1 serv	219	5	2	145	40	3	4
CEREAL BARS								
Kashi TLC (Tasty Little Cereal) Bars, Blackberry Graham	1 bar	110	3	0	125	21	3	2
Kellogg's Nutri-Grain Cereal Bars, fruit filled	1 bar	139	3	0	110	27	1	2

ITEM DESCRIPTION	Serving Size	Calories	Total Fat (g)	Saturated Fat (g)	Sodium (mg)	Carbohydrates (g)	Fiber (g)	Protein (g)
Rice & wheat	1 bar	90	2	0	110	16	0	2
CEREAL, BRAND NAME								
Alpen	1 cup	398	4	1	241	86	10	13
Cream of Rice, cooked w/ water	1 cup	127	0	0	2	28	0	2
Cream of Wheat, instant, cooked w/ water	1 cup	149	1	0	10	32	1	4
Cream of Wheat, Mix 'n Eat, apple, banana & maple flavored	1 packet	132	0	0	242	29	1	2
Cream of Wheat, Mix 'n Eat, plain, cooked w/ water	1 packet	102	0	0	241	21	0	3
Cream of Wheat, quick, cooked w/ water	1 cup	129	0	0	139	27	1	4
Cream of Wheat, reg, cooked w/ water	1 cup	131	1	0	8	28	1	4
Familia	1 cup	473	8	1	61	90	10	12
General Mills Apple Cinnamon Cheerios	3/4 cup	120	2	0	120	25	1	2
General Mills Basic 4	1 cup	210	3	1	320	44	3	4
General Mills Berry Berry Kix	3/4 cup	104	1	0	139	23	1	1
General Mills Berry Burst Cheerios, all flavors	3/4 cup	99	1	0	162	22	2	3
General Mills Boo Berry	1 cup	132	1	0	209	29	0	1
General Mills Cheerios	1 cup	103	2	0	186	21	3	3
General Mills Chocolate Lucky Charms	1 cup	120	1	0	160	26	1	1
General Mills Cinnamon Grahams	3/4 cup	113	1	0	237	26	1	2
General Mills Cinnamon Toast Crunch	3/4 cup	134	3	0	217	25	1	2
General Mills Cocoa Puffs	3/4 cup	108	1	0	144	23	1	1
General Mills Cookie Crisp	1 cup	120	2	0	170	26	1	1
General Mills Cookie Crisp, peanut butter	3/4 cup	130	4	1	135	23	1	2
General Mills Corn Chex	1 cup	114	1	0	289	26	1	2
General Mills Count Chocula	3/4 cup	108	1	0	171	24	1	1
General Mills Country Corn Flakes	1 cup	110	1	0	270	25	1	2
General Mills Fiber One	1/2 cup	60	1	0	105	25	14	2

ITEM DESCRIPTION	Serving Size	Calories	Total Fat (g)	Saturated Fat (g)	Sodium (mg)	Carbohydrates (g)	Fiber (g)	Protein (g)
General Mills Franken Berry	1 cup	132	1	0	209	29	0	1
General Mills French Toast Crunch	3/4 cup	136	3	0	223	24	1	2
General Mills Frosted Cheerios	3/4 cup	110	1	0	200	23	1	2
General Mills Frosted Chex	3/4 cup	110	1	0	180	27	0	1
General Mills Golden Grahams	3/4 cup	120	1	0	270	26	1	1
General Mills Harmony	1-1/4 cup	201	1	0	355	43	2	6
General Mills Honey Nut Cheerios	3/4 cup	110	2	0	190	22	2	3
General Mills Honey Nut Chex	3/4 cup	128	1	0	235	28	0	2
General Mills Honey Nut Clusters	1 cup	218	3	0	290	48	3	4
General Mills Kaboom	1-1/4 cup	120	1	0	190	26	1	1
General Mills Kix	1-1/4 cup	110	1	0	199	25	3	2
General Mills Lucky Charms	3/4 cup	110	1	0	183	22	1	2
General Mills Multi-Bran Chex	3/4 cup	154	1	0	292	40	6	3
General Mills Multi-Grain Cheerios	1 cup	114	1	0	207	25	3	2
General Mills Nature Valley Low Fat Fruit Granola	2/3 cup	212	3	0	207	44	3	4
General Mills Oatmeal Crisp, apple cinnamon	1 cup	210	2	1	270	46	4	4
General Mills Oatmeal Crisp, raisin	1 cup	237	2	1	248	50	4	6
General Mills Oatmeal Crisp, triple berry	1 cup	210	3	1	260	45	5	5
General Mills Oatmeal Crisp, w/ almonds	1 cup	240	5	1	273	46	5	5
General Mills Para Su Familia Raisin Bran	1-1/3 cup	170	1	0	300	42	7	4
General Mills Peanut Butter Toast Crunch	3/4 cup	130	4	1	135	23	1	2
General Mills Raisin Nut Bran	3/4 cup	200	4	1	250	42	5	4
General Mills Reese's Puffs	3/4 cup	126	3	0	193	22	1	2
General Mills Rice Chex	1 cup	103	0	0	240	23	0	2
General Mills Team Cheerios	3/4 cup	100	1	0	180	22	2	2
General Mills Total Corn Flakes	1-1/3 cup	112	0	0	209	26	1	2
General Mills Total Raisin Bran	1 cup	170	1	0	240	42	5	3
General Mills Trix	1 cup	128	2	0	180	28	1	1
General Mills Wheat Chex	3/4 cup	169	1	0	395	38	5	5

ITEM DESCRIPTION	Serving Size	Calories	Total Fat (g)	Saturated Fat (g)	Sodium (mg)	Carbohydrates (g)	Fiber (g)	Protein (g)
General Mills Wheaties	3/4 cup	99	1	0	189	22	3	3
General Mills Wheaties Raisin Bran	1 cup	183	1	0	251	45	5	4
General Mills Whole Grain Total	3/4 cup	100	1	0	190	23	3	2
General Mills Yogurt Burst Cheerios	3/4 cup	120	2	1	190	25	2	2
Health Valley Organic Fiber 7 Flakes	3/4 cup	109	0	0	16	24	4	4
Health Valley Organic Oat Bran Flakes	1 cup	166	1	0	17	37	6	5
Kashi 7 Whole Grain Flakes	1 cup	175	1	0	152	41	6	6
Kashi 7 Whole Grain Honey Puffs	1 cup	114	1	0	6	25	2	3
Kashi 7 Whole Grain Nuggets	1/2 cup	206	2	0	260	47	7	7
Kashi Cinnamon-Raisin Crunch	1 cup	165	1	0	104	41	8	4
Kashi Go Lean	1 cup	148	1	0	86	30	10	14
Kashi Go Lean Crunch!	1 cup	200	3	0	204	36	8	9
Kashi Go Lean Crunch!, honey almond flax	1 cup	202	4	0	138	36	9	9
Kashi Good Friends	1 cup	167	2	0	129	43	12	5
Kashi Granola, Cocoa Beach	1/2 cup	226	9	2	118	34	7	6
Kashi Granola, Mountain Medley	1/2 cup	218	7	1	110	37	6	6
Kashi Granola, Orchard Spice	1/2 cup	222	7	1	129	37	6	6
Kashi Granola, Summer Berry	1/2 cup	214	6	1	132	37	7	7
Kashi Heart to Heart, honey toasted oat	3/4 cup	118	2	0	79	25	5	4
Kashi Heart to Heart, wild blueberry	1 cup	204	3	0	133	42	4	6
Kashi Mighty Bites, cinnamon	1 cup	117	1	0	162	23	3	6
Kashi Mighty Bites, honey crunch	1 cup	116	1	0	159	23	3	6
Kashi Organic Promise Autumn Wheat	1 cup	191	1	0	5	45	6	5
Kashi Organic Promise Cinnamon Harvest	1 cup	184	1	0	5	44	6	4
Kashi Organic Promise Cranberry Sunshine	1 cup	116	1	0	21	26	3	2
Kashi Organic Promise Strawberry Fields	1 cup	118	0	0	200	28	1	3
Kashi Puffs	1 cup	75	1	0	2	15	1	2

ITEM DESCRIPTION	Serving Size	Calories	Total Fat (g)	Saturated Fat (g)	Sodium (mg)	Carbohydrates (g)	Fiber (g)	Protein (g)
Kashi Seven in the Morning	1/2 cup	178	1	0	224	41	6	6
Kellogg's All-Bran Bran Buds	1/3 cup	75	1	0	203	24	13	2
Kellogg's All-Bran Complete Wheat Flakes	3/4 cup	92	1	0	207	23	5	3
Kellogg's All-Bran, original	1/2 cup	81	2	0	75	23	9	4
Kellogg's All-Bran Yogurt Bites	1-1/4 cup	192	3	2	235	44	10	6
Kellogg's Apple Jacks	1 cup	129	0	0	146	30	1	1
Kellogg's Apple Jacks Cereal Straws	3 straws	136	4	2	16	24	0	2
Kellogg's Berry Rice Krispies	1 cup	115	0	0	218	26	0	2
Kellogg's Cocoa Krispies	3/4 cup	118	1	1	197	27	1	2
Kellogg's Cocoa Krispies Cereal Straws	3 straws	136	4	2	16	24	1	2
Kellogg's Corn Flakes	1 cup	101	0	0	202	24	1	2
Kellogg's Corn Flakes, w/ real bananas	3/4 cup	108	2	2	118	22	1	1
Kellogg's Corn Pops	1 cup	117	0	0	120	28	0	1
Kellogg's Cracklin' Oat Bran	3/4 cup	197	7	3	151	35	6	4
Kellogg's Crispix	1 cup	109	0	0	222	25	0	2
Kellogg's Cruncheroos	1 cup	110	2	0	240	22	3	4
Kellogg's Eggo Crunch Cereal, maple syrup	1 cup	124	1	0	158	27	2	2
Kellogg's Froot Loops	1 cup	118	1	1	141	26	1	1
Kellogg's Froot Loops Cereal Straws	3 straws	136	4	2	15	24	0	2
Kellogg's Froot Loops, marshmallow	1 cup	118	1	0	108	27	1	1
Kellogg's Froot Loops, reduced sugar	1-1/4 cup	126	1	0	180	28	1	2
Kellogg's Frosted Flakes	3/4 cup	110	0	0	139	27	1	1
Kellogg's Frosted Flakes, reduced sugar	1 cup	117	0	0	178	28	0	2
Kellogg's Frosted Krispies	3/4 cup	115	0	0	193	27	0	2
Kellogg's Frosted Mini-Wheats, bite size	24 biscuits	203	1	0	5	48	6	6
Kellogg's Frosted Mini-Wheats, bite size maple & brown sugar	24 biscuits	185	1	0	1	43	5	4

ITEM DESCRIPTION	Serving Size	Calories	Total Fat (g)	Saturated Fat (g)	Sodium (mg)	Carbohydrates (g)	Fiber (g)	Protein (g)
Kellogg's Frosted Mini-Wheats, bite size strawberry	24 biscuits	180	1	0	0	43	5	4
Kellogg's Frosted Mini-Wheats, bite size vanilla	24 biscuits	180	1	0	1	43	5	4
Kellogg's Frosted Mini-Wheats, original	5 biscuits	175	1	0	5	42	5	5
Kellogg's Fruit Harvest, apple cinnamon	1 cup	206	3	0	255	43	3	4
Kellogg's Fruit Harvest, banana berry	3/4 cup	119	2	1	136	26	2	2
Kellogg's Fruit Harvest, peach strawberry	3/4 cup	110	0	0	165	26	2	2
Kellogg's Fruit Harvest, strawberry blueberry	3/4 cup	107	0	0	137	25	1	2
Kellogg's Healthy Choice, almond crunch w/raisins	1 cup	198	3	0	215	43	5	5
Kellogg's Honey Crunch Corn Flakes	3/4 cup	116	1	0	210	26	1	2
Kellogg's Honey Smacks	3/4 cup	104	0	0	50	24	1	2
Kellogg's Just Right Fruit & Nut	3/4 cup	194	2	0	243	43	3	4
Kellogg's Just Right, w/crunchy nuggets	1 cup	204	1	0	338	46	3	4
Kellogg's Low Fat Granola, w/o raisins	1/2 cup	190	3	1	107	40	4	4
Kellogg's Low Fat Granola, w/raisins	2/3 cup	230	3	1	148	49	4	5
Kellogg's Mini-Wheats, apple cinnamon	3/4 cup	182	1	0	20	44	5	4
Kellogg's Mini-Wheats, strawberry	24 biscuits	180	1	0	0	43	5	4
Kellogg's Mini-Wheats, strawberry	1 cup	184	1	0	16	44	5	5
Kellogg's Mueslix	2/3 cup	196	3	0	170	40	4	5
Kellogg's Product 19	1 cup	100	0	0	207	25	1	2
Kellogg's Puffed Wheat	3/4 cup	29	0	0	0	7	1	1
Kellogg's Raisin Bran	1 cup	190	1	0	342	46	7	5
Kellogg's Raisin Bran Crunch	1 cup	188	1	0	209	45	4	3
Kellogg's Raisin Mini-Wheats	3/4 cup	188	1	0	3	44	5	5

ITEM DESCRIPTION	Serving Size	Calories	Total Fat (g)	Saturated Fat (g)	Sodium (mg)	Carbohydrates (g)	Fiber (g)	Protein (g)
Kellogg's Rice Krispies	1 1/4 cup	128	0	0	299	28	0	2
Kellogg's Rice Krispies Treats Cereal	3/4 cup	120	1	0	166	25	0	1
Kellogg's Robots	1 cup	113	1	0	157	25	1	2
Kellogg's Scooby-Doo! Berry Bones	1 cup	127	1	0	233	28	1	2
Kellogg's Shredded Wheat Miniatures	30 biscuits	102	1	0	0	24	4	3
Kellogg's Smart Start Strong Heart, antioxidant cereal	1 cup	182	1	0	275	43	3	4
Kellogg's Smart Start Strong Heart, brown sugar	1-1/4 cup	220	2	0	140	47	5	6
Kellogg's Smart Start Strong Heart, original	1-1/4 cup	220	2	0	140	47	5	6
Kellogg's Smorz	1 cup	122	2	1	137	25	1	1
Kellogg's Special K	1 cup	117	0	0	224	22	1	7
Kellogg's Special K, fruit & yogurt	3/4 cup	122	1	0	137	28	2	2
Kellogg's Special K, protein plus	3/4 cup	101	3	1	110	14	5	10
Kellogg's Special K, red berries	1 cup	114	0	0	220	25	1	4
Kellogg's Special K, vanilla almond	3/4 cup	115	1	0	164	25	2	2
Kellogg's SpongeBob Squarepants Cereal	1 cup	118	1	0	121	26	1	2
Kellogg's Star Wars Cereal	1 cup	109	1	0	182	24	2	2
Kellogg's Tiger Power	1 cup	105	1	0	253	21	3	6
Kellogg's Tony's Cinnamon Krunchers	3/4 cup	130	3	1	154	23	0	1
Maltex, cooked w/ water	1 cup	189	1	0	12	39	2	6
Malt-O-Meal Apple Cinnamon Toasty O's	3/4 cup	123	2	0	162	25	2	2
Malt-O-Meal Apple Zings	1 cup	130	1	0	170	29	1	2
Malt-O-Meal Berry Colossal Crunch	3/4 cup	124	2	0	247	26	1	1
Malt-O-Meal Blueberry Muffin Tops Cereal	3/4 cup	133	3	1	124	24	1	1
Malt-O-Meal Chocolate, cooked w/ water	1 serv	118	0	0	8	25	1	3
Malt-O-Meal Cinnamon Toasters	3/4 cup	129	3	1	138	24	1	2

ITEM DESCRIPTION	Serving Size	Calories	Total Fat (g)	Saturated Fat (g)	Sodium (mg)	Carbohydrates (g)	Fiber (g)	Protein (g)
Malt-O-Meal Cocoa Dyno-Bites	3/4 cup	117	1	1	177	26	0	1
Malt-O-Meal Coco Roos	3/4 cup	119	1	0	170	27	1	1
Malt-O-Meal Colossal Crunch	3/4 cup	124	2	0	197	26	0	1
Malt-O-Meal Corn Bursts	1 cup	122	0	0	124	29	1	1
Malt-O-Meal Corn Flakes	1 cup	114	0	0	306	26	1	2
Malt-O-Meal Crispy Rice	1 cup	126	0	0	297	29	0	2
Malt-O-Meal Frosted Flakes	3/4 cup	116	0	0	172	27	1	2
Malt-O-Meal Fruity Dyno-Bites	3/4 cup	109	1	0	173	24	0	1
Malt-O-Meal Golden Puffs	3/4 cup	107	0	0	48	24	1	2
Malt-O-Meal High Fiber Bran Flakes	3/4 cup	113	1	0	195	23	4	3
Malt-O-Meal Honey Buzzers	1 1/3 cup	115	1	0	206	25	1	2
Malt-O-Meal Honey Graham Cereal	3/4 cup	114	1	0	273	25	2	2
Malt-O-Meal Original, cooked w/ water	1 serv	113	0	0	8	23	1	4
Malt-O-Meal Puffed Rice Cereal	1 cup	60	0	0	1	14	0	1
Malt-O-Meal Puffed Wheat Cereal	1 cup	59	0	0	2	12	1	2
Malt-O-Meal Raisin Bran Cereal	1 cup	213	1	0	392	45	8	5
Malt-O-Meal Tootie Fruities	1 cup	128	1	0	148	28	1	2
Maypo, cooked w/ water	1 cup	170	2	0	10	32	6	6
Mother's Cinnamon Oat Crunch	1 cup	228	3	0	251	48	5	6
Mother's Cocoa Bumpers	1 cup	124	1	0	180	29	1	2
Mother's Instant Oatmeal	1/4 cup	144	3	1	1	26	4	5
Mother's Oat Bran	1/2 cup	146	3	1	2	25	6	7
Mother's Peanut Butter Bumpers Cereal	1 cup	133	2	0	266	26	1	3
Mother's Toasted Oat Bran Cereal, brown sugar	3/4 cup	119	2	0	202	24	3	4
Nature's Path, Optimum Slim	1 cup	180	3	0	250	38	11	9
Post 100% Bran Cereal	1/3 cup	83	1	0	121	23	8	4
Post Alpha-Bits Cereal	1 cup	130	1	0	212	27	1	3
Post Bran Flakes	3/4 cup	96	1	0	220	24	5	3
Post Cocoa Pebbles Cereal	3/4 cup	115	1	1	157	25	1	1
Post Frosted Shredded Wheat Spoon Size Cereal	1 cup	183	1	0	10	44	5	4

ITEM DESCRIPTION	Serving Size	Calories	Total Fat (g)	Saturated Fat (g)	Sodium (mg)	Carbohydrates (g)	Fiber (g)	Protein (g)
Post Fruit & Fiber Dates, raisins & walnuts	1 cup	212	3	0	280	42	5	4
Post Fruity Pebbles Cereal	3/4 cup	108	1	0	158	24	0	1
Post Golden Crisp Cereal	3/4 cup	107	0	0	40	25	0	1
Post Grape-Nuts Cereal	1/2 cup	208	1	0	317	46	5	7
Post Grape-Nuts Flakes	3/4 cup	106	1	0	140	24	3	3
Post Honey Bunches of Oats, honey roasted	3/4 cup	118	1	0	180	25	1	2
Post Honey Bunches of Oats, w/ almonds	3/4 cup	126	3	0	187	24	1	2
Post Honeycomb Cereal	1-1/3 cup	115	1	0	215	26	1	2
Post Marshmallow Alpha-Bits Cereal	1 cup	115	1	0	206	25	1	2
Post Oreo O's Cereal	3/4 cup	112	2	0	128	22	2	1
Post Original Shredded Wheat 'n Bran	1-1/4 cup	197	1	0	3	47	8	7
Post Original Shredded Wheat Spoon Size	1 cup	167	1	0	3	41	6	5
Post Raisin Bran Cereal	1 cup	178	1	0	274	43	7	5
Post Selects Banana Nut Crunch Cereal	1 cup	249	6	1	253	44	4	5
Post Selects Blueberry Morning Cereal	1-1/4 cup	211	2	0	266	43	2	4
Post Selects Cranberry Almond Crunch	1 cup	220	3	0	200	45	3	4
Post Selects Great Grains Crunchy Pecan Cereal	2/3 cup	216	6	1	214	38	4	5
Post Selects Great Grains Raisin, Date & Pecan Cereal	2/3 cup	204	5	1	156	40	4	4
Quaker 100% Natural Granola, w/oats & honey	1/2 cup	206	6	4	24	35	3	5
Quaker 100% Natural Granola, w/oats, honey, & raisins	1/2 cup	213	6	4	28	38	3	5
Quaker 100% Natural Granola, w/raisins, low fat	2/3 cup	214	3	1	139	45	3	4
Quaker Apple Zaps	3/4 cup	118	1	0	135	27	1	1

ITEM DESCRIPTION	Serving Size	Calories	Total Fat (g)	Saturated Fat (g)	Sodium (mg)	Carbohydrates (g)	Fiber (g)	Protein (g)
Quaker Cap'n Crunch	3/4 cup	109	2	1	202	23	1	1
Quaker Cap'n Crunch Chocolatey Peanut Butter Crunch Cereal	3/4 cup	112	2	1	141	21	1	2
Quaker Cap'n Crunch Crunch Berries	3/4 cup	105	1	1	182	22	1	1
Quaker Cap'n Crunch Peanut Butter Crunch	3/4 cup	112	2	1	200	21	1	2
Quaker Christmas Crunch	3/4 cup	104	1	1	184	22	1	1
Quaker Cocoa Blasts	1 cup	130	1	0	135	29	1	1
Quaker Cranberry Macadamia Nut Cereal	1 cup	245	6	1	251	46	4	4
Quaker Crunchy Bran	3/4 cup	90	1	1	235	23	5	2
Quaker Fruitangy Oh!s	1 cup	122	1	0	152	27	1	2
Quaker Honey Graham Life Cereal	3/4 cup	119	1	0	156	25	2	3
Quaker Honey Graham Oh!s	3/4 cup	111	2	2	166	23	1	1
Quaker Instant Oatmeal Express, baked apple, cooked w/ water	1 packet	208	3	0	322	42	4	4
Quaker Instant Oatmeal Express, golden brown sugar, cooked w/ water	1 packet	209	3	0	294	42	4	5
Quaker Instant Oatmeal, apples & cinnamon, cooked w/ water	1 packet	130	1	0	165	26	3	3
Quaker Instant Oatmeal, brown sugar cinnamon, cooked w/ water	1 packet	199	4	2	251	38	3	4
Quaker Instant Oatmeal, cinnamon & spice, cooked w/ water	1 packet	177	2	0	249	36	3	4
Quaker Instant Oatmeal, cinnamon roll, cooked w/ water	1 packet	209	3	0	249	41	4	5
Quaker Instant Oatmeal, fruit & cream variety, cooked w/ water	1 packet	139	3	1	181	26	2	3
Quaker Instant Oatmeal, honey nut, cooked w/ water	1 packet	173	4	0	238	31	3	4
Quaker Instant Oatmeal, maple & brown sugar, cooked w/ water	1 packet	157	2	0	253	31	3	4
Quaker Instant Oatmeal, Nutrition for Women, applespice, cooked w/ water	1 packet	178	2	0	319	35	3	5

ITEM DESCRIPTION	Serving Size	Calories	Total Fat (g)	Saturated Fat (g)	Sodium (mg)	Carbohydrates (g)	Fiber (g)	Protein (g)
Quaker Instant Oatmeal, Nutrition for Women, brown sugar, cooked w/ water	1 packet	173	2	0	328	33	3	5
Quaker Instant Oatmeal, raisins & spice, cooked w/ water	1 packet	162	2	0	245	33	3	3
Quaker Instant Oatmeal, vanilla cinnamon, cooked w/ water	1 packet	165	2	0	249	33	3	4
Quaker King Vitamin	1-1/2 cup	120	1	0	259	26	1	2
Quaker Kretschmer Honey Crunch Toasted Wheat Germ	1-2/3 tbsp	52	1	0	2	8	1	4
Quaker Kretschmer Toasted Wheat Bran	1/4 cup	32	1	0	1	10	7	3
Quaker Kretschmer Wheat Germ, reg	1-2/3 tbsp	51	1	0	1	7	2	4
Quaker Life, cinnamon	3/4 cup	119	1	0	153	25	2	3
Quaker Life, original	3/4 cup	119	1	0	164	25	2	3
Quaker Life Vanilla Yogurt Crunch Cereal	1-1/4 cup	210	3	1	248	43	4	5
Quaker Marshmallow Safari	3/4 cup	119	2	0	192	25	1	2
Quaker Oat Bran Cereal	1-1/4 cup	212	3	1	207	43	6	7
Quaker Oatmeal Cereal, brown sugar bliss	1 cup	188	3	1	249	39	4	4
Quaker Oatmeal Squares	1 cup	212	2	1	269	44	4	6
Quaker Oatmeal Squares, cinnamon	1 cup	227	3	0	264	48	5	6
Quaker Puffed Rice	1 cup	54	0	0	1	12	0	1
Quaker Puffed Wheat	1-1/4 cup	55	0	0	1	11	1	2
Quaker Quisp	1 cup	109	2	1	200	23	1	1
Quaker Superman Life Cereal	3/4 cup	112	1	0	167	24	2	3
Quaker Sweet Puffs	1 cup	133	1	0	80	30	1	2
Quaker Toasted Oatmeal Cereal	1 cup	188	2	1	274	39	3	5
Quaker Toasted Oatmeal Cereal, honeynut	1 cup	188	2	1	228	40	3	4
Ralston, cooked w/ water	1 cup	134	1	0	5	28	6	6
Ralston Corn Flakes	1 cup	111	0	0	220	27	1	2
Ralston Crispy Hexagons	1 cup	106	0	0	228	24	0	2
Ralston Crispy Rice	1-1/4 cup	120	0	0	310	29	0	2

ITEM DESCRIPTION	Serving Size	Calories	Total Fat (g)	Saturated Fat (g)	Sodium (mg)	Carbohydrates (g)	Fiber (g)	Protein (g)
Ralston Enriched Bran Flakes	3/4 cup	90	0	0	210	23	5	3
Ralston Tasteeos	1 cup	110	0	0	240	23	3	3
Ralston Waffelos	1 cup	122	1	0	125	26	0	2
Roman Meal Original, w/oats, cooked w/ water & salt	1 cup	170	2	0	540	34	8	7
Weetabix Whole Grain Cereal	1 cup	213	2	0	221	44	7	7
Wheatena, cooked w/ water	1 cup	136	1	0	5	29	7	5
CHAYOTE								
Boiled (1" pcs)	1 cup	38	1	0	2	8	5	1
Fresh (1" pcs)	1 cup	25	0	0	3	6	2	1
CHEESE								
American, pasteurized, processed	3/4 oz slice	79	7	4	313	0	0	5
American, pasteurized, processed, low fat	3/4 oz slice	38	1	1	300	1	0	5
Blue	1 oz	100	8	5	395	1	0	6
Brick	1 oz	105	8	5	159	1	0	7
Brie	1 oz	95	8	5	178	0	0	6
Camembert	1 oz	84	7	4	236	0	0	6
Caraway	1 oz	107	8	5	196	1	0	7
Cheddar	1 oz slice	113	9	6	174	0	0	7
Cheddar, low fat	1 oz slice	48	2	1	171	1	0	7
Cheddar, low sodium	1 oz slice	105	9	6	6	1	0	7
Cheddar or American, pasteurized, processed, fat free	3/4 oz slice	31	0	0	321	3	0	5
Cheddar or American, pasteurized, processed, low sodium	3/4 oz slice	79	7	4	1	0	0	5
Cheshire	1 oz	110	9	6	198	1	0	7
Colby	1 oz slice	110	9	6	169	1	0	7
Colby, low fat	1 oz slice	48	2	1	171	1	0	7
Colby, low sodium	1 oz slice	111	9	6	6	1	0	7
Edam	1 oz	101	8	5	274	0	0	7
Feta	1 oz	75	6	4	316	1	0	4
Fontina	1 oz slice	109	9	5	224	0	0	7
Gjetost	1 oz	132	8	5	170	12	0	3

ITEM DESCRIPTION	Serving Size	Calories	Total Fat (g)	Saturated Fat (g)	Sodium (mg)	Carbohydrates (g)	Fiber (g)	Protein (g)
Goat, hard	1 oz	128	10	7	98	1	0	9
Goat, semisoft	1 oz	103	8	6	146	1	0	6
Goat, soft	1 oz	76	6	4	104	0	0	5
Gouda	1 oz	101	8	5	232	1	0	7
Gruyere	1 oz slice	116	9	5	94	0	0	8
Kraft Free Singles, American, nonfat, pasteurized, processed	1 slice	31	0	0	273	2	0	5
Limburger	1 oz	93	8	5	227	0	0	6
Mexican, queso anejo	1 oz	106	8	5	321	1	0	6
Mexican, queso asadero	1 oz	101	8	5	186	1	0	6
Mexican, queso Chihuahua	1 oz	106	9	5	175	2	0	6
Monterey	1 oz slice	104	8	5	150	0	0	7
Monterey, low fat	1 oz slice	88	6	4	158	0	0	8
Mozzarella, low sodium	1 oz	78	5	3	4	1	0	8
Mozzarella, nonfat	1 oz	42	0	0	211	1	1	9
Mozzarella, part skim milk	1 oz	72	5	3	175	1	0	7
Mozzarella, part skim milk, low moisture	1 oz	86	6	4	150	1	0	7
Mozzarella, whole milk	1 oz	85	6	4	178	1	0	6
Mozzarella, whole milk, low moisture	1 oz	90	7	4	118	1	0	6
Muenster	1 oz slice	103	8	5	176	0	0	7
Muenster, low fat	1 oz slice	105	5	3	168	1	0	7
Neufchatel	1 oz	77	6	4	95	1	0	3
Parmesan, dry grated, reduced fat	1 tbsp	13	1	1	76	0	0	1
Parmesan, grated	1 tbsp	22	1	1	76	0	0	2
Parmesan, hard	1 oz	111	7	5	454	1	0	10
Parmesan, low sodium	1 tbsp	23	2	1	3	0	0	2
Parmesan, shredded	1 tbsp	21	1	1	85	0	0	2
Pimento, pasteurized processed	1 oz	106	9	6	405	0	0	6
Port de Salut	1 oz	100	8	5	151	0	0	7
Provolone	1 oz slice	98	7	5	245	1	0	7
Provolone, reduced fat	1 oz slice	77	5	3	245	1	0	7
Ricotta, part skim milk	1 oz	39	2	1	35	1	0	3

ITEM DESCRIPTION	Serving Size	Calories	Total Fat (g)	Saturated Fat (g)	Sodium (mg)	Carbohydrates (g)	Fiber (g)	Protein (g)
Ricotta, whole milk	1 oz	49	4	2	24	1	0	3
Romano	1 oz	110	8	5	340	1	0	9
Roquefort	1 oz	105	9	5	513	1	0	6
Swiss	1 oz slice	106	8	5	54	2	0	8
Swiss, low fat	1 oz slice	50	1	1	73	1	0	8
Swiss, low sodium	1 oz slice	105	8	5	4	1	0	8
Swiss, pasteurized, processed	3/4 oz slice	70	5	3	288	1	0	5
Swiss, pasteurized, processed, low fat	3/4 oz slice	36	1	1	300	1	0	5
Tilsit	1 oz	96	7	5	213	1	0	7
CHEESE FONDUE	1/2 cup	247	15	9	143	4	0	15
CHEESE FOOD								
American, cold packed	1 oz	94	7	4	274	2	0	6
American, pasteurized, processed	3/4 oz slice	79	7	4	313	1	0	5
Swiss, pasteurized, processed	1 oz	92	7	4	440	1	0	6
CHEESE PUFFS (corn based, low fat)	1 oz	122	3	1	364	21	3	2
CHEESE SAUCE								
Homemade	1 cup	479	36	20	1198	13	0	25
Kraft Cheez Whiz	2 tbsp	75	3	2	597	6	0	6
Ready to serve	1/4 cup	110	8	4	522	4	0	4
CHEESE SPREAD								
Cream cheese base	1 oz	84	8	5	191	1	0	2
Kraft Cheez Whiz	2 tbsp	91	7	4	541	3	0	4
Kraft Velveeta Light	1 oz	62	3	2	444	3	0	5
Kraft Velveeta	1 oz	85	6	4	420	3	0	5
Pasteurized, processed, American	1 oz	82	6	4	381	2	0	5
CHEESE SUBSTITUTE								
American cheddar imitation	1 slice	50	3	2	282	2	0	4
American or cheddar imitation, low cholesterol	1" cube	70	6	1	121	0	0	5
Mozzarella	1 oz	70	3	1	194	7	0	3
CHEESE TWISTS (corn based, low fat)	1 oz	122	3	1	364	21	3	2
CHERIMOYA (fresh, w/o skin)	1 fruit	231	2	0	12	55	7	5

ITEM DESCRIPTION	Serving Size	Calories	Total Fat (g)	Saturated Fat (g)	Sodium (mg)	Carbohydrates (g)	Fiber (g)	Protein (g)
CHERRY JUICE (from concentrate)	1 cup	140	0	0	25	34	0	1
CHERRIES								
Maraschino, canned	1 cherry	8	0	0	0	2	0	0
Sour, red, canned in ex heavy syrup	1 cup	298	0	0	18	76	2	2
Sour, red, canned in heavy syrup	1 cup	233	0	0	18	60	3	2
Sour, red, canned in light syrup	1 cup	189	0	0	18	49	2	2
Sour, red, canned in water	1 cup	88	0	0	17	22	3	2
Sour, red, fresh	1 cup	78	0	0	5	19	3	2
Sour, red, frozen, unsweetened	1 cup	71	1	0	2	17	3	1
Sweet, canned in ex heavy syrup	1 cup	266	0	0	8	68	4	2
Sweet, canned in heavy syrup	1 cup	210	0	0	8	54	4	2
Sweet, canned in juice	1 cup	135	0	0	8	35	4	2
Sweet, canned in light syrup	1 cup	169	0	0	8	44	4	2
Sweet, canned in water	1 cup	114	0	0	2	29	4	2
Sweet, fresh	1 cup	87	0	0	0	22	3	1
Sweet, frozen, sweetened	1 cup	231	0	0	3	58	5	3
CHERRY PIE FILLING								
Cherry pie filling	21 oz can	684	0	0	107	167	4	2
Low calorie	1 cup	140	0	0	32	32	3	2
CHERVIL (dried)	1 tbsp	5	0	0	2	1	0	0
CHESTNUTS								
Chinese, boiled & steamed	1 oz	43	0	0	1	10	0	1
Chinese, dried	1 oz	103	1	0	1	23	0	2
Chinese, fresh	1 oz	64	0	0	1	14	0	1
Chinese, roasted	1 oz	68	0	0	1	15	0	1
European, boiled & steamed	1 oz	37	0	0	8	8	0	1
European, dried, peeled	1 oz	105	1	0	10	22	0	1
European, dried, unpeeled	1 oz	106	1	0	10	22	3	2
European, fresh, peeled	1 oz	56	0	0	1	13	0	0
European, roasted	1 oz	69	1	0	1	15	1	1
Japanese, boiled & steamed	1 oz	16	0	0	1	4	0	0
Japanese, dried	1 oz	102	0	0	10	23	0	1
Japanese, fresh	1 oz	44	0	0	4	10	0	1
Japanese, roasted	1 oz	57	0	0	5	13	0	1

ITEM DESCRIPTION	Serving Size	Calories	Total Fat (g)	Saturated Fat (g)	Sodium (mg)	Carbohydrates (g)	Fiber (g)	Protein (g)
CHICKEN								
Breast, fat free mesquite flavored, slices	2 slices	34	0	0	437	1	0	7
Breast, oven roasted, fat free, slices	2 slices	33	0	0	457	1	0	7
Broiler/fryer, back, meat only, fried	1 back	334	18	5	115	7	0	35
Broiler/fryer, back, meat only, roasted	1 back	191	11	3	77	0	0	23
Broiler/fryer, back, meat only, stewed	1 back	176	9	3	56	0	0	21
Broiler/fryer, back, w/ skin, boneless, fried, battered	1 back	794	53	14	761	25	0	53
Broiler/fryer, back, w/ skin, boneless, fried, w/flour	1 back	477	30	8	130	9	0	40
Broiler/fryer, back, w/ skin, boneless, roasted	1 back	318	22	6	92	0	0	28
Broiler/fryer, back, w/ skin, stewed & chopped	1 cup	413	29	8	102	0	0	35
Broiler/fryer, breast, meat only, fried	1 breast	322	8	2	136	1	0	58
Broiler/fryer, breast, meat only, roasted & chopped	1 cup	231	5	1	104	0	0	43
Broiler/fryer, breast, meat only, stewed & chopped	1 cup	211	4	1	88	0	0	41
Broiler/fryer, breast, w/ skin, boneless, fried, battered	1 breast	728	37	10	770	25	1	70
Broiler/fryer, breast, w/ skin, boneless, fried, w/flour	1 breast	435	17	5	149	3	0	62
Broiler/fryer, breast, w/ skin, roasted & chopped	1 cup	276	11	3	99	0	0	42
Broiler/fryer, breast, w/ skin, stewed & chopped	1 cup	258	10	3	87	0	0	38
Broiler/fryer, dark meat, meat only, fried	1 cup	335	16	4	136	4	0	41
Broiler/fryer, dark meat, meat only, roasted & chopped	1 cup	287	14	4	130	0	0	38

ITEM DESCRIPTION	Serving Size	Calories	Total Fat (g)	Saturated Fat (g)	Sodium (mg)	Carbohydrates (g)	Fiber (g)	Protein (g)
Broiler/fryer, dark meat, meat only, stewed & chopped	1 cup	269	13	3	104	0	0	36
Broiler/fryer, dark meat, w/ skin, boneless, fried, battered	1 chicken	1657	104	28	1640	52	0	121
Broiler/fryer, dark meat, w/ skin, boneless, fried w/ flour	1 chicken	1049	62	17	328	15	0	100
Broiler/fryer, dark meat, w/ skin, boneless, roasted	1 chicken	845	53	15	291	0	0	87
Broiler/fryer, dark meat, w/ skin, boneless, stewed	1 chicken	857	54	15	258	0	0	86
Broiler/fryer, drumstick, meat only, fried	1 drumstick	82	3	1	40	0	0	12
Broiler/fryer, drumstick, meat only, roasted & chopped	1 cup	241	8	2	133	0	0	40
Broiler/fryer, drumstick, meat only, stewed & chopped	1 cup	270	9	2	128	0	0	44
Broiler/fryer, drumstick, w/ skin, boneless, fried, battered	1 drumstick	193	11	3	194	6	0	16
Broiler/fryer, drumstick, w/ skin, boneless, fried w/flour	1 drumstick	120	7	2	44	1	0	13
Broiler/fryer, drumstick, w/ skin, roasted & chopped	1 cup	302	16	4	126	0	0	38
Broiler/fryer, drumstick, w/ skin, stewed & chopped	1 cup	286	15	4	106	0	0	35
Broiler/fryer, leg, meat only, fried	1 leg	196	9	2	90	1	0	27
Broiler/fryer, leg, meat only, roasted & chopped	1 cup	267	12	3	127	0	0	38
Broiler/fryer, leg, meat only, stewed & chopped	1 cup	296	13	4	125	0	0	42
Broiler/fryer, leg, w/ skin, boneless, fried, battered	1 leg	431	26	7	441	14	0	34
Broiler/fryer, leg, w/ skin, boneless, fried w/flour	1 leg	284	16	4	99	3	0	30
Broiler/fryer, leg, w/ skin, roasted & chopped	1 cup	325	19	5	122	0	0	36
Broiler/fryer, leg, w/ skin, stewed & chopped	1 cup	308	18	5	102	0	0	34

ITEM DESCRIPTION	Serving Size	Calories	Total Fat (g)	Saturated Fat (g)	Sodium (mg)	Carbohydrates (g)	Fiber (g)	Protein (g)
Broiler/fryer, light meat, meat only, fried	1 cup	269	8	2	113	1	0	46
Broiler/fryer, light meat, meat only, roasted & chopped	1 cup	242	6	2	108	0	0	43
Broiler/fryer, light meat, meat only, stewed & chopped	1 cup	223	6	2	91	0	0	40
Broiler/fryer, light meat, w/ skin, boneless, fried, battered	1 chicken	1042	58	15	1079	36	0	89
Broiler/fryer, light meat, w/ skin, boneless, fried w/flour	1 chicken	640	31	9	200	5	0	79
Broiler/fryer, light meat, w/ skin, boneless, roasted	1 chicken	586	29	8	198	0	0	77
Broiler/fryer, light meat, w/ skin, boneless, stewed	1 chicken	603	30	8	189	0	0	78
Broiler/fryer, meat & skin & giblets & neck, fried, battered	1 chicken	2991	180	48	2920	93	0	235
Broiler/fryer, meat & skin & giblets & neck, fried w/flour	1 chicken	1926	108	29	609	23	0	202
Broiler/fryer, meat & skin & giblets & neck, roasted	1 chicken	1596	91	25	539	0	0	183
Broiler/fryer, meat & skin & giblets & neck, stewed	1 chicken	1622	93	26	496	0	0	184
Broiler/fryer, meat only, stewed & chopped	1 cup	248	9	3	98	0	0	38
Broiler/fryer, neck, meat only, fried	1 neck	50	3	1	22	0	0	6
Broiler/fryer, neck, meat only, simmered	1 neck	32	1	0	12	0	0	4
Broiler/fryer, neck, w/ skin, boneless, fried, battered	1 neck	172	12	3	144	5	0	10
Broiler/fryer, neck, w/ skin, boneless, fried w/flour	1 neck	120	9	2	30	2	0	9
Broiler/fryer, neck, w/ skin, boneless, simmered	1 neck	94	7	2	20	0	0	7
Broiler/fryer, skin only, fried, battered	1 chicken	1497	110	29	2208	88	0	39
Broiler/fryer, skin only, fried w/ flour	1 chicken	562	48	13	59	10	0	21

ITEM DESCRIPTION	Serving Size	Calories	Total Fat (g)	Saturated Fat (g)	Sodium (mg)	Carbohydrates (g)	Fiber (g)	Protein (g)
Broiler/fryer, skin only, roasted	1 chicken	508	46	13	73	0	0	23
Broiler/fryer, skin only, stewed	1 chicken	523	48	13	81	0	0	22
Broiler/fryer, thigh, meat only, fried	1 thigh	113	5	1	49	1	0	15
Broiler/fryer, thigh, meat only, roasted & chopped	1 cup	293	15	4	123	0	0	36
Broiler/fryer, thigh, meat only, stewed & chopped	1 cup	273	14	4	105	0	0	35
Broiler/fryer, thigh, w/ skin, boneless, fried, battered	1 thigh	238	14	4	248	8	0	19
Broiler/fryer, thigh, w/ skin, boneless, fried w/ flour	1 thigh	162	9	3	55	2	0	17
Broiler/fryer, thigh, w/ skin, boneless, stewed	1 thigh	158	10	3	48	0	0	16
Broiler/fryer, thigh, w/ skin, roasted & chopped	1 cup	346	22	6	118	0	0	35
Broiler/fryer, wing, meat only, fried	1 wing	42	2	1	18	0	0	6
Broiler/fryer, wing, meat only, roasted	1 wing	43	2	0	19	0	0	6
Broiler/fryer, wing, meat only, stewed & chopped	1 cup	253	10	3	102	0	0	38
Broiler/fryer, wing, w/ skin, boneless, fried, battered	1 wing	159	11	3	157	5	0	10
Broiler/fryer, wing, w/ skin, boneless, fried w/flour	1 wing	103	7	2	25	1	0	8
Broiler/fryer, wing, w/ skin, roasted & chopped	1 cup	406	27	8	115	0	0	38
Broiler/fryer, wing, w/ skin, stewed & chopped	1 cup	349	24	7	94	0	0	32
Broiler/fryer, w/ skin, boneless, fried, battered	1 chicken	2693	162	43	2721	88	3	210
Broiler/fryer, w/ skin, boneless, fried w/flour	1 chicken	1689	94	25	528	20	1	179
Broiler/fryer, w/ skin, roasted & chopped	1 cup	335	19	5	115	0	0	38
Broiler/fryer, w/ skin, stewed & chopped	1 cup	307	18	5	94	0	0	35
Canned, meat only, w/ broth	5 oz can	234	11	3	714	0	0	31

ITEM DESCRIPTION	Serving Size	Calories	Total Fat (g)	Saturated Fat (g)	Sodium (mg)	Carbohydrates (g)	Fiber (g)	Protein (g)
Canned, w/o broth	1 cup	377	17	5	277	2	0	52
Capons, giblets, simmered & chopped	1 cup	238	8	3	80	1	0	38
Capons, meat & skin & giblets & neck, roasted	1 capon	3205	165	47	709	1	0	402
Capons, w/ skin, roasted	1 capon	2917	148	42	624	0	0	369
Chicken breast roll, oven roasted	2 oz	75	4	1	494	1	0	8
Chicken roll, light meat	2 slices	63	2	0	604	3	0	9
Chicken spread	1 serv	88	10	2	404	2	0	10
Cornish game hens, meat only, roasted	1 hen	295	9	2	139	0	0	51
Cornish game hens, w/ skin, roasted	1 hen	668	47	13	164	0	0	57
Fajita strips, frozen	1 strip	13	1	0	75	0	0	2
Ground, crumbles, pan browned	3 oz	161	9	3	64	0	0	20
Roasting, dark meat, meat only, roasted & chopped	1 cup	249	12	3	133	0	0	33
Roasting, giblets, simmered & chopped	1 cup	239	8	2	87	1	0	39
Roasting, light meat, meat only, roasted & chopped	1 cup	214	6	2	71	0	0	38
Roasting, meat & skin & giblets & neck, roasted	1 chicken	2358	140	39	761	1	0	257
Roasting, meat & skin, roasted	1 chicken	2141	129	36	701	0	0	230
Roasting, meat only, roasted & chopped	1 cup	234	9	3	105	0	0	35
Stewing, dark meat, meat only, stewed & chopped	1 cup	361	21	6	133	0	0	39
Stewing, giblets, simmered & chopped	1 cup	281	13	4	81	0	0	37
Stewing, light meat, meat only, stewed & chopped	1 cup	298	11	3	81	0	0	46
Stewing, meat only, stewed & chopped	1 cup	332	17	4	109	0	0	43
Stewing, meat, skin, giblets & neck, stewed & chopped	1 cup	342	19	5	107	0	0	40

ITEM DESCRIPTION	Serving Size	Calories	Total Fat (g)	Saturated Fat (g)	Sodium (mg)	Carbohydrates (g)	Fiber (g)	Protein (g)
Stewing, w/ skin, boneless, stewed	1 chicken	1488	99	27	381	0	0	140
Wings, frozen, glazed, BBQ flavored	1 pc	61	4	1	178	1	0	6
Wings, frozen, glazed, BBQ flavored, heated in oven	1 serv	232	14	4	537	3	1	21
Wings, frozen, glazed, BBQ flavored, microwaved	1 serv	184	10	3	619	3	1	19
CHICKEN, BRAND NAME								
Carl Buddig Smoked Slices Chicken, light & dark meat	2 oz	94	6	1	544	0	0	10
Louis Rich Chicken Breast Classic, baked/grilled, Carving Board	1 slice	22	0	0	251	1	0	4
Louis Rich Chicken Breast, oven roasted deluxe	1 serv	28	1	0	333	1	0	5
Louis Rich Chicken, white, oven roasted	1 serv	36	2	0	335	1	0	5
Oscar Mayer Chicken Breast, honey glazed	4 slices	57	1	0	748	2	0	10
Oscar Mayer Chicken Breast, oven roasted, fat free	1 slice	11	0	0	161	0	0	2
CHICKEN BROTH								
Campbell's Red & White, condensed	4 fl oz	20	1	0	770	1	0	1
Canned, condensed	4 fl oz	39	1	0	786	1	0	6
Canned, condensed, prepared w/ water	8 fl oz	39	1	0	776	1	0	5
Canned, low sodium	8 fl oz	38	1	0	72	3	0	5
Canned, reduced sodium	8 fl oz	17	0	0	554	1	0	3
Cube, dry, prepared w/ water	8 fl oz	12	0	0	792	2	0	1
Swanson Chicken Broth	8 fl oz	9	0	0	928	0	0	1
CHICKEN ENTRÉE, BRAND NAME								
Campbell's Supper Bakes Meal Kits, garlic chicken w/ pasta	1/6 box	227	1	1	763	44	2	10
Campbell's Supper Bakes Meal Kits, herb chicken w/ rice	1/6 box	185	1	1	780	40	1	4
Campbell's Supper Bakes Meal Kits, lemon chicken w/ herb rice	1 serv	197	1	1	780	43	2	4

ITEM DESCRIPTION	Serving Size	Calories	Total Fat (g)	Saturated Fat (g)	Sodium (mg)	Carbohydrates (g)	Fiber (g)	Protein (g)
Campbell's Supper Bakes Meal Kits, Southwest-style chicken w/ rice	1/6 box	153	1	0	600	32	2	4
Campbell's Supper Bakes Meal Kits, traditional roast chicken w/ stuffing	1 serv	162	3	1	740	29	2	5
Swanson Chicken a la King	1 can	212	12	3	1371	12	2	14
Swanson Chicken & Dumplings	1 cup	230	10	5	990	24	2	11
Weight Watchers Smart Ones, chicken tenderloins w/ BBQ sauce	1 pkg	242	4	1	638	34	4	17
CHICKEN FAT	1 tbsp	115	13	4	0	0	0	0
CHICKEN STOCK (homemade)	1 cup	86	3	1	343	8	0	6
CHICKEN SUBSTITUTE								
Loma Linda Fried Chik'n w/ Gravy, canned	2 pcs	145	10	1	358	4	2	11
Meatless substitute	1 cup	376	21	3	1191	6	6	40
Meatless substitute, breaded, fried, diced	1 cup	304	17	1	520	11	6	28
Morningstar Farms Chik'n Nuggets, frozen	4 pcs	187	8	1	565	18	2	12
Morningstar Farms Chik Patties Original, frozen	1 patty	140	5	1	593	16	2	8
Morningstar Farms Italian Herb Chik Patties, frozen	1 patty	168	5	1	484	22	2	10
Morningstar Farms Meal Starters Chik'n Strips, frozen	12 strips	139	3	1	507	6	1	23
Morningstar Farms Meatfree Buffalo Wings, frozen	5 pcs	196	8	1	658	20	3	12
Morningstar Farms Original Chik'n Tenders, frozen	2 pcs	189	7	1	578	20	3	12
Morningstar Farms Roasted Herb Chik'n w/ Organic Soy, frozen	1 patty	107	3	0	340	9	2	12
Worthington Chic-Ketts, frozen	1 slice	112	5	1	405	3	2	14
Worthington Diced Chik, canned	1/4 cup	44	0	0	189	2	1	8
Worthington Frichik, canned	2 pcs	144	9	1	361	3	1	12
Worthington Low Fat Frichik, canned	2 pcs	87	2	0	354	4	1	12
CHICORY (fresh)	1 head	9	0	0	1	2	2	0

ITEM DESCRIPTION	Serving Size	Calories	Total Fat (g)	Saturated Fat (g)	Sodium (mg)	Carbohydrates (g)	Fiber (g)	Protein (g)
CHICORY GREENS (fresh, chopped)	1 cup	7	0	0	13	1	1	0
CHICORY ROOTS (fresh)	1 root	44	0	0	30	11	0	1
CHICKPEA FLOUR (besan)	1 cup	356	6	1	59	53	10	21
CHICKPEAS								
Boiled	1 cup	269	4	0	11	45	13	15
Canned	1 cup	286	3	0	718	54	11	12
Fresh	1 cup	728	12	1	48	121	35	39
CHILI								
BBQ w/ beans, ranch style, cooked	1 cup	245	3	0	1834	43	11	13
Beans included, canned	1 cup	287	14	6	1336	30	11	15
Campbell's Chunky Soups Firehouse Hot Spicy Beef Bean Chili	1 cup	233	8	4	870	25	8	15
Con carne, w/ beans, canned	1 cup	298	13	4	1043	28	10	17
Hormel Chili, w/ beans, canned	1 cup	240	4	2	1163	34	8	17
Hormel Chili, w/o beans, canned	1 cup	194	7	2	970	18	3	17
Hormel Vegetarian Chili, w/ beans, canned	1 cup	205	1	0	778	38	10	12
Nalley Chili Con Carne, w/ beans, canned	1 serv	281	8	3	1231	12	13	40
Nestle Chef-Mate Chili, w/ beans, canned	1 cup	420	24	10	1280	34	8	18
Nestle Chef-Mate Chili, w/o beans, canned	1 cup	368	23	8	1400	20	4	23
Old El Paso Chili, w/ beans, canned	1 serv	249	10	2	588	22	10	18
Stagg Classic Chili, w/ beans, canned	1 cup	324	16	7	825	29	7	17
Stagg Country Chili, w/ beans, canned	1 cup	319	16	7	1131	29	6	15
Stagg Dynamite Chili, w/ beans, canned	1 cup	333	15	6	862	31	8	18
Stagg Ranchhouse Chili, w/ beans, canned	1 cup	284	9	3	813	32	9	19
Stagg Silverado Chili, w/ beans, canned	1 cup	227	3	1	864	33	8	18
Worthington Chili, canned	1 cup	283	10	2	1042	25	8	24

ITEM DESCRIPTION	Serving Size	Calories	Total Fat (g)	Saturated Fat (g)	Sodium (mg)	Carbohydrates (g)	Fiber (g)	Protein (g)
CHILI POWDER	1 tbsp	24	1	0	76	4	3	1
CHITTERLINGS								
(pork, variety meat, simmered)	3 oz	198	17	8	15	0	0	11
CHIVES								
Freeze-dried	1 tbsp	1	0	0	0	0	0	0
Fresh, chopped	1 tbsp	1	0	0	0	0	0	0
CHOCOLATE								
Baking, M&M's Milk Chocolate Mini Baking Bits	1/2 oz	70	3	2	10	10	0	1
Baking, M&M's Semisweet Chocolate Mini Baking Bits	1/2 oz	72	4	2	0	9	1	1
Baking, Mexican, squares	1 tablet	85	3	2	1	15	1	1
Dark	1 oz	155	9	5	7	17	2	1
Dark, 45-59% cacao solid	1 oz	154	9	5	7	18	2	1
Dark, 60-69% cacao solid	1 oz	164	11	6	3	15	2	2
Dark, 70-85% cacao solid	1 oz	170	12	7	6	13	3	2
Sweet	1 oz	143	10	6	5	17	2	1
CHOCOLATE CHIPS								
Milk chocolate	1 cup	899	50	31	133	100	6	13
Semisweet	1 cup	805	50	30	18	106	10	7
Semisweet, made w/ butter	1 cup	811	50	30	19	108	10	7
White chocolate	1 cup	916	55	33	153	101	0	10
CHOCOLATE DRINK MIX								
Reduced calorie, dairy powder prepared w/ water & ice	1 serv	70	1	0	148	11	2	5
Powder, prepared w/ whole milk	1 cup	225	9	5	159	30	1	9
Powder, w/ added nutrients, prepared w/ whole milk	1 serv	234	8	5	136	31	0	9
Whey & milk based	1 cup	120	1	1	222	26	2	2
CHOCOLATE-HAZELNUT SPREAD	2 tbsp	200	11	11	15	23	2	2
CHOCOLATE MILK								
Commercial	1 cup	208	8	5	150	26	2	8
Commercial, low fat	1 cup	158	3	2	152	26	1	8
Commercial, reduced fat	1 cup	190	5	3	165	30	2	7
CHOCOLATE MOUSSE (homemade)	1/2 cup	454	32	18	77	32	1	8

ITEM DESCRIPTION	Serving Size	Calories	Total Fat (g)	Saturated Fat (g)	Sodium (mg)	Carbohydrates (g)	Fiber (g)	Protein (g)
CHOCOLATE SYRUP								
Fudge	2 tbsp	133	3	2	131	24	1	2
Hershey's Genuine Chocolate FlavorLite Syrup	2 tbsp	50	0	0	35	12	0	0
Hershey's Genuine Chocolate Flavor Syrup	2 tbsp	50	0	0	35	12	0	0
Prepared w/ whole milk	1 cup	254	8	5	133	36	1	9
Regular	2 tbsp	109	0	0	28	25	1	1
CHRYSANTHEMUM								
Leaves, fresh, chopped	1 cup	12	0	0	60	2	2	2
Garland, boiled (1" pcs)	1 cup	20	0	0	53	4	2	2
Garland, fresh (1" pcs)	1 cup	6	0	0	30	1	1	1
CILANTRO (fresh)	5 sprigs	1	0	0	3	0	0	0
CINNAMON (ground)	1 tbsp	19	0	0	1	6	4	0
CISCO (smoked)	3 oz	150	10	1	409	0	0	14
CITRUS FRUIT JUICE DRINK (frozen concentrate, prepared w/ water)	8 fl oz	114	0	0	10	28	0	1
CLAM & TOMATO JUICE (canned)	5.5 oz	80	0	0	601	18	1	1
CLAMS								
Breaded & fried	3 oz	172	9	2	309	9	0	12
Canned, drained	3 oz	126	2	0	95	4	0	22
Canned, liquid	3 oz	2	0	0	183	0	0	0
Cooked in moist heat	3 oz	126	2	0	95	4	0	22
CLEMENTINES (fresh, whole)	1 fruit	35	0	0	1	9	1	1
CLOVES (ground)	1 tbsp	21	1	0	16	4	2	0
COCOA								
Cocoa, hot, homemade	1 cup	192	6	4	110	27	3	9
Hershey's European Style Cocoa, powder, unsweetened	1 tbsp	84	1	0	0	3	1	1
Nestle Rich Chocolate	1 envelope	80	3	2	170	15	1	1
Nestle Rich Chocolate, w/ marshmallows	1 envelope	80	3	3	160	15	1	1
Powder, high fat, plain	1 tbsp	16	1	1	1	3	2	1
Powder, prepared w/ water	6 fl oz	113	1	1	150	24	1	2
Powder, unsweetened	1 tbsp	12	1	0	1	3	2	1

ITEM DESCRIPTION	Serving Size	Calories	Total Fat (g)	Saturated Fat (g)	Sodium (mg)	Carbohydrates (g)	Fiber (g)	Protein (g)
Powder w/aspartame, prepared w/ water	6 fl oz	56	0	0	138	11	1	2
Swiss Miss, no sugar added, powder	1 envelope	57	0	0	131	11	1	2
COCOA BUTTER OIL	1 tbsp	120	14	8	0	0	0	0
COCONUT CREAM								
Canned, sweetened	1 cup	1057	48	46	107	158	1	3
Fresh liquid from grated meat	1 cup	792	83	74	10	16	5	9
COCONUT MEAT								
Dried, creamed	1 oz	194	20	17	10	6	0	2
Dried, sweetened, flaked, canned	1 cup	341	24	22	15	32	4	3
Dried, sweetened, flaked, packaged	1 cup	388	24	22	242	44	8	3
Dried, sweetened, shredded	1 cup	466	33	29	244	44	4	3
Dried, toasted	1 oz	168	13	12	10	13	0	2
Dried, unsweetened	1 oz	187	18	16	10	7	5	2
Fresh, shredded	1 cup	283	27	24	16	12	7	3
COCONUT MILK								
Canned liquid from grated meat & water	1 cup	445	48	43	29	6	0	5
Fresh liquid from grated meat & water	1 cup	552	57	51	36	13	5	6
Frozen liquid	1 cup	485	50	44	29	13	0	4
COCONUT OIL	1 tbsp	117	14	12	0	0	0	0
COCONUT WATER	1 cup	46	0	0	252	9	3	2
COD								
Atlantic, canned, solids & liquid	3 oz	89	1	0	185	0	0	19
Atlantic, cooked in dry heat	3 oz	89	1	0	66	0	0	19
Atlantic, dried & salted	1 oz	82	1	0	1992	0	0	18
Pacific, cooked in dry heat	3 oz	89	1	0	77	0	0	20
COD LIVER OIL	1 tbsp	123	14	3	0	0	0	0
COFFEE								
Brewed, prepared w/ water	8 fl oz	2	0	0	5	0	0	0
Espresso, restaurant	1 fl oz	1	0	0	4	0	0	0
Instant, decaffeinated, prepared w/ water	6 fl oz	4	0	0	7	1	0	0

ITEM DESCRIPTION	Serving Size	Calories	Total Fat (g)	Saturated Fat (g)	Sodium (mg)	Carbohydrates (g)	Fiber (g)	Protein (g)
Instant, reg, prepared w/ water	6 fl oz	4	0	0	7	1	0	0
Instant, w/chicory, prepared w/ water	6 fl oz	5	0	0	13	1	0	0
Instant, w/ sugar, cappuccino flavor	4 tsp	53	1	0	23	11	0	0
Instant, w/ sugar, French flavor	4 tsp	63	3	1	72	9	0	1
Instant, w/ sugar, mocha flavor	2 tbsp	60	2	1	41	10	0	1
COFFEE LIQUEUR								
53 proof	1 fl oz	113	0	0	3	16	0	0
63 proof	1 fl oz	107	0	0	3	11	0	0
34 proof, w/cream	1 fl oz	102	5	3	29	7	0	1
COFFEE SUBSTITUTE								
Natural Touch Kaffree Roma, powder	1 tsp, rounded	7	0	0	3	2	0	0
Prepared w/ water	6 fl oz	11	0	0	9	2	1	0
Prepared w/ whole milk	6 fl oz	120	6	4	91	10	0	6
COLESLAW	1 tbsp	62	5	1	114	4	0	0
Coleslaw, reduced fat	1 tbsp	56	3	1	272	7	0	0
COLLARDS								
Boiled, chopped	1 cup	49	1	0	30	9	5	4
Fresh, chopped	1 cup	11	0	0	7	2	1	1
Frozen, boiled, chopped	1 cup	61	1	0	85	12	5	5
CONCH (baked or broiled, slices)	1 cup	165	2	0	194	2	0	33
COOKIES								
Animal Crackers	1	11	0	0	10	2	0	0
Arrowroot	1	22	1	0	18	4	0	0
Butter, commercial	1	23	1	1	18	3	0	0
Chocolate chip, commercial, higher fat, (2.25" dia)	1	48	2	1	32	7	0	1
Chocolate chip, commercial, lower fat	1	45	2	0	38	7	0	1
Chocolate chip, commercial, soft	1	55	3	1	33	8	0	1
Chocolate chip, homemade, made w/ butter (2.25" dia)	1	78	5	2	55	9	0	1
Chocolate chip, homemade, made w/ margarine (2.25" dia)	1	78	5	1	58	9	0	1
Chocolate chip, refrigerated dough	1 oz	126	6	2	59	17	0	1

ITEM DESCRIPTION	Serving Size	Calories	Total Fat (g)	Saturated Fat (g)	Sodium (mg)	Carbohydrates (g)	Fiber (g)	Protein (g)
Chocolate chip, refrigerated dough, baked (2.25" dia)	1	59	3	1	28	8	0	1
Chocolate sandwich, w/ creme filling, chocolate coated	1	82	4	1	55	11	1	1
Chocolate sandwich, w/ creme filling, reg	1	54	2	1	58	8	0	1
Chocolate sandwich, w/ extra creme filling	1	65	3	1	46	9	0	1
Chocolate wafers	1	26	1	0	35	4	0	0
Coconut macaroons, homemade (2" dia)	1	97	3	3	59	17	0	1
Fig bars	1	56	1	0	56	11	1	1
Fortune	1	30	0	0	22	7	0	0
Fudge, cake type	1	73	1	0	40	16	1	1
Gingersnaps	1	29	1	0	46	5	0	0
Graham crackers, chocolate coated (2.5" sq)	1	68	3	2	41	9	0	1
Graham crackers, plain, honey, or cinnamon (2.5" sq)	1	30	1	0	42	5	0	0
Ladyfingers, w/ lemon juice & rind	1	40	1	0	16	7	0	1
Ladyfingers, w/o lemon juice & rind	1	40	1	0	16	7	0	1
Marshmallow, chocolate-coated (1.75" dia)	1	55	2	1	22	9	0	1
Molasses (3.5" dia)	1	138	4	1	147	24	0	2
Oatmeal, commercial (3.5" dia)	1	112	5	1	96	17	1	2
Oatmeal, commercial, fat free (3.5" dia)	1	113	0	0	75	20	2	1
Oatmeal, commercial, soft	1	61	2	1	52	10	0	1
Oatmeal, homemade, w/o raisins (2-5/8" dia)	1	67	3	1	90	10	0	1
Oatmeal, homemade, w/ raisins (2-5/8" dia)	1	65	2	0	81	10	0	1
Oatmeal, refrigerated dough	1 oz	120	5	1	83	17	1	2
Oatmeal, refrigerated dough, baked	1	57	3	1	39	8	0	1
Peanut butter, commercial	1	72	4	1	62	9	0	1
Peanut butter, commercial, soft	1	69	4	1	50	9	0	1
Peanut butter, homemade	1	95	5	1	104	12	0	2
Peanut butter, refrigerated dough	1 oz	130	7	2	113	15	0	2
Peanut butter, refrigerated dough, baked	1	60	3	1	52	7	0	1
Peanut butter sandwich	1	67	3	1	52	9	0	1
Raisin, soft	1	60	2	1	51	10	0	1

ITEM DESCRIPTION	Serving Size	Calories	Total Fat (g)	Saturated Fat (g)	Sodium (mg)	Carbohydrates (g)	Fiber (g)	Protein (g)
Shortbread, pecan, commercial (2" dia)	1	76	5	1	39	8	0	1
Shortbread, plain, commercial (1-5/8" sq)	1	40	2	0	36	5	0	0
Sugar, commercial	1	72	3	1	54	10	0	1
Sugar, homemade, made w/ margarine (3" dia)	1	66	3	1	69	8	0	1
Sugar, refrigerated dough	1 oz	124	6	1	120	17	0	1
Sugar, refrigerated dough, baked	1	73	3	1	70	10	0	1
Sugar wafers w/creme filling (3.5" X 1")	1	46	2	0	13	6	0	0
Tea biscuits	1	22	1	0	19	4	0	0
Vanilla sandwich w/creme filling (1.75" dia)	1	48	2	0	35	7	0	0
Vanilla wafers, higher fat	1	28	1	0	18	4	0	0
Vanilla wafers, lower fat	1	28	1	0	19	4	0	0
COOKIES, BRAND NAME								
Archway Home Style Cookies, apple filled, oatmeal	1 serv	98	3	1	83	17	0	1
Archway Home Style Cookies, apricot filled	1 serv	100	3	1	80	16	1	1
Archway Home Style Cookies, chocolate chip drop	1 serv	102	4	1	98	16	0	1
Archway Home Style Cookies, chocolate chip ice box	1 serv	119	6	2	65	16	1	1
Archway Home Style Cookies, coconut macaroon	1 serv	101	5	4	53	13	1	1
Archway Home Style Cookies, cookie jar hermits	1 serv	98	2	1	164	18	1	1
Archway Home Style Cookies, dark molasses	1 serv	114	4	1	155	19	0	1
Archway Home Style Cookies, date filled, oatmeal	1 serv	100	3	1	83	17	1	1
Archway Home Style Cookies, Dutch cocoa	1 serv	103	4	1	92	17	1	1
Archway Home Style Cookies, fat free, devil's food	1 serv	68	0	0	79	16	1	1
Archway Home Style Cookies, fat free, oatmeal raisin	1 serv	108	0	0	179	25	1	1

ITEM DESCRIPTION	Serving Size	Calories	Total Fat (g)	Saturated Fat (g)	Sodium (mg)	Carbohydrates (g)	Fiber (g)	Protein (g)
Archway Home Style Cookies, frosty lemon	1 serv	112	4	2	95	17	0	1
Archway Home Style Cookies, fruit & honey bar	1 serv	106	3	1	107	18	1	1
Archway Home Style Cookies, gourmet apple 'n raisin	1 serv	113	4	1	137	17	1	1
Archway Home Style Cookies, gourmet oatmeal pecan	1 serv	132	6	2	97	17	1	2
Archway Home Style Cookies, gourmet rocky road	1 serv	129	6	1	79	18	1	1
Archway Home Style Cookies, iced molasses	1 serv	118	4	1	148	19	0	1
Archway Home Style Cookies, iced oatmeal	1 serv	122	5	1	106	19	1	1
Archway Home Style Cookies, oatmeal	1 serv	105	4	1	98	17	1	1
Archway Home Style Cookies, oatmeal raisin	1 serv	106	3	1	88	18	1	1
Archway Home Style Cookies, old fashioned molasses	1 serv	106	3	1	146	18	0	1
Archway Home Style Cookies, old fashioned windmill	1 serv	94	4	1	94	14	0	1
Archway Home Style Cookies, peanut butter	1 serv	101	5	1	85	12	1	2
Archway Home Style Cookies, pecan ice box	1 serv	120	6	1	76	15	0	1
Archway Home Style Cookies, raspberry filled	1 serv	100	3	1	84	16	1	1
Archway Home Style Cookies, reduced fat ginger snaps	1 serv	136	4	1	130	24	0	1
Archway Home Style Cookies, Ruth's Golden Oatmeal	1 serv	121	5	1	109	18	1	2
Archway Home Style Cookies, Ruth's Oatmeal	1 serv	111	4	1	114	17	1	2
Archway Home Style Cookies, sugar	1 serv	99	3	1	154	17	0	1
Archway Home Style Cookies, sugar free, chocolate chip	1 serv	117	5	2	64	16	0	1

ITEM DESCRIPTION	Serving Size	Calories	Total Fat (g)	Saturated Fat (g)	Sodium (mg)	Carbohydrates (g)	Fiber (g)	Protein (g)
Archway Home Style Cookies, sugar free, oatmeal	1 serv	106	5	1	74	16	1	1
Keebler Chocolate Graham Selects	1 serv	144	5	1	111	22	0	2
Keebler Golden Vanilla Wafers	1 serv	147	6	1	120	22	0	2
Little Debbie Nut Bar, wafer w/peanut butter, chocolate covered	1 serv	312	19	4	127	31	0	5
Nabisco Chips Ahoy Chocolate Chip Cookies	3	160	8	2.5	105	21	1	2
Nabisco Graham Crackers	1 serv	119	3	0	185	21	1	2
Nabisco Oreo Crunchies, cookie crumb topping	1 serv	52	2	0	58	8	0	1
Nabisco Oreo Sandwich Cookie	2	160	7	2	160	25	1	1
Pepperidge Farm Bordeaux	4	130	5	3.5	95	19	0	1
Pepperidge Farm Milano	3	180	10	5	80	21	1	2
Pillsbury Chocolate Chip Cookies, refrigerated dough	1 serv	135	7	2	85	17	1	1
CORIANDER								
Leaves, dried	1 tbsp	5	0	0	4	1	0	0
Leaves, fresh	1/4 cup	1	0	0	2	0	0	0
Seed	1 tbsp	15	1	0	2	3	2	1
CORN								
White	1 cup	184	8	1	58	123	0	16
Yellow	1 cup	184	8	1	58	123	12	16
CORN & CANOLA OIL	1 tbsp	124	14	1	0	0	0	0
CORN BRAN	1 cup	170	1	0	5	65	60	6
CORNBREAD								
Dry mix, prepared	1 pc	188	6	2	467	29	1	4
Homemade, made w/ 2% milk	1 pc	173	5	1	428	28	0	4
CORN CAKES (very low sodium)	1 cake	35	0	0	3	8	0	1
CORN CHIPS (BBQ flavor, w/ enriched masa flour)	1 oz	148	9	1	216	16	0	2
CORNED BEEF								
Carl Buddig Cooked Corned Beef, chopped, pressed	2 oz serv	81	4	2	765	1	0	11
Hormel Corned Beef Hash, canned	1 cup	387	24	10	1003	22	3	21

ITEM DESCRIPTION	Serving Size	Calories	Total Fat (g)	Saturated Fat (g)	Sodium (mg)	Carbohydrates (g)	Fiber (g)	Protein (g)
Loaf, jellied	1 slice	43	2	1	267	0	0	6
Nestle Chef-Mate Corned Beef Hash, canned	1 cup	455	30	14	1619	28	3	21
Substitute, Worthington Meatless Corned Beef, frozen	1 slice	46	3	0	144	2	1	4
CORN FLOUR								
Degermed, unenriched, yellow	1 cup	472	2	0	1	104	2	7
Masa, white	1 cup	416	4	1	6	87	11	11
Masa, yellow	1 cup	416	4	1	6	87	0	11
Whole grain, blue	100 grams	364	5	0	5	74	9	10
Whole grain, white	1 cup	422	5	1	6	90	9	8
Whole grain, yellow	1 cup	422	5	1	6	90	9	8
CORNMEAL								
Degermed, white	1 cup	587	3	0	11	126	6	12
Degermed, yellow	1 cup	587	3	0	11	126	6	12
Self-rising, bolted, plain, yellow	1 cup	407	4	1	1521	86	8	10
Self-rising, bolted, w/ wheat flour, white	1 cup	592	5	1	2242	125	11	14
Self-rising, degermed, white	1 cup	490	2	0	1860	103	10	12
Self-rising, degermed, yellow	1 cup	490	2	0	1860	103	10	12
Whole grain, white	1 cup	442	4	1	43	94	9	10
Whole grain, yellow	1 cup	442	4	1	43	94	9	10
CORN MUFFIN MIX	1 oz	119	3	1	315	20	2	2
CORNNUTS								
BBQ flavor	1 oz	124	4	1	277	20	2	3
Nacho flavor	1 oz	124	4	1	180	20	2	3
Plain	1 oz	126	4	1	156	20	2	2
CORN OIL (all purpose)	1 tbsp	120	14	2	0	0	0	0
CORN PUDDING (homemade)	1 cup	328	13	6	702	43	3	11
CORN SALAD (fresh)	1 cup	12	0	0	2	2	0	1
CORNSTARCH	1 cup	488	0	0	12	117	1	0
CORN, SWEET								
White, canned, cream style, reg	1/2 cup	92	1	0	365	23	2	2

ITEM DESCRIPTION	Serving Size	Calories	Total Fat (g)	Saturated Fat (g)	Sodium (mg)	Carbohydrates (g)	Fiber (g)	Protein (g)
White, canned, vacuum packed, no salt	1/2 cup	83	1	0	3	20	2	3
White, canned, vacuum packed, reg	1/2 cup	83	1	0	286	20	2	3
White, canned, whole kernel	1/2 cup	66	1	0	265	15	2	2
White, canned, whole kernel, no salt	1/2 cup	82	1	0	15	20	1	2
White, canned, whole kernel, reg	1/2 cup	82	1	0	273	20	2	2
White, fresh (6" long)	1 ear	63	1	0	11	14	2	2
White, frozen, kernels, boiled	1/2 cup	66	0	0	4	16	2	2
Yellow, boiled (6" long)	1 ear	96	1	0	0	22	2	3
Yellow, canned, cream style, no salt	1/2 cup	92	1	0	4	23	2	2
Yellow, canned, cream style, reg	1/2 cup	92	1	0	365	23	2	2
Yellow, canned in brine, reg	1/2 cup	82	1	0	273	20	2	2
Yellow, canned, no salt	1/2 cup	82	1	0	15	20	2	2
Yellow, canned, vacuum packed, no salt	1/2 cup	83	1	0	3	20	2	3
Yellow, canned, vacuum packed, reg	1/2 cup	83	1	0	286	20	2	3
Yellow, canned, whole kernel	1/2 cup	66	1	0	265	15	2	2
Yellow, fresh	1/2 cup	66	1	0	12	15	2	2
Yellow, frozen, kernels, boiled	1/2 cup	66	1	0	1	16	2	2
CORN SYRUP								
Dark	1 tbsp	57	0	0	31	16	0	0
High fructose	1 tbsp	53	0	0	0	14	0	0
Light	1 tbsp	62	0	0	14	17	0	0
COTTAGE CHEESE								
Creamed, small curd	1/2 cup	110	5	2	410	4	0	13
Creamed, w/fruit	1/2 cup	110	4	3	389	5	0	12
Low fat, 1% milkfat	1/2 cup	81	1	1	459	3	0	14
Low fat, 1% milkfat, lactose reduced	1/2 cup	84	1	1	250	4	1	14
Low fat, 1% milkfat, no sodium	1/2 cup	81	1	1	15	3	0	14
Low fat, 2% milkfat	1/2 cup	97	3	1	373	4	0	13
Nonfat, dry, large or small curd	1/2 cup	52	0	0	239	5	0	8

ITEM DESCRIPTION	Serving Size	Calories	Total Fat (g)	Saturated Fat (g)	Sodium (mg)	Carbohydrates (g)	Fiber (g)	Protein (g)
COTTONSEED FLOUR								
Low fat	1 oz	94	0	0	10	10	0	14
Part defatted	1 cup	337	6	1	33	38	3	39
Part defatted, meal	1 oz	104	1	0	10	11	0	14
COTTONSEED OIL (all purpose)	1 tbsp	120	14	4	0	0	0	0
COUSCOUS (cooked)	1 cup	176	0	0	8	36	2	6
COWPEAS								
Catjang, boiled	1 cup	200	1	0	32	35	6	14
Catjang, fresh	1 cup	573	3	1	97	100	18	40
Common, boiled	1 cup	200	1	0	7	36	11	13
Common, canned, plain	1 cup	185	1	0	718	33	8	11
Common, canned w/pork	1 cup	199	4	1	840	40	8	7
Common, fresh	1 cup	561	2	1	27	100	18	39
Fresh	1 cup	131	1	0	6	27	7	4
Fresh, boiled	1 cup	160	1	0	7	34	8	5
Frozen, boiled	1 cup	224	1	0	8	40	11	14
Leafy tips, boiled, chopped	1 cup	12	0	0	3	1	0	2
Leafy tips, fresh, chopped	1 cup	10	0	0	3	2	0	1
Young pods w/seeds, boiled	1 cup	32	0	0	3	7	0	2
Young pods w/seeds, fresh	1 cup	41	0	0	4	9	0	3
CRAB								
Alaska King, cooked in moist heat	3 oz	82	1	0	911	0	0	16
Blue, canned	1 cup	134	2	0	450	0	0	28
Blue, crab cakes	1 cake	93	5	1	198	0	0	12
Blue, flaked, cooked in moist heat	1 cup	120	2	0	329	0	0	24
Dungeness, cooked in moist heat	3 oz	94	1	0	321	1	0	19
Imitation Alaska King, made from surimi	3 oz	81	0	0	715	13	0	6
Queen, cooked in moist heat	3 oz	98	1	0	587	0	0	20
CRABAPPLES (fresh, slices)	1 cup	84	0	0	1	22	0	0
CRACKER MEAL	1 cup	440	2	0	32	93	3	11
CRACKERS								
Cheese, low sodium (1" sq)	1	5	0	0	5	1	0	0
Cheese, regular (1" sq)	1	5	0	0	10	1	0	0

ITEM DESCRIPTION	Serving Size	Calories	Total Fat (g)	Saturated Fat (g)	Sodium (mg)	Carbohydrates (g)	Fiber (g)	Protein (g)
Cheese, sandwich type, w/peanut butter filling	1 sandwich	32	2	0	46	4	0	1
Crispbread, rye	1 crispbread	37	0	0	26	8	2	1
Matzo, egg	1 matzo	109	1	0	6	22	1	3
Matzo, egg & onion	1 matzo	109	1	0	80	22	1	3
Matzo, plain	1 matzo	111	0	0	1	23	1	3
Matzo, whole wheat	1 matzo	98	0	0	1	22	3	4
Melba toast, plain	1 toast	20	0	0	41	4	0	1
Melba toast, plain, w/o salt	1 toast	20	0	0	1	4	0	1
Melba toast, rye (includes pumpernickel)	1 toast	19	0	0	45	4	0	1
Melba toast, wheat	1 toast	19	0	0	42	4	0	1
Milk	1 cracker	50	2	0	65	8	0	1
Oyster	5 crackers	21	0	0	56	4	0	0
Oyster, low salt	5 crackers	21	0	0	32	4	0	0
Oyster, unsalted	5 crackers	21	0	0	32	4	0	0
Ritz Crackers	1 cracker	16	1	0	29	2	0	0
Rusk toast	1 rusk	41	1	0	25	7	0	1
Rye, sandwich, w/cheese filling	1 sandwich	34	2	0	73	4	0	1
Rye, wafers, plain	1 cracker	37	0	0	87	9	3	1
Rye, wafers, seasoned (triple crackers)	1 triple	84	2	0	195	16	5	2
Saltines	5 crackers	63	1	0	167	11	0	2
Saltines, fat free, low sodium	5 crackers	59	0	0	95	12	0	2
Saltines, low salt	5 crackers	63	1	0	95	11	0	1
Saltines, unsalted tops	5 crackers	65	2	0	115	11	0	1
Sandwich, w/cheese filling	1 sandwich	33	1	0	98	4	0	1
Sandwich, w/peanut butter filling	1 sandwich	35	2	0	50	4	0	1
Wheat	1 cup, crushed	393	17	4	660	54	4	7
Wheat, low salt	1 cup, crushed	14	1	0	8	2	0	0
Wheat, sandwich, w/cheese filling	1 sandwich	35	2	0	64	4	0	1
Wheat, sandwich, w/peanut butter filling	1 sandwich	35	2	0	56	4	0	1

ITEM DESCRIPTION	Serving Size	Calories	Total Fat (g)	Saturated Fat (g)	Sodium (mg)	Carbohydrates (g)	Fiber (g)	Protein (g)
Whole wheat	1 cracker	18	1	0	26	3	0	0
Whole wheat, low salt	1 cracker	18	1	0	10	3	0	0
CRANBERRIES								
Dried, sweetened	1/3 cup	123	1	0	1	33	2	0
Fresh	1 cup	46	0	0	2	12	5	0
CRANBERRY-APPLE JUICE								
Bottled	8 fl oz	154	0	0	5	39	0	0
Low calorie	8 fl oz	46	0	0	12	11	0	0
CRANBERRY-APRICOT JUICE (bottled)	8 fl oz	157	0	0	5	40	0	0
CRANBERRY BEANS								
Boiled	1 cup	241	1	0	2	43	18	17
Canned	1 cup	216	1	0	863	39	16	14
Fresh	1 cup	653	2	1	12	117	48	45
CRANBERRY-GRAPE JUICE (bottled)	8 fl oz	137	0	0	7	34	0	0
CRANBERRY JUICE (unsweetened)	1 cup	116	0	0	5	31	0	1
CRANBERRY JUICE COCKTAIL								
Bottled	8 fl oz	137	0	0	5	34	0	0
Frozen concentrate, prepared w/ water	8 fl oz	111	0	0	9	28	0	0
CRANBERRY-ORANGE RELISH (canned)	1 cup	490	0	0	88	127	0	1
CRANBERRY SAUCE (canned, sweetened)	1 cup	418	0	0	80	108	3	1
CRAYFISH								
Farmed, cooked in moist heat	3 oz	74	1	0	82	0	0	15
Wild, cooked in moist heat	3 oz	70	1	0	80	0	0	14
CREAM								
Half & half	1 tbsp	20	2	1	6	1	0	0
Light	1 tbsp	29	3	2	6	1	0	0
CREAM CHEESE								
Cream cheese	1 tbsp	50	5	3	47	1	0	1
Low fat	1 tbsp	30	2	1	70	1	0	1
CREAM OF TARTAR	1 tsp	8	0	0	2	2	0	0

ITEM DESCRIPTION	Serving Size	Calories	Total Fat (g)	Saturated Fat (g)	Sodium (mg)	Carbohydrates (g)	Fiber (g)	Protein (g)
CREAM PUFFS								
Homemade, shell & custard filling	1 puff	335	20	5	443	30	1	9
Homemade, shell only	1 puff	239	17	4	368	15	0	6
CREAM SUBSTITUTE								
Liquid, light	1 fl oz	21	1	0	18	3	0	0
Powder, light	1 packet	13	0	0	7	2	0	0
CRÈME DE MENTHE (72 proof)	1 fl oz	125	0	0	2	14	0	0
CRESS								
Garden, boiled	1 cup	31	1	0	11	5	1	3
Garden, fresh	1 cup	16	0	0	7	3	1	1
CROAKER (Atlantic, breaded & fried)	3 oz	188	11	3	296	6	0	15
CROISSANTS								
Apple	1 med	145	5	3	156	21	1	4
Butter	1 med	231	12	7	424	26	1	5
Cheese	1 med	236	12	6	316	27	1	5
CROOKNECK & STRAIGHTNECK SQUASH								
Boiled, slices	1 cup	36	1	0	0	8	3	2
Canned, w/o salt, slices	1 cup	28	0	0	11	6	3	1
Fresh, slices	1 cup	25	0	0	3	5	2	1
Frozen, boiled, slices	1 cup	48	0	0	12	11	3	2
CROUTONS								
Pepperidge Farm Classic Style Croutons, seasoned	1 serv	33	1	0	97	4	0	1
Plain	1 cup	122	2	0	209	22	1	4
Seasoned	1 cup	186	7	2	495	25	2	4
CUCUMBER								
Peeled, fresh, slices	1 cup	14	0	0	2	3	1	1
w/peel, fresh, slices	1 cup	16	0	0	2	4	1	1
CUMIN SEED	1 tbsp	22	1	0	10	3	1	1
CUPCAKES (chocolate, w/frosting)	1 cupcake	131	2	0	178	29	2	2
CURRANTS								
European black, fresh	1 cup	71	0	0	2	17	0	2
Red & white, fresh	1 cup	63	0	0	1	15	5	2
Zante, dried	1 cup	408	0	0	12	107	10	6

ITEM DESCRIPTION	Serving Size	Calories	Total Fat (g)	Saturated Fat (g)	Sodium (mg)	Carbohydrates (g)	Fiber (g)	Protein (g)
CURRY POWDER	1 tbsp	20	1	0	3	4	2	1
CUSK (cooked in dry heat)	3 oz	95	1	0	34	0	0	21
CUTTLEFISH (cooked in moist heat)	3 oz	134	1	0	632	1	0	28
DAIQUIRI								
Canned	1 fl oz	38	0	0	12	5	0	0
Homemade	1 fl oz	56	0	0	2	2	0	0
DANDELION GREENS								
Boiled, chopped	1 cup	35	1	0	46	7	3	2
Fresh, chopped	1 cup	25	0	0	42	5	2	1
DANISH PASTRY								
Almond (4.25" dia)	1 pastry	280	16	4	236	30	1	5
Cheese	1 pastry	266	16	5	320	26	1	6
Cinnamon (4.25" dia)	1 pastry	262	15	4	241	29	1	5
Fruit (4.25" dia)	1 pastry	263	13	3	251	34	1	4
Kellogg's Pop-Tarts Pastry Swirls, apple cinnamon	1 pastry	256	11	3	190	37	1	3
Kellogg's Pop-Tarts Pastry Swirls, cheese	1 pastry	252	11	3	180	37	0	3
Kellogg's Pop-Tarts Pastry Swirls, strawberry	1 pastry	254	11	3	170	37	1	3
Lemon	1 pastry	263	13	2	251	34	1	4
DATES								
Deglet Noor	1 date	20	0	0	0	5	1	0
Medjool	1 date	66	0	0	0	18	2	0
DILL SEED	1 tbsp	20	1	0	1	4	1	1
DILL WEED								
Dried	1 tbsp	8	0	0	6	2	0	1
Sprigs, fresh	5 sprigs	0	0	0	1	0	0	0
DOLPHINFISH (cooked in dry heat)	3 oz	93	1	0	96	0	0	20
DOUGHNUTS								
Cake type, chocolate, sugared or glazed (3" dia)	1	175	8	2	143	24	1	2
Cake type, plain (3.25" dia)	1	226	13	4	301	25	1	3
Cake type, plain, chocolate coated or frosted (3" dia)	1	194	11	6	178	22	1	2

ITEM DESCRIPTION	Serving Size	Calories	Total Fat (g)	Saturated Fat (g)	Sodium (mg)	Carbohydrates (g)	Fiber (g)	Protein (g)
Cake type, plain, sugared or glazed (3" dia)	1	192	10	3	181	23	1	2
Cake type, wheat, sugared or glazed (3" dia)	1	162	9	1	160	19	1	3
Holes, glazed	1	52	2	1	50	7	0	1
French crullers, glazed (3" dia)	1	169	8	2	141	24	0	1
Honey buns, glazed, enriched (4" x 3")	1	259	12	4	252	33	1	4
Honey buns, glazed, unenriched (3.25" dia)	1	242	14	3	205	27	1	4
Old fashioned, plain (3.25" dia)	1	226	13	4	301	25	1	3
Yeast leavened, glazed, enriched (3" dia)	1	124	6	2	120	16	1	2
Yeast leavened, glazed, unenriched (3.25" dia)	1	242	14	3	205	27	1	4
Yeast leavened, w/ creme filling (3-1/2" x 2-1/2")	1	307	21	5	263	26	1	5
Yeast leavened, w/ jelly filling (3-1/2" x 2-1/2")	1	289	16	4	249	33	1	5
DOVE cooked (includes squab), diced	1 cup	307	18	5	80	0	0	33
DRUM (freshwater, cooked in dry heat)	3 oz	130	5	1	82	0	0	19
DUCK								
Meat only, roasted, chopped	1 cup	281	16	6	91	0	0	33
w/ skin, roasted, chopped	1 cup	472	40	14	83	0	0	27
DUCK EGGS (whole, fresh)	1	130	10	3	102	1	0	9
DUCK FAT	1 tbsp	113	13	4	0	0	0	0
DURIAN (fresh or frozen, chopped)	1 cup	357	13	0	5	66	9	4
ECLAIRS								
Custard filled, w/ chocolate glaze, homemade	1	262	16	4	337	24	1	6
Weight Watchers, frozen	1	142	4	1	177	24	1	3
EDAMAME (frozen)	1 cup	189	8	1	9	15	8	17
EEL (boneless, cooked in dry heat)	3 oz	201	13	3	55	0	0	20
EGG CUSTARD								
Baked, homemade	1/2 cup	148	6	3	86	15	0	7
Dry mix, prepared w/ 2% milk	100 grams	111	3	1	89	17	0	4

ITEM DESCRIPTION	Serving Size	Calories	Total Fat (g)	Saturated Fat (g)	Sodium (mg)	Carbohydrates (g)	Fiber (g)	Protein (g)
EGGNOG								
Eggnog	8 fl oz	343	19	11	137	34	0	10
Mix prepared w/ whole milk	8 fl oz	258	8	5	150	39	0	8
EGGPLANT								
Boiled, cubed	1 cup	35	0	0	1	9	3	1
Fresh, cubed	1 cup	20	0	0	2	5	3	1
Pickled	1 cup	67	1	0	2277	13	3	1
EGG ROLLS								
Chicken, refrigerated, heated	1	158	4	1	448	23	2	8
Pork, refrigerated, heated	1	189	6	1	446	25	2	8
Vegetable, refrigerated, heated	1	153	4	1	438	25	2	5
EGG ROLL WRAPPERS	1	93	0	0	183	19	1	3
EGGS								
Cooked, omelet	1 lg	96	7	2	98	0	0	6
Dried	1 tbsp	30	2	1	26	0	0	2
Fresh	1 lg	72	5	2	70	0	0	6
Fried	1 lg	90	7	2	94	0	0	6
Hard-boiled	1 lg	78	5	2	62	1	0	6
Poached	1 lg	71	5	2	147	0	0	6
Scrambled	1 lg	102	7	2	171	1	0	7
EGG SUBSTITUTE								
Frozen	1/4 cup	96	7	1	119	2	0	7
Liquid	1 tbsp	13	1	0	28	0	0	2
Powder	7/10 oz	89	3	1	160	4	0	11
EGG YOLK								
Fresh	1 lg	54	5	2	8	1	0	3
Frozen	1/2 lb	688	58	18	152	3	0	35
Frozen, sugared	1/2 lb	697	52	16	152	25	0	31
ELDERBERRIES (fresh)	1 cup	106	1	0	9	27	10	1
ENCHILADA SAUCE (Pace)	1 serv	24	0	0	520	5	1	1
ENDIVE (fresh)	1 head	87	1	0	113	17	16	6
ENERGY DRINK, BRAND NAME								
Red Bull	8.3 fl oz	115	0	0	214	28	0	1
Red Bull, sugar free	8.3 fl oz	12	0	0	210	2	0	1

ITEM DESCRIPTION	Serving Size	Calories	Total Fat (g)	Saturated Fat (g)	Sodium (mg)	Carbohydrates (g)	Fiber (g)	Protein (g)
ENGLISH MUFFINS								
Apple-cinnamon, toasted	1	144	1	0	192	29	2	5
Mixed grain, toasted	1	156	1	0	276	31	2	6
Plain, toasted	1	140	1	0	248	27	2	5
Raisin-cinnamon, toasted	1	144	1	0	192	29	2	5
Sourdough, toasted	1	140	1	0	248	27	2	5
Thomas' English Muffins	1 serv	132	1	0	197	26	0	5
Wheat, toasted	1	160	1	0	216	25	3	5
Whole wheat, toasted	1	135	1	0	422	27	5	6
FALAFEL (homemade)	1 patty	57	3	0	50	5	0	2
FAVA BEANS								
Boiled	1 cup	187	1	0	8	33	9	13
Canned	1 cup	182	1	0	1160	32	10	14
Fresh beans	1 cup	512	2	0	20	87	38	39
Fresh, in pod	1 cup	111	1	0	32	22	0	10
FENNEL								
Bulb, fresh, slices	1 cup	27	0	0	45	6	3	1
Seed, whole	1 tbsp	20	1	0	5	3	2	1
FENUGREEK (seed)	1 tbsp	36	1	0	7	6	3	3
FIGS								
Canned in ex heavy syrup	1 cup	279	0	0	3	73	0	1
Canned in heavy syrup	1 cup	228	0	0	3	59	6	1
Canned in light syrup	1 cup	174	0	0	3	45	6	1
Canned in water	1 cup	131	0	0	2	35	5	1
Dried, stewed	1 cup	277	1	0	10	71	11	4
Dried, uncooked	1 fruit	21	0	0	1	5	1	0
Fresh, whole	1 lg	47	0	0	1	12	2	0
FISH BROTH	1 cup	39	1	0	776	1	0	5
FISH OIL								
Menhaden	1 tbsp	123	14	4	0	0	0	0
Menhaden, fully hydrogenated	1 tbsp	113	13	12	0	0	0	0
FISH SAUCE	1 tbsp	6	0	0	1390	1	0	1
FISH STOCK (homemade)	1 cup	40	2	0	363	0	0	5

ITEM DESCRIPTION	Serving Size	Calories	Total Fat (g)	Saturated Fat (g)	Sodium (mg)	Carbohydrates (g)	Fiber (g)	Protein (g)
FISH STICKS								
Frozen, preheated	1 stick	70	4	1	118	6	0	3
Meatless	1 stick	81	5	1	137	3	2	6
FLATFISH								
(flounder & sole, cooked in dry heat)	3 oz	99	1	0	89	0	0	21
FLAXSEED								
Oil	1 tbsp	120	14	1	0	0	0	0
Seeds, whole	1 tbsp	55	4	0	3	3	3	2
FLOUNDER								
(flounder & sole cooked in dry heat)	3 oz	99	1	0	89	0	0	21
FRANKFURTERS								
Beef (5" long x 3/4" dia)	1	148	13	5	513	2	0	5
Beef & pork	1	137	12	5	504	1	0	5
Beef & pork, low fat	1	88	6	2	716	3	0	6
Beef, low fat	1	133	11	5	593	1	0	7
Beef, pork, & turkey, fat free	1	62	1	0	455	6	0	7
Chicken	1 link	100	7	2	380	1	0	7
Low sodium	1	180	16	7	177	1	0	7
Meat & poultry, low fat	1 cup, slices	182	4	1	1406	12	0	22
Pork	1 link	204	18	7	620	0	0	10
Turkey	1	100	8	2	485	2	0	6
FRANKFURTERS, BRAND NAME								
Butcher Boy Meats Turkey Franks	1 serv	134	10	3	651	3	0	8
Hebrew National Beef Franks	1 serv	150	14	6	460	1	0	6
Hebrew National Beef reduced fat	1 serv	110	9	3.5	490	2	0	5
Hormel Wrangler Beef Franks	1	162	14	6	557	1	0	7
Louis Rich Franks, turkey & chicken	1 serv	85	6	2	511	2	0	5
Oscar Mayer Little Wieners, pork & turkey	1 serv	177	16	6	592	1	0	6
Oscar Mayer Wieners, beef	1 serv	147	14	6	461	1	0	5
Oscar Mayer Wieners, beef, bun length	1 link	185	17	7	584	2	0	6
Oscar Mayer Wieners, beef, fat free	1 serv	39	0	0	464	3	0	7
Oscar Mayer Wieners, beef, light	1 serv	110	8	4	615	2	0	6

ITEM DESCRIPTION	Serving Size	Calories	Total Fat (g)	Saturated Fat (g)	Sodium (mg)	Carbohydrates (g)	Fiber (g)	Protein (g)
Oscar Mayer Wieners, light pork, turkey & beef	1 serv	111	8	3	591	2	0	7
Oscar Mayer Wieners, pork & turkey	1 link	147	13	4	445	1	0	5
Oscar Mayer Wieners, turkey & cheese	1 serv	143	13	5	514	1	0	5
FRANKFURTERS SUBSTITUTE								
Frankfurter, meatless	1	163	10	1	330	5	3	14
Loma Linda Big Franks, canned	1 link	111	6	1	217	3	2	11
Loma Linda Linketts, canned	1 link	73	4	1	140	2	1	7
Loma Linda Little Links, canned	2 links	102	6	1	217	3	2	9
Loma Linda Low Fat Big Franks, canned	1 link	79	2	0	245	3	2	12
Morningstar Farms America's Original Veggie Dog, frozen	1 link	75	1	0	609	7	2	11
Morningstar Farms Meatless Corn Dogs, frozen	1 pc	162	4	1	466	22	3	8
Morningstar Farms Meatless Mini Corn Dogs, frozen	4 pcs	174	5	1	515	22	3	10
Morningstar Farms Veggie Corn Dogs, frozen	1 pc	164	5	1	522	22	2	8
Worthington Super Links, canned	1 link	105	7	1	340	3	1	7
FRENCH BEANS								
Boiled	1 cup	228	1	0	11	43	17	12
Fresh	1 cup	631	4	0	33	118	46	35
FRENCH TOAST								
Frozen	1 pc	126	4	1	292	19	1	4
Homemade, w/ 2% milk	1 slice	149	7	2	311	16	0	5
FROSTING								
Chocolate, creamy, ready to eat	2 tbsp	163	7	2	75	26	0	0
Coconut, ready to eat	16 oz pkg	2000	111	40	901	243	12	7
Cream cheese, ready to eat	2 tbsp	137	6	2	63	22	0	0
Vanilla, creamy, ready to eat	16 oz pkg	1931	75	14	850	314	0	0
White, fluffy, dry mix, prepared w/ water	1 pkg	769	0	0	491	197	0	5
FROZEN BREAKFAST ITEMS								
Breakfast burrito, ham & cheese, frozen	1 serv	212	7	2	405	28	1	10

ITEM DESCRIPTION	Serving Size	Calories	Total Fat (g)	Saturated Fat (g)	Sodium (mg)	Carbohydrates (g)	Fiber (g)	Protein (g)
Cinnamon swirl French toast w/ sausage, frozen	1 serv	415	23	7	502	38	2	13
Scrambled eggs & sausage w/ hashed brown potatoes, frozen	1 serv	361	27	7	772	17	1	13
FROZEN YOGURT								
Chocolate	1/2 cup	110	3	2	55	19	1	3
Chocolate, nonfat milk, sweetened w/o sugar	1/2 cup	100	1	0	75	18	1	4
Chocolate, soft serve	1/2 cup	115	4	3	71	18	2	3
Flavors other than chocolate	1/2 cup	110	3	2	55	19	0	3
Vanilla, soft serve	1/2 cup	117	4	2	63	17	0	3
FRUIT & VEGETABLE JUICE DRINK (w/ added nutrients)	8 fl oz	72	0	0	52	18	0	0
FRUIT COCKTAIL								
Canned in ex heavy syrup	1 cup	229	0	0	16	60	3	1
Canned in ex light syrup	1 cup	111	0	0	10	29	3	1
Canned in heavy syrup	1 cup	181	0	0	15	47	2	1
Canned in heavy syrup, drained	1 cup	150	0	0	13	40	4	1
Canned in juice	1 cup	109	0	0	9	28	2	1
Canned in light syrup	1 cup	138	0	0	15	36	2	1
Canned in water	1 cup	76	0	0	9	20	2	1
FRUIT DRINKS								
Fruit-flavored drink mix powder, low calorie, w/ aspartame	1 tsp	17	0	0	32	7	0	0
Fruit-flavored drink mix, powder, unsweetened	2 tbsp	56	0	0	682	23	0	0
FRUIT LEATHER								
Betty Crocker Fruit Roll Ups, berry flavored	2 rolls	104	1	0	89	24	0	0
Pieces	1 pkg	97	1	0	109	22	0	0
Rolls	1 lg	78	1	0	67	18	0	0
FRUIT PUNCH								
Canned	8 fl oz	117	0	0	94	30	0	0
Frozen concentrate	1 fl oz	56	0	0	3	14	0	0

ITEM DESCRIPTION	Serving Size	Calories	Total Fat (g)	Saturated Fat (g)	Sodium (mg)	Carbohydrates (g)	Fiber (g)	Protein (g)
Frozen concentrate, prepared w/ water	8 fl oz	114	0	0	12	29	0	0
Juice drink, frozen concentrate	1 fl oz	62	0	0	4	15	0	0
Juice drink, frozen concentrate, prepared w/ water	8 fl oz	98	0	0	12	24	0	0
Powder, w/o sodium, prepared w/ water	8 fl oz	97	0	0	18	25	0	0
FRUIT SALAD								
Canned in ex heavy syrup	1 cup	228	0	0	13	59	3	1
Canned in heavy syrup	1 cup	186	0	0	15	49	3	1
Canned in juice	1 cup	124	0	0	12	32	3	1
Canned in light syrup	1 cup	146	0	0	15	38	3	1
Canned in water	1 cup	74	0	0	7	19	3	1
Tropical, canned in heavy syrup	1 cup	221	0	0	5	57	3	1
FUDGE								
Chocolate marshmallow, homemade	1 pc	91	4	2	17	14	0	0
Chocolate, homemade	1 pc	70	2	1	8	13	0	0
Peanut butter, homemade	1 pc	62	1	0	19	12	0	1
GARBANZO BEANS								
Boiled	1 cup	269	4	0	11	45	13	15
Canned	1 cup	286	3	0	718	54	11	12
Fresh	1 cup	728	12	1	48	121	35	39
GARLIC								
Fresh	1 tsp	4	0	0	0	1	0	0
Powder	1 tbsp	28	0	0	2	6	1	1
GEFILTE FISH (sweet)	1 pc	35	1	0	220	3	0	4
GELATIN DESSERT								
Dry mix, prepared w/ water	1/2 cup	84	0	0	101	19	0	2
Dry mix, w/ aspartame, prepared w/ water	1/2 cup	23	0	0	56	5	0	1
GIN								
80 proof	1 fl oz	64	0	0	0	0	0	0
86 proof	1 fl oz	70	0	0	0	0	0	0
90 proof	1 fl oz	73	0	0	0	0	0	0
94 proof	1 fl oz	76	0	0	0	0	0	0

ITEM DESCRIPTION	Serving Size	Calories	Total Fat (g)	Saturated Fat (g)	Sodium (mg)	Carbohydrates (g)	Fiber (g)	Protein (g)
GINGER (ground)	1 tbsp	19	0	0	2	4	1	0
GINGER ROOT (fresh)	1 tsp	2	0	0	0	0	0	0
GINKGO NUTS								
Canned	1 oz	31	0	0	87	6	3	1
Dried	1 oz	99	1	0	4	21	0	3
Fresh	1 oz	52	0	0	2	11	0	1
GOAT MILK	1 cup	168	10	7	122	11	0	9
GOOSE								
Eggs, fresh	1 egg	266	19	5	199	2	0	20
Fat	1 tbsp	115	13	4	0	0	0	0
Meat & skin, roasted, chopped	1 cup	427	31	10	98	0	0	35
Meat only, roasted	1/2 goose	1407	75	27	449	0	0	171
GOOSEBERRIES								
Canned in light syrup	1 cup	184	1	0	5	47	6	2
Fresh	1 cup	66	1	0	2	15	7	1
GRANOLA (homemade)	1 cup	597	29	5	30	65	11	18
GRANOLA BARS								
Coconut, chocolate coated	1 oz bar	151	9	6	43	16	2	1
Fruit filled, nonfat	1 oz bar	97	0	0	5	22	2	2
Hard, almond	1 oz bar	140	7	4	73	18	1	2
Hard, chocolate chip	1 oz bar	124	5	3	98	20	1	2
Hard, peanut	1 oz bar	136	6	1	79	18	1	3
Hard, peanut butter	1 oz bar	137	7	1	80	18	1	3
Hard, plain	1 oz bar	132	6	1	82	18	2	3
Oats, fruits & nut	1 oz bar	113	2	0	71	22	2	2
Soft, chocolate chip	1 oz bar	117	5	2	50	20	1	2
Soft, chocolate chip, graham & marshmallow	1 oz bar	120	4	3	88	20	1	2
Soft, chocolate chip, milk chocolate coated	1 oz bar	130	7	4	56	18	1	2
Soft, nut & raisin	1 oz bar	127	6	3	71	18	2	2
Soft, peanut butter	1 oz bar	119	4	1	115	18	1	3
Soft, peanut butter & chocolate chip	1 oz bar	121	6	2	92	17	1	3

ITEM DESCRIPTION	Serving Size	Calories	Total Fat (g)	Saturated Fat (g)	Sodium (mg)	Carbohydrates (g)	Fiber (g)	Protein (g)
Soft, peanut butter, milk chocolate coated	1 oz bar	144	9	5	55	15	1	3
Soft, plain	1 oz bar	124	5	2	78	19	1	2
Soft, raisin	1 oz bar	125	5	3	79	19	1	2
GRAPE DRINK (canned)	8 fl oz	152	0	0	40	39	0	0
GRAPE JUICE								
Canned or bottled	8 fl oz	152	0	0	13	37	0	1
Frozen concentrate, prepared w/ water	1 cup	128	0	0	5	32	0	0
Unsweetened	1 cup	152	0	0	13	37	1	1
GRAPE LEAVES								
Canned	1 leaf	3	0	0	114	0	0	0
Fresh	1 leaf	3	0	0	0	1	0	0
GRAPEFRUIT								
Pink & red, California & Arizona, fresh	1/2 fruit	46	0	0	1	12	0	1
Pink & red, Florida, fresh	1/2 fruit	37	0	0	0	9	1	1
Sections, canned in juice	1 cup	92	0	0	17	23	1	2
Sections, canned in light syrup	1 cup	152	0	0	5	39	1	1
Sections, canned in water	1 cup	88	0	0	5	22	1	1
White, California, fresh	1/2 fruit	44	0	0	0	11	0	1
White, Florida, fresh	1/2 fruit	38	0	0	0	10	0	1
GRAPEFRUIT JUICE								
Pink	1 cup	96	0	0	2	23	0	1
White	1 cup	96	0	0	2	23	0	1
White, canned, sweetened	1 cup	115	0	0	5	28	0	1
White, canned, unsweetened	1 cup	94	0	0	2	22	0	1
White, frozen concentrate, unsweetened, prepared w/ water	1 cup	101	0	0	2	24	0	1
GRAPES								
American type	1 cup	62	0	0	2	16	1	1
Canned in heavy syrup	1 cup	195	0	0	13	50	2	1
Canned in water	1 cup	98	0	0	15	25	2	1
European red or green	1 cup	104	0	0	3	27	1	1

ITEM DESCRIPTION	Serving Size	Calories	Total Fat (g)	Saturated Fat (g)	Sodium (mg)	Carbohydrates (g)	Fiber (g)	Protein (g)
GRAPESEED OIL	1 tbsp	120	14	1	0	0	0	0
GRAVY								
Au jus, canned	1/4 cup	10	0	0	30	1	0	1
Au jus, dry	1 tsp	9	0	0	348	1	0	0
Beef, canned	1/4 cup	31	1	1	326	3	0	2
Brown, dry	1 tbsp	22	1	0	291	4	0	1
Campbell's Au Jus Gravy	1/4 cup	5	0	0	230	0	0	1
Campbell's Beef Gravy	1/4 cup	25	1	0	270	3	0	1
Campbell's Brown Gravy, w/onions	1/4 cup	25	1	0	330	4	0	0
Campbell's Chicken Gravy	1/4 cup	40	3	1	260	3	0	0
Campbell's Country Style Cream Gravy	1/4 cup	45	3	1	190	3	0	1
Campbell's Country Style Sausage Gravy	1/4 cup	70	6	2	270	3	0	2
Campbell's Golden Pork Gravy	1/4 cup	45	3	2	310	3	0	1
Campbell's Mushroom Gravy	1/4 cup	20	1	0	280	3	0	0
Campbell's Turkey Gravy	1/4 cup	25	1	0	270	3	0	1
Chicken, canned	1/4 cup	47	3	1	343	3	0	1
Chicken, dry	1 tbsp	30	1	0	332	5	0	1
Franco-American Slow Roast Beef Gravy	1/4 cup	25	1	1	310	3	0	1
Franco-American Slow Roast Chick Gravy	1/4 cup	20	1	0	240	3	0	1
Franco-American Slow Roast Turkey Gravy	1/4 cup	25	1	0	320	4	0	1
Heinz Home Style Beef Gravy	1/4 cup	22	1	0	335	4	0	1
Meat or poultry, low sodium, prepared	1/4 cup	31	1	1	11	4	0	2
Mushroom, canned	1/4 cup	50	3	0	570	5	0	1
Pork, dry, powder	1 serv	25	1	0	359	4	0	1
Turkey, canned	1/4 cup	30	1	0	343	3	0	2
Turkey, dry	1 serv	26	1	0	307	5	0	1
GREAT NORTHERN BEANS								
Boiled	1 cup	209	1	0	4	37	12	15

ITEM DESCRIPTION	Serving Size	Calories	Total Fat (g)	Saturated Fat (g)	Sodium (mg)	Carbohydrates (g)	Fiber (g)	Protein (g)
Canned	1 cup	299	1	0	10	55	13	19
Fresh	1 cup	620	2	1	26	114	37	40
GRENADINE SYRUP	1 tbsp	54	0	0	5	13	0	0
GRITS								
Quaker Instant Grits, cheddar cheese flavor, prepared w/ water	1 packet	102	2	0	508	20	1	2
Quaker Instant Grits, country bacon flavor, prepared w/ water	1 packet	97	0	0	413	21	1	3
Quaker Instant Grits, plain, prepared w/ water	1 cup	167	0	0	514	37	2	4
White, reg & quick, cooked w/ water	1 cup	143	0	0	5	31	1	3
Yellow, reg & quick, cooked w/ water	1 cup	143	0	0	5	31	1	3
GROUND CHERRIES (fresh)	1 cup	74	1	0	0	16	0	3
GROUPER (cooked in dry heat)	3 oz	100	1	0	45	0	0	21
GUANABANA NECTAR (canned)	1 cup	148	0	0	20	37	0	0
GUAVA NECTAR (canned)	1 cup	143	0	0	18	37	3	0
GUAVAS								
Fresh	1 fruit	37	1	0	1	8	3	1
Strawberry, fresh	1 fruit	4	0	0	2	1	0	0
Sauce, cooked	1 cup	86	0	0	10	23	9	1
GUM								
Bubble, Bazooka	1 pc	15	0	0	0	4	0	0
Chewing gum	1 stick	7	0	0	0	2	0	0
Chewing gum, sugarless	1 pc	5	0	0	0	2	0	0
HADDOCK								
Cooked in dry heat	3 oz	95	1	0	74	0	0	21
Smoked, boneless	1 oz	33	0	0	216	0	0	7
HALIBUT								
Atlantic & Pacific, cooked in dry heat	3 oz	119	3	0	59	0	0	23
Greenland, cooked in dry heat	3 oz	203	15	3	88	0	0	16
HAM								
Boneless, ex lean (approx 5% fat), roasted	3 oz	123	5	2	1023	1	0	18
Boneless, reg (approx 11% fat), roasted	3 oz	151	8	3	1275	0	0	19

ITEM DESCRIPTION	Serving Size	Calories	Total Fat (g)	Saturated Fat (g)	Sodium (mg)	Carbohydrates (g)	Fiber (g)	Protein (g)
Carl Buddig Smoked Slices	2 oz	93	5	2	787	1	0	11
Chopped, canned	1 oz	68	5	2	387	0	0	5
Chopped, from fresh	1 oz	50	3	1	372	1	0	5
Ex lean & reg, canned, roasted	3 oz	142	7	2	908	0	0	18
Ex lean (approx 4% fat), canned, roasted	3 oz	116	4	1	965	0	0	18
Ex lean, slices	1 slice, oval	29	1	0	286	0	0	5
Honey-smoked	2 oz	69	1	1	510	4	0	10
Hormel Cure 81	1 serv	89	3	1	872	0	0	15
Loaf or roll, w/ cheese	1 slice	67	5	2	302	1	0	4
Minced	1 oz	75	6	2	353	1	0	5
Oscar Mayer Ham, 96% fat free	1 slice	22	1	0	258	0	0	3
Oscar Mayer Ham & Cheese Loaf	1 serv	66	5	2	327	1	0	4
Oscar Mayer Ham, boiled	1 slice	22	1	0	283	0	0	3
Oscar Mayer Ham, chopped	1 slice	50	3	1	350	1	0	5
Oscar Mayer Ham, honey	1 slice	23	1	0	262	1	0	4
Oscar Mayer Ham, smoked	1 slice	21	1	0	255	0	0	3
Reg (approx 11% fat)	1 slice	46	2	1	365	1	0	5
Reg (approx 13% fat), canned, roasted	3 oz	142	13	4	800	0	0	17
Salad spread	1 tbsp	32	2	1	137	2	0	1
Spread, w/ cheese	1 tbsp	37	3	1	180	0	0	2
Whole, lean & fat, roasted	3 oz	207	14	5	1009	0	0	18
HAZELNUT OIL	1 tbsp	120	14	1	0	0	0	0
HAZELNUTS OR FILBERTS								
Raw	1 oz	178	17	1	0	5	3	4
Blanched	1 oz	178	17	1	0	5	3	4
Dry roasted, w/o salt	1 oz	183	18	1	0	5	3	4
Oscar Mayer	1 serv	52	4	1	300	0	0	4
HEARTS OF PALM (canned)	1 cup	41	1	0	622	7	4	4
HEAVY CREAM	1 tbsp	52	6	3	6	0	0	0
HERRING								
Atlantic, cooked in dry heat	3 oz	173	10	2	98	0	0	20
Atlantic, kippered, boneless	1 oz	62	4	1	260	0	0	7
Atlantic, pickled, boneless	1 oz	74	5	1	247	3	0	4

ITEM DESCRIPTION	Serving Size	Calories	Total Fat (g)	Saturated Fat (g)	Sodium (mg)	Carbohydrates (g)	Fiber (g)	Protein (g)
Pacific, cooked in dry heat	3 oz	213	15	4	81	0	0	18
HERRING OIL	1 tbsp	123	14	3	0	0	0	0
HICKORY NUTS (dried)	1 cup	788	77	8	1	22	8	15
HOISIN SAUCE	1 tbsp	35	1	0	258	7	0	1
HOMINY								
Canned, white	1 cup	119	1	0	346	24	4	2
Canned, yellow	1 cup	115	1	0	336	23	4	2
Quaker Hominy, white, quick, dry	1/4 cup	128	1	0	1	29	2	3
Quaker Hominy, white, reg, dry	1/4 cup	142	1	0	1	32	2	4
Quaker Hominy, yellow, quick, dry	1/4 cup	125	1	0	1	29	2	3
HONEY	1 tbsp	64	0	0	1	17	0	0
HONEYDEW (fresh, diced)	1 cup	61	0	0	31	15	1	1
HONEY LOAF (pork & beef)	1 slice	35	1	0	370	3	0	3
HORSERADISH (prepared)	1 tbsp	7	0	0	47	2	1	0
HUBBARD SQUASH								
Baked, cubed	1 cup	102	1	0	16	22	0	5
Boiled, mashed	1 cup	71	1	0	12	15	7	3
Fresh, cubed	1 cup	46	1	0	8	10	0	2
HUMMUS								
Commercial	1 tbsp	25	1	0	57	2	1	1
Homemade	1 tbsp	27	1	0	36	3	1	1
HUSH PUPPIES	1 cup	512	21	3	1015	70	4	12
ICE CREAM								
Bar, chocolate or caramel covered, w/ nuts	1 bar	171	11	7	50	17	0	2
Blue Bunny Premium Chocolate	1/2 cup	150	70	4.5	45	16	0	4
Blue Bunny Reduced Fat Vanilla	1/2 cup	110	5	3	65	16	2	3
Breyers Ice Cream, 98% fat free, chocolate	1/2 cup	92	1	1	51	21	4	3
Breyers Ice Cream, 98% fat free, vanilla	1/2 cup	93	1	1	50	21	4	2
Breyers Ice Cream, all natural, light, chocolate	1/2 cup	137	5	3	51	20	1	4
Breyers Ice Cream, all natural, light, mint chocolate chip	1/2 cup	133	5	3	46	19	0	3

ITEM DESCRIPTION	Serving Size	Calories	Total Fat (g)	Saturated Fat (g)	Sodium (mg)	Carbohydrates (g)	Fiber (g)	Protein (g)
Breyers Ice Cream, all natural, light, vanilla	1/2 cup	110	3	2	48	17	0	3
Breyers Ice Cream, all natural, light, vanilla, chocolate & strawberry	1/2 cup	109	3	2	47	18	0	3
Breyers Ice Cream, no sugar added, butter pecan	1/2 cup	122	7	3	112	14	1	3
Breyers Ice Cream, no sugar added, chocolate caramel	1/2 cup	107	4	3	55	18	1	3
Breyers Ice Cream, no sugar added, vanilla	1/2 cup	99	4	3	46	15	0	3
Breyers Ice Cream, no sugar added, vanilla, chocolate & strawberry	1/2 cup	97	4	3	46	15	1	3
Chocolate	1/2 cup	143	7	4	50	19	1	3
Chocolate, light	1 serv	137	5	3	48	17	1	3
Chocolate, light, no sugar added	1/2 cup	109	4	3	54	18	1	3
Chocolate, low carb	1/2 cup	127	8	5	50	10	3	3
Chocolate, rich	1/2 cup	189	13	8	42	15	1	3
Edy's Grand Chocolate	1/2 cup	150	8	4.5	35	17	1	3
Edy's Slow Churned Chocolate	1/2 cup	100	4	2	30	15	0	3
French vanilla, soft serve	1/2 cup	191	11	6	52	19	1	4
Healthy Choice, praline & caramel	1/2 cup	121	2	1	63	23	1	3
Klondike Slim-a-Bear, chocolate cone	1 cone	177	3	1	126	36	3	3
Klondike Slim-a-Bear, chocolate sandwich	1 sandwich	135	2	1	120	28	3	4
Klondike Slim-a-Bear, fudge bar, 98% fat free, no sugar added	3.5 oz bar	92	1	1	89	22	4	3
Klondike Slim-a-Bear, mint sandwich	1 sandwich	134	1	0	122	28	3	4
Klondike Slim-a-Bear, vanilla cone	1 cone	175	3	1	126	35	3	3
Klondike Slim-a-Bear, vanilla sandwich	1 sandwich	135	1	0	122	28	3	4
Vanilla, light	1/2 cup	125	4	2	56	20	0	4
Vanilla, light, no sugar added	1/2 cup	105	5	3	65	15	1	3
Vanilla, low carb	1/2 cup	125	8	4	32	10	3	2

ITEM DESCRIPTION	Serving Size	Calories	Total Fat (g)	Saturated Fat (g)	Sodium (mg)	Carbohydrates (g)	Fiber (g)	Protein (g)
Vanilla, rich	1/2 cup	266	17	11	65	24	0	4
ICE CREAM CONES								
Cake or wafer	1 cone	17	0	0	6	3	0	0
Sugar	1 cone	40	0	0	32	8	0	1
ICE POPS								
Creamsicle Pops, no sugar added	1 pop	25	0	0	18	6	0	1
Creamsicle Pops, sugar free	1 pop	20	1	1	2	5	3	1
Fudgesicle Bars, fat free	1 pop	65	0	0	48	14	1	3
Fudgesicle Pops, no sugar added	1 serv	88	1	0	86	19	1	3
Popsicle Scribblers	1.2 oz pop	27	0	0	4	7	0	0
Popsicles, sugar free, orange, cherry & grape	1-3/4 oz pop	12	0	0	6	3	0	0
Regular	1-3/4 oz pop	41	0	0	4	10	0	0
Sweetened w/low calorie sweetener	1-3/4 oz pop	13	0	0	6	3	0	0
ICED TEA, BRAND NAME								
Arizona Iced Tea, w/ lemon	8 fl oz	89	0	0	9	22	0	0
Lipton Brisk Iced Tea, w/ lemon	8 fl oz	86	0	0	51	22	0	0
Nestle Cool Nestea Iced Tea w/ lemon	8 fl oz	88	0	0	51	22	0	0
Snapple Lemon Iced Tea	8 fl oz	80	0	0	5	21	0	0
ICES								
Frozen fruit & juice bars	3 oz bar	80	0	0	4	19	1	1
Italian, restaurant prepared	1/2 cup	61	0	0	5	16	0	0
Lime	1/2 cup	127	0	0	22	32	0	0
Pineapple-coconut	1/2 cup	112	3	2	35	24	1	0
JACKFRUIT								
Canned in syrup	1 cup	164	0	0	20	43	2	1
Fresh, slices	1 cup	155	0	0	5	40	3	2
JAMS & PRESERVES								
Apricot	1 tbsp	48	0	0	8	13	0	0
Dietetic, any flavor	1 tbsp	18	0	0	0	8	0	0
Flavors other than apricot	1 tbsp	56	0	0	6	14	0	0
JAVA PLUM (Jambolan), fresh	3 fruit	5	0	0	1	1	0	0

ITEM DESCRIPTION	Serving Size	Calories	Total Fat (g)	Saturated Fat (g)	Sodium (mg)	Carbohydrates (g)	Fiber (g)	Protein (g)
JELLIES								
Jellies	1 tbsp	56	0	0	6	15	0	0
Red sugar, homemade	1 tbsp	34	0	0	0	9	0	0
JELLYFISH (dried, salted)	1 cup	21	1	0	5620	0	0	3
JICAMA (fresh, slices)	1 cup	46	0	0	5	11	6	1
JUICE DRINKS, BRAND NAME								
V8 Splash, berry blend	8 oz	70	0	0	51	18	0	0
V8 Splash, diet berry blend	8 oz	10	0	0	34	3	0	0
V8 Splash, fruit medley	8 oz	80	0	0	51	19	0	0
V8 Splash, mango peach	8 oz	80	0	0	39	20	0	0
V8 Splash, strawberry kiwi	8 oz	70	0	0	51	18	0	0
V8 Splash, tropical blend	8 oz	70	0	0	51	18	0	0
V8 Splash, tropical blend, diet	8 oz	10	0	0	36	3	0	0
V8 Splash Smoothies, strawberry banana	8 oz	91	0	0	71	20	0	3
V8 Splash Smoothies, tropical colada	8 oz	101	0	0	49	21	1	3
V8 Vegetable Juice, 100% vegetable juice	8 oz	51	0	0	481	10	2	2
V8 Vegetable Juice, essential antioxidants	8 oz	51	0	0	481	11	2	2
V8 Vegetable Juice, low sodium	8 oz	51	0	0	141	10	2	2
V8 Vegetable Juice, spicy hot V8	8 oz	49	0	0	620	10	2	2
V8 V- Fusion Juices, acai berry	8 oz	111	0	0	69	27	0	0
V8 V- Fusion Juices, peach mango	8 oz	121	0	0	69	28	0	1
V8 V- Fusion Juices, strawberry banana	8 oz	121	0	0	69	29	0	1
V8 V- Fusion Juices, tropical	8 oz	121	0	0	81	28	0	1
JUTE								
Potherb, boiled	1 cup	32	0	0	10	6	2	3
Potherb, fresh	1 cup	10	0	0	2	2	0	1
KALE								
Boiled, chopped	1 cup	36	1	0	30	7	3	2
Fresh, chopped	1 cup	34	0	0	29	7	1	2
Frozen, boiled, chopped	1 cup	39	1	0	20	7	3	4
Scotch, boiled, chopped	1 cup	36	1	0	58	7	2	2

ITEM DESCRIPTION	Serving Size	Calories	Total Fat (g)	Saturated Fat (g)	Sodium (mg)	Carbohydrates (g)	Fiber (g)	Protein (g)
Scotch, fresh, chopped	1 cup	28	0	0	47	6	1	2
KAMUT (cooked)	1 cup	251	2	0	0	52	0	11
KANPYO (dried gourd strips)	1 strip	16	0	0	1	4	0	1
KIDNEY BEANS								
California red, boiled	1 cup	219	0	0	7	40	17	16
California red, fresh	1 cup	607	0	0	20	110	46	45
Liquid from stewed kidney beans	1 cup	113	8	3	5	7	0	4
Red, boiled	1 cup	225	1	0	4	40	13	15
Red, canned	1 cup	215	1	0	660	40	14	13
Red, fresh	1 cup	620	2	0	22	113	28	41
Royal red, boiled	1 cup	218	0	0	9	39	17	17
Royal red, fresh	1 cup	605	1	0	24	107	46	47
Sprouted, fresh	1 cup	53	1	0	11	8	0	8
KIWI FRUIT (fresh, w/o skin)	1 fruit	56	0	0	3	13	3	1
KOHLRABI								
Boiled, slices	1 cup	48	0	0	35	11	2	3
Fresh	1 cup	36	0	0	27	8	5	2
KUMQUATS (fresh)	1 fruit	13	0	0	2	3	1	0
LAMB								
Australian, composite of retail cuts, 1/8" fat, cooked	3 oz	218	14	7	65	0	0	21
Australian, composite of retail cuts, lean, 1/8" fat, cooked	3 oz	218	8	3	68	0	0	23
Australian, foreshank, 1/8" fat, braised	3 oz	218	4	2	85	0	0	23
Australian, leg, center slice, bone in, 1/8" fat, broiled	3 oz	183	10	5	55	0	0	22
Australian, leg, shank half, 1/8" fat, roasted	3 oz	196	12	5	57	0	0	21
Australian, leg, sirloin chops, boneless, 1/8" fat, broiled	3 oz	200	12	5	54	0	0	22
Australian, leg, sirloin half, boneless, 1/8" fat, roasted	3 oz	239	16	8	66	0	0	21
Australian, leg, whole shank & sirloin, 1/8" fat, roasted	3 oz	207	13	6	60	0	0	21
Australian, loin, 1/8" fat, broiled	3 oz	186	10	5	66	0	0	22

ITEM DESCRIPTION	Serving Size	Calories	Total Fat (g)	Saturated Fat (g)	Sodium (mg)	Carbohydrates (g)	Fiber (g)	Protein (g)
Australian, rib, 1/8" fat, roasted	3 oz	235	17	8	65	0	0	19
Australian, shoulder, arm, 1/8" fat, braised	3 oz	264	17	8	62	0	0	25
Australian, shoulder, blade, 1/8" fat, broiled	3 oz	247	19	9	75	0	0	18
Australian, shoulder, whole arm & blade, 1/8" fat, cooked	3 oz	252	18	9	72	0	0	20
Domestic, composite of retail cuts, 1/4" fat, USDA Choice, cooked	3 oz	250	18	8	61	0	0	21
Domestic, composite of retail cuts, 1/8" fat, USDA Choice, cooked	3 oz	230	15	6	61	0	0	22
Domestic, cubed for stew, leg & shoulder, 1/4" fat, braised	3 oz	190	7	3	60	0	0	29
Domestic, cubed for stew, leg & shoulder, 1/4" fat, broiled	3 oz	158	6	2	65	0	0	24
Domestic, foreshank, 1/4" fat, USDA Choice, braised	3 oz	207	11	5	61	0	0	24
Domestic, foreshank, 1/8" fat, braised	3 oz	207	11	5	61	0	0	24
Domestic, leg, shank half, 1/4" fat, USDA Choice, roasted	3 oz	191	11	4	55	0	0	22
Domestic, leg, shank half, 1/8" fat, USDA Choice, roasted	3 oz	184	10	4	55	0	0	23
Domestic, leg, sirloin half, 1/4" fat, USDA Choice, roasted	3 oz	248	18	7	58	0	0	21
Domestic, leg, sirloin half, 1/8" fat, USDA Choice, roasted	3 oz	241	17	7	58	0	0	21
Domestic, leg, whole shank & sirloin, 1/4" fat, USDA Choice, roasted	3 oz	219	14	6	56	0	0	22
Domestic, leg, whole shank & sirloin, 1/8" fat, USDA Choice, roasted	3 oz	206	12	5	57	0	0	22
Domestic, loin, 1/4" fat, USDA Choice, broiled	3 oz	269	20	8	65	0	0	21
Domestic, loin, 1/4" fat, USDA Choice, roasted	3 oz	263	20	9	54	0	0	19
Domestic, loin, 1/8" fat, USDA Choice, broiled	3 oz	252	18	7	66	0	0	22

ITEM DESCRIPTION	Serving Size	Calories	Total Fat (g)	Saturated Fat (g)	Sodium (mg)	Carbohydrates (g)	Fiber (g)	Protein (g)
Domestic, loin, 1/8" fat, USDA Choice, roasted	3 oz	246	18	8	54	0	0	20
Domestic, rib, 1/4" fat, USDA Choice, broiled	3 oz	307	25	11	65	0	0	19
Domestic, rib, 1/4" fat, USDA Choice, roasted	3 oz	305	25	11	62	0	0	18
Domestic, rib, 1/4" fat, USDA Choice, broiled	3 oz	289	23	10	65	0	0	20
Domestic, rib, 1/8" fat, USDA Choice, roasted	3 oz	290	23	10	63	0	0	19
Domestic, shoulder, arm, 1/4" fat, USDA Choice, braised	3 oz	294	20	8	61	0	0	26
Domestic, shoulder, arm, 1/4" fat, USDA Choice, broiled	3 oz	239	17	7	65	0	0	21
Domestic, shoulder, arm, 1/4" fat, USDA Choice, roasted	3 oz	237	17	7	55	0	0	19
Domestic, shoulder, arm, 1/8" fat, broiled	3 oz	229	15	7	66	0	0	21
Domestic, shoulder, arm, 1/8" fat, USDA Choice, braised	3 oz	286	19	8	61	0	0	26
Domestic, shoulder, arm, 1/8" fat, USDA Choice, roasted	3 oz	227	16	7	55	0	0	19
Domestic, shoulder, blade, 1/4" fat, USDA Choice, braised	3 oz	293	21	9	64	0	0	24
Domestic, shoulder, blade, 1/4" fat, USDA Choice, broiled	3 oz	236	17	7	70	0	0	20
Domestic, shoulder, blade, 1/4" fat, USDA Choice, roasted	3 oz	239	18	7	56	0	0	19
Domestic, shoulder, blade, 1/8" fat, USDA Choice, braised	3 oz	288	20	8	64	0	0	25
Domestic, shoulder, blade, 1/8" fat, USDA Choice, broiled	3 oz	227	16	6	71	0	0	20
Domestic, shoulder, blade, 1/8" fat, USDA Choice, roasted	3 oz	230	16	7	57	0	0	19
Domestic, shoulder, whole arm & blade, 1/4" fat, USDA Choice, braised	3 oz	292	21	9	64	0	0	24
Domestic, shoulder, whole arm & blade, 1/4" fat, USDA Choice, broiled	3 oz	236	16	7	66	0	0	21

ITEM DESCRIPTION	Serving Size	Calories	Total Fat (g)	Saturated Fat (g)	Sodium (mg)	Carbohydrates (g)	Fiber (g)	Protein (g)
Domestic, shoulder, whole arm & blade, 1/4" fat, USDA Choice, roasted	3 oz	235	17	7	56	0	0	19
Domestic, shoulder, whole arm & blade, 1/8" fat, USDA Choice, braised	3 oz	287	20	8	63	0	0	25
Domestic, shoulder, whole arm & blade, 1/8" fat, USDA Choice, broiled	3 oz	228	16	6	70	0	0	20
Domestic, shoulder, whole arm & blade, 1/8" fat, USDA Choice, roasted	3 oz	229	16	7	56	0	0	19
Ground, broiled	3 oz	241	17	7	69	0	0	21
Quarters, boiled, chopped	1 cup	58	1	0	52	9	4	6
LARD	1 tbsp	115	13	5	0	0	0	0
LASAGNA (vegetable, frozen, baked)	1 cup	314	14	5	796	32	4	16
LEEKS								
Boiled	1 leek	38	0	0	12	9	1	1
Freeze-dried	1 tbsp	1	0	0	0	0	0	0
Fresh	1 leek	54	0	0	18	13	2	1
LEMONADE								
Frozen concentrate, pink, prepared w/ water	8 fl oz	99	0	0	10	26	0	0
Frozen concentrate, yellow, prepared w/ water	8 fl oz	99	0	0	10	26	0	0
Lemonade-flavor drink, powder, prepared w/ water	8 fl oz	66	0	0	33	17	0	0
Powder, low calorie, w/ aspartame, prepared w/ water	8 fl oz	7	0	0	10	2	0	0
Powder, prepared w/ water	8 fl oz	98	0	0	8	26	0	0
LEMON GRASS (citronella, fresh)	1 tbsp	5	0	0	0	1	0	0
LEMON JUICE								
Canned or bottled	2 tbsp	6	0	0	6	2	0	0
Fresh	2 tbsp	8	0	0	0	3	0	0
Frozen, unsweetened	2 tbsp	7	0	0	0	2	0	0
LEMONS								
Fresh, sections	1 cup	61	1	0	4	20	6	2
Fresh, whole	1 fruit	22	0	0	3	12	5	1
Peel, fresh	1 tbsp	3	0	0	0	1	1	0

ITEM DESCRIPTION	Serving Size	Calories	Total Fat (g)	Saturated Fat (g)	Sodium (mg)	Carbohydrates (g)	Fiber (g)	Protein (g)
LENTILS								
Boiled	1 cup	230	1	0	4	40	16	18
Sprouted, fresh	1 cup	82	0	0	8	17	0	7
LETTUCE								
Bibb, shredded	1 cup	7	0	0	3	1	1	1
Boston, shredded	1 cup	7	0	0	3	1	1	1
Cos, shredded	1 cup	8	0	0	4	2	1	1
Green leaf, shredded	1 cup	5	0	0	10	1	0	0
Iceberg, shredded	1 cup	10	0	0	7	2	1	1
Red leaf, shredded	1 cup	4	0	0	7	1	0	0
Romaine, shredded	1 cup	8	0	0	4	2	1	1
LIGHT CREAM								
(whipped)	1 cup	350	37	23	41	4	0	3
LIMA BEANS								
Boiled	1/2 cup	105	0	0	14	20	5	6
Boiled, baby	1/2 cup	115	0	0	3	21	7	7
Boiled, large	1/2 cup	108	0	0	2	20	7	7
Canned, no salt	1/2 cup	88	0	0	5	17	5	5
Canned, w/ salt	1/2 cup	88	0	0	312	17	5	5
Fresh	1/2 cup	88	1	0	6	16	4	5
Fresh, baby	1/2 cup	338	1	0	13	63	21	21
Fresh, large	1/2 cup	301	1	0	16	56	17	19
Frozen, boiled, baby	1/2 cup	94	0	0	26	18	5	6
LIMEADE (frozen concentrate, prepared w/ water)	8 fl oz	128	0	0	7	34	0	0
LIME JUICE								
Canned or bottled, unsweetened	1 fl oz	6	0	0	5	2	0	0
Fresh	1 fl oz	8	0	0	1	3	0	0
LIMES fresh (2" dia)	1 fruit	20	0	0	1	7	2	0
LING (cooked in dry heat)	3 oz	94	1	0	147	0	0	21
LINGCOD (cooked in dry heat)	3 oz	93	1	0	65	0	0	19
LITCHIS								
Dried	1 fruit	7	0	0	0	2	0	0
Fresh	1 fruit	6	0	0	0	2	0	0

ITEM DESCRIPTION	Serving Size	Calories	Total Fat (g)	Saturated Fat (g)	Sodium (mg)	Carbohydrates (g)	Fiber (g)	Protein (g)
LIVERWURST SPREAD	1/4 cup	168	14	5	385	3	1	7
LOBSTER								
Northern, cooked in moist heat	3 oz	83	1	0	323	1	0	17
Spiny, cooked in moist heat	3 oz	122	2	0	193	3	0	22
LOGANBERRIES (frozen)	1 cup	81	0	0	1	19	8	2
LOQUATS (fresh)	1 lg	9	0	0	0	2	0	0
LOTUS ROOT								
Boiled	1/2 cup	40	0	0	27	10	2	1
Fresh (9 1/2" long)	1 root	85	0	0	46	20	6	3
MACADAMIA NUTS								
Dry roasted	1 cup	948	100	16	5	18	11	10
Dry roasted, w/ salt	1 cup	945	100	16	350	17	11	10
Fresh	1 cup	962	102	16	7	19	12	11
MACE (ground)	1 tbsp	25	2	1	4	3	1	0
MACKEREL								
Atlantic, cooked in dry heat	3 oz	223	15	4	71	0	0	20
Jack, canned, drained	1 cup	296	12	4	720	0	0	44
King, cooked in dry heat	3 oz	114	2	0	173	0	0	22
Pacific & Jack, cooked in dry heat	3 oz	171	9	2	94	0	0	22
Salted, cooked	1 cup	415	34	10	6052	0	0	25
Spanish, cooked in dry heat	3 oz	134	5	2	56	0	0	20
MALABAR SPINACH (cooked)	1 bunch	4	0	0	9	0	0	0
MALT (beverage)	1 cup	88	0	0	31	19	0	0
MALTED DRINK MIX								
Chocolate, powder, prepared w/ whole milk	8 fl oz	225	9	5	159	30	1	9
Powder, prepared w/ whole milk	8 fl oz	233	10	5	209	27	0	10
MALT SYRUP	1 tbsp	76	0	0	8	17	0	1
MANGO								
Nectar, canned	1 cup	128	0	0	13	33	1	0
Fresh	1 fruit	135	1	0	4	35	4	1
MANGOSTEEN								
(canned in syrup, drained)	1 cup	143	1	0	14	35	4	1
MAPLE SYRUP	1 tbsp	52	0	0	2	13	0	0

ITEM DESCRIPTION	Serving Size	Calories	Total Fat (g)	Saturated Fat (g)	Sodium (mg)	Carbohydrates (g)	Fiber (g)	Protein (g)
MARGARINE								
20% fat	1 tbsp	26	3	0	110	0	0	0
20% fat, no salt	1 tbsp	22	3	0	0	0	0	0
48% fat , tub	1 tbsp	59	7	1	90	0	0	0
60% fat, stick	1 tbsp	77	9	2	112	0	0	0
60% fat, stick, no salt	1 tbsp	75	8	2	0	0	0	0
60% fat, stick, tub, bottle	1 tbsp	75	8	1	112	0	0	0
60% fat, tub or bottle, unsalted	1 tbsp	75	8	2	4	0	0	0
70% fat, soybean & part hydrogenated soybean oil, stick	1 tbsp	87	10	2	98	0	0	0
80% fat, composite, stick, unsalted	1 tbsp	102	11	2	0	0	0	0
80% fat, composite, stick, w/ salt	1 tbsp	100	11	2	132	0	0	0
80% fat, composite, tub, unsalted	1 tbsp	101	11	2	4	0	0	0
80% fat, composite, tub, w/ salt	1 tbsp	101	11	2	93	0	0	0
80% fat, corn & soybean oils, stick	1 tbsp	100	11	2	92	0	0	0
Fat free, tub	1 tbsp	7	0	0	85	1	0	0
Hard, soybean oils	1 tbsp	101	11	2	133	0	0	0
Hard, sunflower, soybean & cottonseed oils	1 tbsp	101	11	2	133	0	0	0
Liquid, soybean & cottonseed oils	1 tbsp	102	11	2	111	0	0	0
Margarine-butter blend, soybean oil & butter	1 tbsp	101	11	2	89	0	0	0
No salt	1 tbsp	101	11	2	0	0	0	0
Salted	1 tbsp	101	11	2	133	0	0	0
MARGARINE SUBSTITUTE								
Benecol Light Spread	1 tbsp	50	5	1	94	1	0	0
Smart Balance Light Buttery Spread	1 tbsp	47	5	1	81	0	0	0
Smart Balance Omega Plus Spread	1 tbsp	85	9	3	102	0	0	0
Smart Balance Regular Buttery Spread	1 tbsp	85	9	3	90	0	0	0
Spread, 37% fat, unspecified oils	1 tbsp	51	6	1	88	0	0	1
Spread, 40% fat, reduced calorie, made w/ yogurt, salted	1 tbsp	46	5	1	88	0	0	0

ITEM DESCRIPTION	Serving Size	Calories	Total Fat (g)	Saturated Fat (g)	Sodium (mg)	Carbohydrates (g)	Fiber (g)	Protein (g)
Spread, 40% fat, reduced calorie, stick, salted	1 tbsp	50	6	1	139	0	0	0
Spread, 60% fat, vegetable oil, tub	1 tbsp	75	8	2	110	0	0	0
Spread, 67-70% fat, vegetable oil, tub	1 tbsp	85	10	2	75	0	0	0
Spread, 70% fat, liquid, salted	1 tbsp	87	10	1	139	0	0	0
Spread, fat free, liquid, salted	1 tbsp	6	0	0	125	0	0	0
Spread, made w/ yogurt, stick, salted	1 tbsp	88	10	2	83	0	0	0
Spread, stick or tub, sweetened	1 tbsp	75	7	1	76	2	0	0
MARINARA SAUCE	1/2 cup	111	3	1	535	18	3	2
Low sodium	1/2 cup	111	3	1	38	18	3	2
MARJORAM (dried)	1 tbsp	5	0	0	1	1	1	0
MARSHMALLOWS	1 reg	23	0	0	6	6	0	0
Marshmallow topping	1 oz	91	0	0	23	22	0	0
MAYONNAISE								
Cholesterol free	1 tbsp	103	12	2	73	0	0	0
Diet or reduced calorie, cholesterol free	1 tbsp	49	5	1	107	1	0	0
Diet, cholesterol free	1 tbsp	57	5	1	105	4	0	0
Kraft Mayo, fat free	1 tbsp	11	0	0	120	2	0	0
Kraft Mayo, light	1 tbsp	50	5	1	120	1	0	0
Low calorie	1 tbsp	38	3	0	100	3	0	0
Low sodium, low calorie or diet	1 tbsp	32	3	0	15	2	0	0
Light	1 tbsp	49	5	1	101	1	0	0
Reg, w/ salt	1 tbsp	59	5	1	107	4	0	0
Soybean & safflower oil, w/ salt	1 tbsp	99	11	1	78	0	0	0
Soybean oil, w/o salt	1 tbsp	99	11	2	4	0	0	0
Soybean oil, w/ salt	1 tbsp	99	11	2	78	0	0	0
MAYONNAISE SUBSTITUTE								
Fat free	1 tbsp	13	0	0	126	2	0	0
Imitation, milk cream	1 tbsp	15	1	0	76	2	0	0
Imitation, soybean	1 tbsp	35	3	0	75	2	0	0
Imitation, soybean, no cholesterol	1 tbsp	68	7	1	50	2	0	0
Kraft Miracle Whip Free, nonfat	1 tbsp	13	0	0	126	2	0	0

ITEM DESCRIPTION	Serving Size	Calories	Total Fat (g)	Saturated Fat (g)	Sodium (mg)	Carbohydrates (g)	Fiber (g)	Protein (g)
Kraft Miracle Whip, light	1 tbsp	37	3	0	131	2	0	0
Made w/ tofu	1 tbsp	48	5	0	116	0	0	1
MENHADEN								
Fish oil	1 tbsp	123	14	4	0	0	0	0
Fish oil, fully hydrogenated	1 tbsp	113	13	12	0	0	0	0
MILK								
Canned, condensed, sweetened	1 cup	982	27	17	389	166	0	24
Canned, evaporated	1 cup	338	19	12	267	25	0	17
Canned, evaporated, nonfat	1 cup	200	1	0	294	29	0	19
Dry, nonfat, instant	1 cup	243	0	0	373	35	0	24
Dry, nonfat, reg	1 cup	434	1	1	642	62	0	43
Dry, whole	1 cup	635	34	21	475	49	0	34
Imitation, non-soy	1 cup	112	5	1	134	13	0	4
Low fat, 1% milkfat	1 cup	102	2	2	107	12	0	8
Low sodium	1 cup	149	8	5	7	11	0	8
Nonfat, calcium fortified, fat free or skim	1 cup	86	0	0	127	12	0	8
Reduced fat, 2% milkfat	1 cup	122	5	3	100	11	0	8
Whole, 3.25% milkfat	1 cup	146	8	5	98	11	0	8
MILKFISH (cooked in dry heat)	3 oz	162	7	0	78	0	0	22
MILK SHAKES								
Thick, chocolate	8 fl oz	270	6	4	252	48	1	7
Thick, vanilla	8 fl oz	254	7	4	216	40	0	9
MILLET								
Millet, cooked	1 cup	207	2	0	3	41	2	6
Millet, puffed	1 cup	74	1	0	1	17	1	3
Millet, fresh	1 cup	756	8	1	10	146	17	22
MISO	1 cup	547	17	3	10252	73	15	32
MIXED FRUIT								
Peaches, cherries, raspberries, grapes, & boysenberries, frozen, sweetened	10 oz pkg	278	1	0	9	69	5	4
Peaches, pears, & pineapple, canned in heavy syrup	1 cup	184	0	0	10	48	3	1

ITEM DESCRIPTION	Serving Size	Calories	Total Fat (g)	Saturated Fat (g)	Sodium (mg)	Carbohydrates (g)	Fiber (g)	Protein (g)
Prunes, apricots, & pears, dried	11 oz pkg	712	1	0	53	188	23	7
MIXED NUTS								
Dry roasted, w/ peanuts, w/o salt	1 cup	814	70	9	16	35	12	24
Dry roasted, w/ peanuts, w/ salt	1 cup	814	70	9	917	35	12	24
Oil roasted, w/o peanuts, w/o salt	1 cup	886	81	13	16	32	8	22
Oil roasted, w/ peanuts, w/o salt	1 cup	876	80	12	16	30	14	24
Oil roasted, w/o peanuts, w/ salt	1 cup	886	81	13	441	32	8	22
Oil roasted, w/ peanuts, w/ salt	1 cup	876	80	12	595	30	13	24
MIXED VEGETABLES								
Canned	1 cup	88	1	0	549	17	9	3
Canned, drained	1 cup	80	0	0	243	15	5	4
Canned, no salt	1 cup	67	0	0	47	13	6	3
Frozen, boiled	10 oz pkg	179	0	0	96	36	12	8
MOCHA MIX (w/ whitener & low calorie sweetener)	1 tsp, dry	16	1	1	32	5	0	1
MOLASSES	1 tbsp	58	0	0	7	15	0	0
MOLE SAUCE (dry mix, prepared)	1 cup	1513	110	0	3085	111	27	20
MONKFISH (cooked in dry heat)	3 oz	82	2	0	20	0	0	16
MORTADELLA (beef, pork)	1 slice	47	4	1	187	0	0	2
MOTH BEANS								
Boiled	1 cup	207	1	0	18	37	0	14
Fresh	1 cup	672	3	1	59	121	0	45
MOUSSE (homemade, chocolate)	1/2 cup	454	32	18	77	32	1	8
MUFFINS								
Betty Crocker Wild Blueberry Muffin, from mix	1 serv	128	2	0	186	26	0	2
Blueberry, commercial (2.75" dia)	1	259	13	2	208	33	1	3
Blueberry, commercial, low fat	1	181	3	1	224	36	3	3
Blueberry, homemade, made w/ 2% milk	1	162	6	1	251	23	0	4
Blueberry, toaster type	1	103	3	0	158	18	1	2
Corn, commercial, small	1	201	6	1	344	34	2	4
Corn, homemade, made w/ 2% milk, small	1	180	7	1	333	25	0	4

ITEM DESCRIPTION	Serving Size	Calories	Total Fat (g)	Saturated Fat (g)	Sodium (mg)	Carbohydrates (g)	Fiber (g)	Protein (g)
Corn, toaster type	1	114	4	1	142	19	1	2
Krusteaz Almond Poppyseed Muffin, from mix	1 serv	167	4	1	236	30	1	2
Oat bran, small	1	178	5	1	259	32	3	5
Plain, homemade, made w/ 2% milk	1	169	7	1	266	24	2	4
Wheat bran, toaster type w/ raisins	1	106	3	0	178	19	3	2
MULBERRIES (fresh)	10 fruit	6	0	0	2	1	0	0
MULLET (striped, cooked in dry heat)	3 oz	128	4	1	60	0	0	21
MULTIGRAIN CHIPS								
SunChips Multigrain Snack, French onion	1 oz	141	6	1	132	19	2	2
SunChips Multigrain Snack, harvest cheddar	1 oz	139	6	1	153	18	2	2
SunChips Multigrain Snack, original	1 oz	139	6	1	93	19	2	2
MUNG BEANS								
Boiled	1 cup	212	1	0	4	39	15	14
Fresh	1 cup	718	2	1	31	130	34	49
Sprouted, boiled	1 cup	26	0	0	12	5	1	3
Sprouted, canned	1 cup	15	0	0	175	3	1	2
Sprouted, fresh	1 cup	31	0	0	6	6	2	3
Sprouted, stir-fried	1 cup	62	0	0	11	13	2	5
MUSHROOMS								
Boiled	1 cup, pcs	44	1	0	3	8	3	3
Brown, Italian, or cremini, fresh, slices	1 cup	19	0	0	4	3	0	2
Canned	1 cup	39	0	0	663	8	4	3
Cloud ears, dried	1 cup	80	0	0	10	20	20	3
Enoki, fresh	1 lg	2	0	0	0	0	0	0
Maitake, fresh, diced	1 cup	26	0	0	1	5	2	1
Oyster, fresh	1 large	64	1	0	27	10	3	5
Portabella, grilled, slices	1 cup	42	1	0	12	6	3	5
Portabella, fresh, diced	1 cup	22	0	0	5	4	1	2
Shiitake	1 cup, pcs	81	0	0	6	21	3	2
Shiitake, dried	1 mushroom	11	0	0	0	3	0	0

ITEM DESCRIPTION	Serving Size	Calories	Total Fat (g)	Saturated Fat (g)	Sodium (mg)	Carbohydrates (g)	Fiber (g)	Protein (g)
Shiitake, stir-fried, slices	1 cup	47	0	0	5	7	4	3
Straw, canned	1 cup	58	1	0	699	8	5	7
White, fresh	1 cup, pcs	15	0	0	4	2	1	2
White, stir-fried, slices	1 cup	28	0	0	13	4	2	4
MUSSELS								
Blue, cooked in moist heat	3 oz	146	4	1	314	6	0	20
Blue, fresh	1 med	14	0	0	46	1	0	2
MUSTARD (yellow, prepared)	1 tsp	3	0	0	57	0	0	0
MUSTARD GREENS								
Boiled, chopped	1 cup	21	0	0	22	3	3	3
Fresh, chopped	1 cup	15	0	0	14	3	2	2
Frozen, boiled, chopped	1 cup	28	0	0	38	5	4	3
MUSTARD OIL	1 tbsp	124	14	2	0	0	0	0
MUSTARD SEED (yellow)	1 tbsp	53	3	0	1	4	2	3
MUSTARD SPINACH								
Boiled, chopped	1 cup	29	0	0	25	5	4	3
Fresh, chopped	1 cup	33	0	0	32	6	4	3
NATTO	1 cup	371	19	3	12	25	9	31
NAVY BEANS								
Boiled	1 cup	255	1	0	0	47	19	15
Canned	1 cup	296	1	0	1174	54	13	20
Fresh	1 cup	701	3	0	10	126	51	46
Fresh, sprouted	1 cup	70	1	0	14	14	0	6
NECTARINES (fresh, whole)	1 sml	57	0	0	0	14	2	1
NOODLES								
Cellophane, dehydrated	1 cup	491	0	0	14	121	1	0
Chinese restaurant noodles, flat, crunchy	1 cup	234	14	2	170	23	0	5
Chow mein	1 cup	237	14	2	198	26	2	4
Egg	1 cup	221	3	1	8	40	2	7
Egg, w/ salt	1 cup	221	3	0	264	40	2	7
Long rice & mung bean, dehydrated	1 cup	491	0	0	14	121	1	0
Rice	1 cup	192	0	0	33	44	2	2
Soba	1 cup	113	0	0	68	24	0	6

ITEM DESCRIPTION	Serving Size	Calories	Total Fat (g)	Saturated Fat (g)	Sodium (mg)	Carbohydrates (g)	Fiber (g)	Protein (g)
Somen	1 cup	231	0	0	283	48	0	7
Spinach egg	1 cup	211	3	1	19	39	4	8
NUTMEG								
Ground	1 tbsp	37	3	2	1	3	1	0
Butter oil	1 tbsp	120	14	12	0	0	0	0
NUTRITIONAL SUPPLEMENT (Ensure Plus, liquid nutrition)	1 cup	355	11	2	239	50	0	13
NUTS IN SYRUP TOPPING	2 tbsp	184	9	1	17	24	1	2
OAT BRAN								
Cooked	1 cup	88	2	0	2	25	6	7
Fresh	1 cup	231	7	1	4	62	14	16
OAT OIL	1 tbsp	120	14	3	0	0	0	0
OCEAN PERCH (Atlantic, cooked in dry heat)	3 oz	103	2	0	82	0	0	20
OCTOPUS (cooked in moist heat)	3 oz	139	2	0	391	4	0	25
OILS (corn, peanut, & olive)	1 tbsp	124	14	2	0	0	0	0
OKRA								
Boiled, slices	1/2 cup	18	0	0	5	4	2	1
Fresh	1 cup	31	0	0	8	7	3	2
Frozen, boiled, slices	1/2 cup	26	0	0	3	5	3	2
OLIVE LOAF								
Pork	1 slice	66	5	2	416	3	0	3
Oscar Mayer, chicken, pork, & turkey	1 serv	74	6	2	369	2	0	3
OLIVE OIL (salad or cooking)	1 tbsp	119	14	2	0	0	0	0
OLIVES								
Pickled, canned or bottled	1 olive	4	0	0	42	0	0	0
Ripe, canned, jumbo to colossal	1 jumbo	7	1	0	75	0	0	0
Ripe, canned, small to extra large	1 lg	5	0	0	38	0	0	0
ONION POWDER	1 tbsp	24	0	0	4	6	0	1
ONION RINGS (Breaded, heated in oven) (3-4" dia)	10 rings	289	19	6	266	27	1	4
ONIONS								
Boiled	1 cup	92	0	0	6	21	3	3
Canned, chopped	1 cup	43	0	0	831	9	3	2

ITEM DESCRIPTION	Serving Size	Calories	Total Fat (g)	Saturated Fat (g)	Sodium (mg)	Carbohydrates (g)	Fiber (g)	Protein (g)
Dehydrated flakes	1/4 cup	49	0	0	3	12	1	1
Fresh, chopped	1 cup	64	0	0	6	15	3	2
Frozen, chopped, boiled	1/2 cup	29	0	0	13	7	2	1
Frozen, whole, boiled	1 cup	59	0	0	17	14	3	1
Sweet, fresh	1 onion	106	0	0	26	25	3	3
Yellow, sauteed, chopped	1 cup	115	9	0	10	7	2	1
Young green	1 stalk	3	0	0	0	1	0	0
ORANGE & APRICOT JUICE DRINK (canned)	8 fl oz	128	0	0	5	32	0	1
ORANGE DRINK								
Breakfast drink	8 fl oz	108	0	0	5	27	1	0
Breakfast drink, frozen concentrate w/ juice & pulp, prepared w/ water	8 fl oz	112	0	0	25	28	0	0
Breakfast drink, powder, prepared w/ water	6 fl oz	100	0	0	10	26	0	0
Canned	8 fl oz	122	0	0	7	31	0	0
Orange juice drink	8 fl oz	134	0	0	5	33	0	0
ORANGE-GRAPEFRUIT JUICE (canned, unsweetened)	1 cup	106	0	0	7	25	0	1
ORANGE JUICE								
California, chilled, including juice from concentrate	1 cup	110	1	0	2	25	0	2
Canned, unsweetened	1 cup	117	0	0	10	27	1	2
Fresh	1 cup	112	1	0	2	26	1	2
Frozen concentrate, unsweetened, prepared w/ water	1 cup	112	0	0	2	27	1	2
ORANGE MARMALADE	1 tbsp	49	0	0	11	13	0	0
ORANGE ROUGHY (cooked in dry heat)	3 oz	89	1	0	59	0	0	19
ORANGES								
Fresh, all varieties (2-5/8" dia)	1 fruit	62	0	0	0	15	3	1
Fresh, California, Valencia (2-5/8" dia)	1 fruit	59	0	0	0	14	3	1
Fresh, Florida (2-5/8" dia)	1 fruit	65	0	0	0	16	3	1
Fresh, navel (2-7/8" dia)	1 fruit	69	0	0	1	18	3	1
Peel only, fresh	1 tbsp	6	0	0	0	2	1	0
ORANGE-STRAWBERRY-BANANA JUICE	1 cup	117	0	0	9	29	1	1

ITEM DESCRIPTION	Serving Size	Calories	Total Fat (g)	Saturated Fat (g)	Sodium (mg)	Carbohydrates (g)	Fiber (g)	Protein (g)
OREGANO (dried, ground)	1 tsp	6	0	0	0	1	0	0
OYSTERS								
Eastern, breaded & fried	3 oz	167	11	3	354	10	0	7
Eastern, canned, drained	1 cup	112	4	1	181	6	0	11
Eastern, farmed, cooked in dry heat	3 oz	67	2	1	139	6	0	6
Eastern, farmed, fresh	3 oz	50	1	0	151	5	0	4
Eastern, wild, cooked in dry heat	3 oz	61	2	0	207	4	0	7
Eastern, wild, cooked in moist heat	3 oz	116	4	1	359	7	0	12
Eastern, wild, fresh	3 oz	116	2	1	179	3	0	6
Pacific, cooked in moist heat	3 oz	139	4	1	180	8	0	16
Pacific, fresh	3 oz	69	2	0	90	4	0	8
OYSTER SAUCE	1 tbsp	9	0	0	492	2	0	0
OYSTER STEW (Campbell's Red & White, condensed)	1/2 cup	79	6	4	910	5	0	2
PALM KERNEL OIL	1 tbsp	117	14	11	0	0	0	0
PALM OIL	1 tbsp	120	14	7	0	0	0	0
PAM COOKING SPRAY	1 spray	2	0	0	0	0	0	0
PANCAKES								
Blueberry, homemade (4" dia)	1	84	4	1	157	11	0	2
Buttermilk, homemade (4" dia)	1	86	4	1	198	11	0	3
Kellogg's Eggo Buttermilk Pancakes	1	90	3	1	205	15	0	2
Plain, dry mix, complete, prepared (4" dia)	1	74	1	0	239	14	1	2
Plain, dry mix, plus egg (4" dia)	1	83	3	1	192	11	1	3
Plain, frozen	1	92	2	0	207	16	1	2
Plain, frozen, microwavable	1	91	2	0	215	17	1	2
Plain, homemade (4" dia)	1	86	4	1	167	11	0	2
Whole wheat, dry mix, plus egg (4" dia)	1	92	3	1	252	13	1	4
PANCAKE SYRUP								
Cane, 15% maple	1 tbsp	56	0	0	21	14	0	0
Corn, refiner & sugar	1 tbsp	64	0	0	14	17	0	0
Reduced calorie	1 tbsp	25	0	0	27	7	0	0
Regular	1 tbsp	47	0	0	16	12	0	0

ITEM DESCRIPTION	Serving Size	Calories	Total Fat (g)	Saturated Fat (g)	Sodium (mg)	Carbohydrates (g)	Fiber (g)	Protein (g)
With 2% maple	1 tbsp	53	0	0	12	14	0	0
With butter	1 tbsp	59	0	0	20	15	0	0
PAPAYA								
Nectar, canned	1 cup	142	0	0	12	36	2	0
Fresh, cubed	1 cup	55	0	0	4	14	3	1
PAPRIKA	1 tbsp	20	1	0	2	4	3	1
PARSLEY								
Dried	1 tbsp	4	0	0	7	1	1	0
Freeze-dried	1 tbsp	1	0	0	2	0	0	0
Fresh	1 tbsp	1	0	0	2	0	0	0
PARSNIPS								
Boiled, slices	1 cup	111	0	0	16	27	6	2
Fresh, slices	1 cup	100	0	0	13	24	7	2
PASSION FRUIT								
Purple, fresh	1 fruit	17	0	0	5	4	2	0
Juice, purple, fresh	1 cup	126	0	0	15	34	1	1
Juice, yellow, fresh	1 cup	148	0	0	15	36	1	2
PASTA								
Corn	1 cup	176	1	0	0	39	7	4
Fresh, refrigerated, plain	2 oz	75	1	0	3	14	0	3
Fresh, refrigerated, spinach	2 oz	74	1	0	3	14	0	3
Homemade, made w/ egg	2 oz	74	1	0	47	13	0	3
Homemade, made w/o egg	2 oz	71	1	0	42	14	0	2
Macaroni, elbows	1 cup	221	1	0	1	43	3	8
Macaroni, protein fortified, small shells	1 cup	189	0	0	6	36	0	9
Macaroni, vegetable, spirals	1 cup	172	0	0	8	36	6	6
Macaroni, whole wheat, elbows	1 cup	174	1	0	4	37	4	7
Spaghetti, cooked	1 cup	221	1	0	1	43	3	8
Spaghetti, protein fortified, cooked	1 cup	230	0	0	7	44	2	11
Spaghetti, spinach, cooked	1 cup	182	1	0	20	37	0	6
Spaghetti, whole wheat, cooked	1 cup	174	1	0	4	37	6	7
Tortellini, w/cheese filling	3/4 cup	249	6	3	279	38	2	11
Vermicelli, made from soy	1 cup	463	0	0	6	115	6	0

ITEM DESCRIPTION	Serving Size	Calories	Total Fat (g)	Saturated Fat (g)	Sodium (mg)	Carbohydrates (g)	Fiber (g)	Protein (g)
PASTA ENTRÉE								
Chef Boyardee Beefaroni, canned	1 cup	236	7	3	959	35	1	8
Chef Boyardee Beef Ravioli, tomato & meat sauce	1 cup	224	7	3	910	33	1	8
Chef Boyardee Mini Beef Ravioli, tomato & meat sauce	1 cup	232	8	3	935	31	3	8
Chef Boyardee Spaghetti & Meatballs, tomato sauce, canned	1 serv	257	10	4	925	31	4	11
Healthy Choice Beef Macaroni, frozen	1 serv	211	2	1	444	33	5	14
Hodgson Mill Whole Wheat Macaroni & Cheese, mix	1 serv	263	3	1	428	48	5	10
Kraft Macaroni & Cheese, mix	1 serv	259	3	1	561	48	2	11
Lipton Alfredo Egg Noodles, creamy sauce, mix	1 cup	389	11	4	1646	58	0	14
Macaroni & cheese, canned	1 serv	200	6	2	1027	28	1	8
Pasta w/sliced franks in tomato sauce, canned	1 serv	262	12	4	1215	30	2	9
Spaghettios A to Z's	1 serv	176	1	0	879	36	3	6
Spaghettios A to Z's, w/meatballs	1 serv	257	9	4	990	33	3	11
Spaghettios Original	1 serv	179	0	0	630	37	3	6
Spaghettios Raviolios, beef ravioli, meat sauce	1 serv	267	8	4	1091	38	4	11
Spaghettios, w/ meatballs	1 serv	239	8	4	660	32	4	11
Spaghettios, w/ sliced franks	1 serv	234	10	5	930	27	5	9
Spaghetti, w/ meatballs, canned	1 cup	273	13	5	1035	28	0	11
Spaghetti w/ meat sauce, frozen	1 serv	255	3	1	473	43	5	14
PASTRAMI								
Beef, 98% fat free	1 slice	9	0	0	96	0	0	2
Carl Buddig Smoked Beef, chopped, pressed	2 oz	80	4	2	602	1	0	11
PÂTÉ								
Chicken liver, canned	1 tbsp	26	2	1	50	1	0	2
Foie gras, goose liver, canned, smoked	1 tbsp	60	6	2	91	1	0	1
Liver, canned	1 tbsp	41	4	1	91	0	0	2

ITEM DESCRIPTION	Serving Size	Calories	Total Fat (g)	Saturated Fat (g)	Sodium (mg)	Carbohydrates (g)	Fiber (g)	Protein (g)
Truffle flavor	2 oz	183	16	6	452	4	0	6
PEACH NECTAR (canned)	1 cup	134	0	0	17	35	2	1
PEACHES								
Canned in ex heavy syrup, slices	1 cup	252	0	0	21	68	3	1
Canned in ex light syrup, slices	1 cup	104	0	0	12	27	3	1
Canned in heavy syrup	1 cup	194	0	0	16	52	3	1
Canned in heavy syrup, drained	1 cup	171	0	0	13	44	5	1
Canned in juice	1 cup	110	0	0	10	29	3	2
Canned in light syrup, slices	1 cup	136	0	0	13	37	3	1
Canned in water, slices	1 cup	59	0	0	7	15	3	1
Dehydrated, stewed	1 cup	322	1	0	10	83	0	5
Dehydrated, uncooked	1 cup	377	1	0	12	96	0	6
Dried, stewed, w/o sugar	1 cup	199	1	0	5	51	7	3
Dried, stewed, w/ sugar	1 cup	278	1	0	5	72	7	3
Dried, uncooked, halves	1 cup	382	1	0	11	98	13	6
Fresh (2-1/2" dia)	1 fruit	51	0	0	0	12	2	1
Frozen, slices, sweetened, thawed	1 cup	235	0	0	15	60	5	2
Spiced, canned in heavy syrup	1 cup	182	0	0	10	49	3	1
PEANUT BUTTER								
Chunky, w/o salt	2 tbsp	188	16	3	5	7	3	8
Chunky, w/ salt	2 tbsp	188	16	3	156	7	3	8
Creamy	2 tbsp	201	18	3	117	6	2	8
Reduced sodium	2 tbsp	202	16	2	65	7	2	8
Smooth, w/o salt	2 tbsp	188	16	3	5	6	2	8
Smooth, w/ salt	2 tbsp	188	16	3	147	6	2	8
PEANUT FLOUR								
Defatted	1 cup	196	0	0	108	21	10	31
Low fat	1 cup	257	13	2	1	19	10	20
PEANUT OIL	1 tbsp	124	14	2	0	0	0	0
PEANUTS								
All types, boiled, w/ salt	1 oz	290	6	1	213	6	3	4
All types, dry roasted, w/o salt	1 oz	166	14	2	2	6	3	4
All types, dry roasted, w/ salt	1 oz	166	14	2	230	6	2	7
All types, fresh	1 cup	828	72	10	26	24	12	38

ITEM DESCRIPTION	Serving Size	Calories	Total Fat (g)	Saturated Fat (g)	Sodium (mg)	Carbohydrates (g)	Fiber (g)	Protein (g)
All types, oil roasted, w/o salt, chopped	1 cup	773	66	9	8	25	9	35
All types, oil roasted, w/ salt, chopped	1 cup	863	76	13	461	22	14	40
Spanish, fresh	1 cup	832	72	11	32	23	14	38
Spanish, oil roasted, w/o salt	1 cup	851	72	11	9	26	13	41
Spanish, oil roasted, w/ salt	1 cup	851	72	11	637	26	13	41
Valencia, fresh	1 cup	832	69	11	1	31	13	37
Valencia, oil roasted, w/o salt	1 cup	848	74	11	9	23	13	39
Valencia, oil roasted, w/ salt	1 cup	848	74	11	1112	23	13	39
Virginia, fresh	1 cup	822	71	9	15	24	12	37
Virginia, oil roasted, w/o salt	1 cup	827	70	9	9	28	13	37
Virginia, oil roasted, w/ salt	1 cup	827	70	9	619	28	13	37
PEANUT SPREAD (reduced sugar)	2 tbsp	202	17	3	139	4	2	8
PEAR NECTAR (canned)	1 cup	150	0	0	10	39	2	0
PEARS								
Asian, fresh (2 1/2" dia)	1 fruit	51	0	0	0	13	4	1
Canned in ex heavy syrup, halves	1 cup	258	0	0	13	67	4	1
Canned in ex light syrup, halves	1 cup	116	0	0	5	30	4	1
Canned in heavy syrup	1 cup	197	0	0	13	51	4	1
Canned in heavy syrup, drained	1 cup	149	0	0	10	38	5	0
Canned in juice, halves	1 cup	124	0	0	10	32	4	1
Canned in light syrup, halves	1 cup	143	0	0	13	38	4	0
Canned in water, halves	1 cup	71	0	0	5	19	4	0
Dried, stewed, w/o sugar, halves	1 cup	324	1	0	8	86	16	2
Dried, stewed, w/ sugar, halves	1 cup	392	1	0	8	104	16	2
Dried, uncooked, halves	1 cup	472	1	0	11	125	14	3
Fresh, whole	1 sml	86	0	0	1	23	5	1
PEAS								
Boiled	1/2 cup	34	0	0	3	6	2	3
Frozen, boiled	1/2 cup	34	0	0	4	7	2	3
Green, boiled	1/2 cup	67	0	0	2	13	4	4
Green, canned, seasoned	1/2 cup	57	0	0	290	11	2	4
Green, canned, w/o salt	1/2 cup	66	0	0	11	12	4	4

ITEM DESCRIPTION	Serving Size	Calories	Total Fat (g)	Saturated Fat (g)	Sodium (mg)	Carbohydrates (g)	Fiber (g)	Protein (g)
Green, canned, w/o salt, drained	1/2 cup	59	0	0	2	11	3	4
Green, canned, w/ salt	1/2 cup	60	1	0	255	10	4	4
Green, fresh	1/2 cup	59	0	0	4	10	4	4
Green, frozen, boiled	1/2 cup	62	0	0	58	11	4	4
PEAS & CARROTS								
Canned, w/o salt	1/2 cup	48	0	0	5	11	4	3
Canned, w/ salt	1/2 cup	48	0	0	332	11	3	3
Frozen, boiled	1/2 cup	38	0	0	54	8	2	2
PEAS & ONIONS								
Canned	1/2 cup	31	0	0	265	5	1	2
Frozen, boiled	1/2 cup	40	0	0	33	8	2	2
PECANS								
Chopped	1 cup	753	78	7	0	15	11	10
Dry roasted, w/o salt	1 oz	201	21	2	0	4	3	3
Dry roasted, w/ salt	1 oz	201	21	2	109	4	3	3
Oil roasted, w/o salt	1 cup	786	83	8	1	14	10	10
Oil roasted, w/ salt	1 cup	787	83	8	432	14	10	10
PECTIN (unsweetened, dry mix)	1-3/4 oz pkg	162	0	0	100	45	4	0
PEPEAO (dried)	1 cup	72	0	0	17	19	0	1
PEPPER								
Black	1 tbsp	16	0	0	3	4	2	1
Red or cayenne	1 tbsp	17	1	0	2	3	1	1
White	1 tbsp	21	0	0	0	5	2	1
PEPPER SAUCE								
Hot sauce	1 tsp	1	0	0	124	0	0	0
Hot chili, green, canned	1 tbsp	3	0	0	4	1	0	0
Hot chili, red, canned	1 tbsp	3	0	0	4	1	0	0
PEPPERED LOAF (pork & beef)	1 slice	42	2	1	432	1	0	5
PEPPERMINT (fresh)	2 tbsp	2	0	0	1	0	0	0
PEPPERONI (pork, beef)	1 oz	138	12	4	463	0	0	6
PEPPERS								
Ancho, dried	1 pepper	48	1	0	7	9	4	2
Banana, fresh (4" long)	1 pepper	9	0	0	4	2	1	1
Hot chili, green, canned, w/o seeds	1 pepper	15	0	0	856	4	1	1

ITEM DESCRIPTION	Serving Size	Calories	Total Fat (g)	Saturated Fat (g)	Sodium (mg)	Carbohydrates (g)	Fiber (g)	Protein (g)
Hot chili, green, fresh	1 pepper	18	0	0	3	4	1	1
Hot chili, red, canned, w/o seeds	1 pepper	15	0	0	856	4	1	1
Hot chili, red, fresh	1 pepper	18	0	0	4	4	1	1
Hot chili, sun-dried	1 pepper	3	0	0	1	1	0	0
Hungarian, fresh	1 pepper	8	0	0	0	2	0	0
Jalapeño, canned, chopped	1 cup	37	1	0	2273	6	4	1
Jalapeño, fresh, slices	1 cup	27	1	0	1	5	3	1
Pace Diced Green Chilies	2 tbsp	8	0	0	100	2	1	0
Pace Jalapeños Nacho Sliced Peppers	2 tbsp	4	0	0	300	1	1	0
Pasilla, dried	1 pepper	24	1	0	6	4	2	1
Serrano, fresh, chopped	1 cup	34	0	0	10	7	4	2
Sweet, green, boiled, chopped	1 cup	38	0	0	3	9	2	1
Sweet, green, canned, halves	1 cup	25	0	0	1917	5	2	1
Sweet, green, freeze-dried	1 tbsp	1	0	0	1	0	0	0
Sweet, green, fresh, chopped	1 cup	30	0	0	4	7	3	1
Sweet, red, boiled, strips	1 cup	38	0	0	3	9	2	1
Sweet, red, canned, halves	1 cup	25	0	0	1917	5	2	1
Sweet, red, freeze-dried	1 tbsp	1	0	0	1	0	0	0
Sweet, red, fresh, chopped	1 cup	46	0	0	6	9	3	1
Sweet, red, frozen, boiled, chopped	1 cup	22	0	0	5	4	0	1
Sweet, yellow, fresh	1 lg	50	0	0	4	12	2	2
PERCH (cooked in dry heat)	3 oz	99	1	0	67	0	0	21
PERSIMMONS								
Japanese, dried	1 fruit	93	0	0	1	25	5	0
Japanese, fresh	1 fruit	118	0	0	2	31	6	1
Native, fresh	1 fruit	32	0	0	0	8	0	0
PHEASANT (cooked, chopped)	1 cup	346	17	5	60	0	0	45
PHYLLO DOUGH	1 sheet	57	1	0	92	10	0	1
PICANTE SAUCE								
Pace Organic Picante Sauce	2 tbsp	8	0	0	220	2	1	0
Pace Picante Sauce	2 tbsp	8	0	0	250	2	1	0
PICKLE RELISH								
Hamburger	1 tbsp	19	0	0	164	5	1	0

ITEM DESCRIPTION	Serving Size	Calories	Total Fat (g)	Saturated Fat (g)	Sodium (mg)	Carbohydrates (g)	Fiber (g)	Protein (g)
Hot dog	1 tbsp	14	0	0	164	4	0	0
Sweet	1 tbsp	20	0	0	122	5	0	0
PICKLES								
Chowchow, sweet, w/ cauliflower, onion & mustard	1 cup	296	2	0	1291	65	4	4
Cucumber, dill, low sodium	1 med	12	0	0	12	3	1	0
Cucumber, dill or kosher dill (4" long)	1 pickle	16	0	0	1181	4	2	1
Cucumber, sour (4" long)	1 pickle	15	0	0	1631	3	2	0
Cucumber, sour, low sodium (4" long)	1 pickle	15	0	0	24	3	2	0
Cucumber, sweet, gherkin (3" long)	1 pickle	32	0	0	160	7	0	0
Cucumber, sweet, low sodium	1 med	43	0	0	6	12	0	0
PICO DE GALLO (Pace)	2 tbsp	10	0	0	150	3	0	0
PIE								
Apple, commercial (9" dia)	1/8 pie	296	14	5	332	43	2	2
Apple, homemade (9" dia)	1/8 pie	411	19	5	327	58	0	4
Banana cream, homemade (9" dia)	1/8 pie	387	20	5	346	47	1	6
Banana cream, prepared from no-bake mix (9" dia)	1/8 pie	231	12	6	267	29	1	3
Blueberry, commercial (9" dia)	1/8 pie	290	13	2	406	44	1	2
Blueberry, homemade (9" dia)	1/8 pie	360	17	4	272	49	0	4
Cherry, commercial (9" dia)	1/8 pie	325	14	3	308	50	1	3
Cherry, fried (5" x 3.75")	1 pie	404	21	3	479	55	3	4
Cherry, homemade (9" dia)	1/8 pie	486	22	5	344	69	0	5
Chocolate cream, commercial (8" dia)	1/6 pie	344	22	6	154	38	2	3
Chocolate mousse, prepared from no-bake mix (9" dia)	1/8 pie	247	15	8	437	28	0	3
Coconut cream, commercial (7" dia)	1/8 pie	143	8	3	122	18	1	1
Coconut cream, prepared from no-bake mix (9" dia)	1/8 pie	259	17	8	309	27	1	3
Coconut custard, commercial (8" dia)	1/6 pie	270	14	6	348	31	2	6
Dutch apple, commercial (9" dia)	1/8 pie	380	15	3	262	58	2	3

ITEM DESCRIPTION	Serving Size	Calories	Total Fat (g)	Saturated Fat (g)	Sodium (mg)	Carbohydrates (g)	Fiber (g)	Protein (g)
Egg custard, commercial (8" dia)	1/6 pie	220	12	2	252	22	2	6
Fruit, fried (5" x 3.75")	1 pie	404	21	3	479	55	3	4
Lemon fried (5" x 3.75")	1 pie	404	21	3	479	55	3	4
Lemon meringue, commercial (8" dia)	1/6 pie	303	10	2	165	53	1	2
Lemon meringue, homemade (9" dia)	1/8 pie	362	16	4	307	50	0	5
Mince, homemade (9" dia)	1/8 pie	477	18	4	419	79	4	4
Peach (8" dia)	1/6 pie	261	12	2	316	38	1	2
Pecan, commercial	1 slice	541	22	4	319	79	3	6
Pecan, homemade (9" dia)	1/8 pie	503	27	5	320	64	0	6
Pumpkin, commercial	1 slice	323	13	3	310	46	2	5
Pumpkin, homemade (9" dia)	1/8 pie	316	14	5	349	41	0	7
Vanilla cream, homemade (9" dia)	1/8 pie	350	18	5	328	41	1	6
PIE CRUST								
Chocolate cookie, commercial	1 crust	882	41	9	916	117	5	11
Chocolate wafer, chilled, homemade (9" dia)	1 crust	1128	69	15	1499	121	3	11
Deep dish, frozen, baked	1 crust	1053	64	18	794	106	5	12
Graham cracker, baked, homemade (9" dia)	1 crust	1037	52	11	1199	137	3	9
Graham cracker, chilled, homemade (9" dia)	1 crust	1181	60	12	1366	156	4	10
Graham cracker, commercial (9" dia)	1 crust	915	45	9	762	117	3	9
Nabisco Nilla Pie Crust	1 serv	144	8	1	63	18	0	1
Refrigerated, reg, baked	1 crust	1004	57	22	936	116	3	7
Standard, baked, from mix (9" dia)	1 crust	802	49	12	1166	81	3	11
Standard, baked, homemade (9" dia)	1 crust	949	62	16	976	86	3	12
Standard, frozen, enriched (9" dia)	1 crust	783	44	14	720	87	5	10
Standard, frozen, unenriched (9" dia)	1 crust	649	41	6	818	63	1	6
Vanilla wafer, chilled, homemade (9" dia)	1 crust	935	64	13	906	88	0	7

ITEM DESCRIPTION	Serving Size	Calories	Total Fat (g)	Saturated Fat (g)	Sodium (mg)	Carbohydrates (g)	Fiber (g)	Protein (g)
PIGEON PEAS								
Mature seeds, boiled	1 cup	203	1	0	8	39	11	11
Mature seeds, fresh	1 cup	703	3	1	35	129	31	44
Immature seeds, boiled	1 cup	170	2	0	8	30	9	9
Immature seeds, fresh	1 cup	209	3	1	8	37	8	11
PIKE								
Northern, cooked in dry heat	3 oz	96	1	0	42	0	0	21
Walleye, cooked in dry heat	3 oz	101	1	0	55	0	0	21
PILINUTS (dried)	1 cup	863	95	37	4	5	0	13
PIMENTO (canned)	1 tbsp	3	0	0	2	1	0	0
PIMENTO LOAF								
Pork & pickles	1 slice	86	6	2	496	3	1	4
Oscar Mayer Pickle Pimiento Loaf, chicken	1 serv	75	6	2	357	3	0	3
PIÑA COLADA								
Canned	1 fl oz	77	2	2	23	9	0	0
Homemade	1 fl oz	55	1	1	2	7	0	0
PINEAPPLE								
Canned in ex heavy syrup, chunks	1 cup	216	0	0	3	56	2	1
Canned in heavy syrup, chunks	1 cup	198	0	0	3	51	2	1
Canned in juice, chunks	1 cup	149	0	0	2	39	2	1
Canned in juice, drained, chunks	1 cup	109	0	0	2	28	2	1
Canned in light syrup, chunks	1 cup	131	0	0	3	34	2	1
Canned in water, chunks	1 cup	79	0	0	2	20	2	1
Fresh, ex sweet varieties, chunks	1 cup	84	0	0	2	22	2	1
Fresh, traditional varieties, chunks	1 cup	74	0	0	2	19	0	1
Frozen, sweetened, chunks	1 tbsp	211	0	0	5	54	3	1
PINEAPPLE & GRAPEFRUIT JUICE DRINK (canned)	8 fl oz	118	0	0	35	29	0	1
PINEAPPLE & ORANGE JUICE DRINK (canned)	8 fl oz	125	0	0	8	30	0	3
PINEAPPLE JUICE								
Frozen concentrate, unsweetened, prepared w/ water	1 cup	130	0	0	3	32	1	1

ITEM DESCRIPTION	Serving Size	Calories	Total Fat (g)	Saturated Fat (g)	Sodium (mg)	Carbohydrates (g)	Fiber (g)	Protein (g)
Unsweetened, canned	1 cup	133	0	0	5	32	1	1
PINEAPPLE TOPPING	2 tbsp	106	0	0	18	28	0	0
PINE NUTS (dried)	1 cup	909	92	7	3	18	5	18
PINK BEANS								
Boiled	1 cup	252	1	0	3	47	9	15
Fresh	1 cup	720	2	1	17	135	27	44
PINTO BEANS								
Boiled	1 cup	245	1	0	2	45	15	15
Canned	1 cup	206	2	0	706	37	11	12
Fresh	1 cup	670	2	0	23	121	30	41
Frozen, boiled	10 oz pkg	460	1	0	236	88	24	26
PISTACHIO NUTS								
Dry roasted, w/o salt	1 cup	700	56	7	12	34	13	26
Dry roasted, w/ salt	1 cup	696	56	7	496	33	13	26
Fresh	1 cup	682	54	7	1	34	13	25
PITA BREAD white (6-1/2" dia)	1 pita	165	1	0	322	33	1	5
PITANGA (Surinam cherry, fresh)	1 fruit	2	0	0	0	1	0	0
PIZZA								
Cheese, reg crust, frozen, baked	15.1 oz pizza	1211	56	19	2020	131	10	47
Cheese, rising crust, frozen, baked	19.7 oz pizza	1547	52	23	3308	196	15	74
Meat & vegetable, reg crust, frozen, baked	22.9 oz pizza	1777	93	31	3574	162	14	73
Meat & vegetable, rising crust, frozen, baked	14.3 oz pizza	1125	49	18	2656	119	10	52
Pepperoni, reg crust, frozen, baked	1 pizza	1267	65	21	2645	122	9	48
PIZZA SAUCE (canned)	1/4 cup	34	1	0	117	5	1	1
PLANTAIN CHIPS	1 oz	158	10	3	111	16	1	0
PLANTAINS								
Cooked, mashed	1 cup	232	0	0	10	62	5	2
Fresh	1 med	218	1	0	7	57	4	2
PLUMS								
Canned in ex heavy syrup	1 cup	264	0	0	50	69	3	1

ITEM DESCRIPTION	Serving Size	Calories	Total Fat (g)	Saturated Fat (g)	Sodium (mg)	Carbohydrates (g)	Fiber (g)	Protein (g)
Canned in heavy syrup	1 cup	230	0	0	49	60	2	1
Canned in heavy syrup, drained	1 cup	163	0	0	35	42	3	1
Canned in juice	1 cup	146	0	0	3	38	2	1
Canned in light syrup	1 cup	159	0	0	50	41	2	1
Canned in water	1 cup	102	0	0	2	27	2	1
Fresh (2-1/8" dia)	1 fruit	30	0	0	0	8	1	0
PLUM SAUCE	1 tbsp	35	0	0	102	8	0	0
POI	1 cup	269	0	0	29	65	1	1
POKE								
Boiled	1 cup	33	1	0	30	5	2	4
Fresh	1 cup	37	1	0	37	6	3	4
POLLOCK (Atlantic, cooked in dry heat)	3 oz	100	1	0	94	0	0	21
POMEGRANATE JUICE (bottled)	1 cup	134	1	0	22	33	0	0
POMEGRANATES fresh (4" dia)	1 fruit	234	3	0	8	53	11	5
POMPANO (Florida, cooked in dry heat)	3 oz	179	10	4	65	0	0	20
POPCORN								
Air popped	2/3 cup	110	1	0	2	22	4	4
Caramel coated, fat free	2/3 cup	108	0	0	81	26	1	1
Caramel coated, w/o peanuts	2/3 cup	122	4	1	58	22	2	1
Caramel coated, w/ peanuts	2/3 cup	113	2	0	84	23	1	2
Cheese flavor	2/3 cup	149	9	2	252	15	3	3
Microwave, butter, w/ palm oil	2/3 cup	150	9	4	219	16	3	2
Microwave, butter, w/ partially hydrogenated oil	2/3 cup	149	8	2	219	16	3	2
Microwave, low fat, low sodium	2/3 cup	122	3	0	139	21	4	4
Oil popped	2/3 cup	142	12	2	300	13	2	2
Oil popped, low fat	2/3 cup	108	2	0	178	22	4	3
Oil popped, unsalted	2/3 cup	148	8	1	1	16	3	3
Unpopped kernels	1 oz	106	1	0	2	21	4	3
POPCORN CAKES	1 cake	38	0	0	29	8	0	1
POPOVERS (dry mix, enriched)	1 oz	105	1	0	257	20	0	3
POPPYSEEDS	1 tbsp	46	4	0	2	2	2	2
POPPYSEED OIL	1 tbsp	120	14	2	0	0	0	0

PORK

ITEM DESCRIPTION	Serving Size	Calories	Total Fat (g)	Saturated Fat (g)	Sodium (mg)	Carbohydrates (g)	Fiber (g)	Protein (g)
Back ribs, roasted	3 oz	315	25	9	86	0	0	21
Canned	1 can	1598	106	34	1736	5	0	158
Composite of retail cuts, cooked	3 oz	315	15	5	53	0	0	23
Composite of retail cuts, lean, cooked	3 oz	315	8	3	50	0	0	25
Cured, bacon, broiled, pan fried or roasted	1 slice	43	3	1	185	0	0	3
Cured, bacon, broiled, pan fried or roasted, low sodium	1 slice	43	3	1	82	0	0	3
Cured, Canadian-style bacon, grilled	1 slice	43	2	1	363	0	0	6
Cured, feet, pickled	3 oz	315	9	3	476	0	0	10
Cured, shoulder, arm picnic, roasted	3 oz	315	18	7	911	0	0	17
Cured, shoulder, blade roll, roasted	3 oz	315	20	7	827	0	0	15
Ground, cooked	3 oz	315	18	7	62	0	0	22
Hormel Always Tender, center cut chops	1 serv	187	11	4	423	1	0	21
Hormel Always Tender, loin	1 serv	162	8	3	401	1	0	21
Hormel Always Tender, loin filets, lemon & garlic	1 serv	132	5	2	661	2	0	20
Hormel Always Tender, tenderloin, peppercorn	1 serv	123	4	1	665	2	0	19
Hormel Always Tender, tenderloin, teriyaki	1 serv	133	3	1	463	5	0	20
Leg, rump half, roasted	3 oz	214	12	4	53	0	0	25
Leg, shank half, roasted	3 oz	246	17	6	50	0	0	22
Leg, whole, roasted	3 oz	232	15	5	51	0	0	23
Loin, blade chops, braised	3 oz	275	22	8	47	0	0	19
Loin, blade chops, broiled	3 oz	272	21	8	60	0	0	19
Loin, blade chops, pan fried	3 oz	291	24	9	57	0	0	18
Loin, blade roast, roasted	3 oz	275	21	8	26	0	0	20
Loin, center loin chops, braised	3 oz	210	12	5	50	0	0	24
Loin, center loin chops, broiled	3 oz	178	9	3	47	0	0	22
Loin, center loin chops, pan fried	3 oz	235	14	5	68	0	0	25
Loin, center loin roast, roasted	3 oz	199	11	4	54	0	0	22
Loin, center rib chops, braised	3 oz	212	13	5	34	0	0	23

ITEM DESCRIPTION	Serving Size	Calories	Total Fat (g)	Saturated Fat (g)	Sodium (mg)	Carbohydrates (g)	Fiber (g)	Protein (g)
Loin, center rib chops, broiled	3 oz	189	11	4	47	0	0	21
Loin, center rib chops, pan fried	3 oz	225	14	5	42	0	0	22
Loin, center rib roast, roasted	3 oz	217	13	5	41	0	0	23
Loin, country-style ribs, braised	3 oz	232	15	5	49	0	0	23
Loin, country-style ribs, roasted	3 oz	279	22	8	44	0	0	20
Loin, sirloin chops, braised	3 oz	208	13	5	43	0	0	22
Loin, sirloin chops, broiled	3 oz	220	14	5	58	0	0	23
Loin, sirloin chops, lean, broiled	3 oz	164	6	2	48	0	0	26
Loin, sirloin roast, lean, roasted	3 oz	173	8	2	50	0	0	24
Loin, sirloin roast, roasted	3 oz	196	11	3	48	0	0	23
Loin, tenderloin, broiled	3 oz	171	7	2	54	0	0	25
Loin, tenderloin, roasted	3 oz	125	3	1	48	0	0	22
Loin, top loin chops, braised	3 oz	198	11	4	36	0	0	24
Loin, top loin chops, broiled	3 oz	167	8	3	37	0	0	23
Loin, top loin chops, pan fried	3 oz	218	13	5	47	0	0	25
Loin, top loin roast, roasted	3 oz	163	8	2	39	0	0	22
Oriental style, dehydrated	1 cup	135	14	5	151	0	0	3
Pickled pork hocks	100 grams	171	11	3	1050	0	0	19
Shoulder, arm picnic, braised	3 oz	280	20	7	75	0	0	24
Shoulder, arm picnic, roasted	3 oz	269	20	7	60	0	0	20
Shoulder, blade, Boston roast, roasted	3 oz	229	16	6	57	0	0	20
Shoulder, blade, Boston steak, broiled	3 oz	220	14	5	59	0	0	22
Shoulder, Boston butt, blade steak, braised	3 oz	315	15	6	49	0	0	21
Shoulder breast, broiled	1 pc	604	17	5	202	0	0	106
Shoulder, petite tender, broiled	1 pc	143	4	1	49	0	0	25
Spareribs, braised	3 oz	337	26	9	79	0	0	25
Spareribs, roasted	3 oz	315	26	8	77	0	0	18
Various meats & by-products, feet, simmered	3 oz	197	14	4	62	0	0	19
Various meats & by-products, liver, braised	3 oz	140	4	1	42	3	0	22
Various meats & by-products, tail, simmered	3 oz	337	30	11	21	0	0	14

ITEM DESCRIPTION	Serving Size	Calories	Total Fat (g)	Saturated Fat (g)	Sodium (mg)	Carbohydrates (g)	Fiber (g)	Protein (g)
PORK ENTRÉE								
Campbell's Pork & Beans	1 serv	138	1	1	439	25	7	6
Supper Bakes, Savory Pork Chops w/ Herb Stuffing	1 serv	153	1	0	780	31	2	5
PORK FAT (cooked)	1 oz	180	19	7	8	0	0	3
PORK SKINS								
BBQ flavor	1 oz	153	9	3	756	0	0	16
Plain	1 oz	154	9	3	521	0	0	17
POTATO CHIPS								
Baked, white, restructured	1 cup	159	6	1	312	24	2	2
BBQ	1 oz	139	9	2	213	15	1	2
Cheese	1 oz	141	8	2	225	16	2	2
Cheese, made from dried potatoes	1 oz	156	10	3	214	14	1	2
Fat free, salted	1 oz	107	0	0	182	24	2	3
Fat free, w/ Olestra	1 oz	78	0	0	157	18	2	2
Fat free, w/ Olestra, made from dried potatoes	1 oz	72	0	0	122	16	2	1
Light	1 oz	134	6	1	139	19	2	2
Light, made from dried potatoes	1 oz	142	7	2	117	18	1	1
Plain, made from dried potatoes	1 oz	158	11	3	110	15	1	1
Sour cream & onion, made from dried potatoes	1 oz	155	10	3	204	15	0	2
Plain, salted	1 oz	155	11	3	149	14	1	2
Plain, unsalted	1 oz	152	10	3	2	15	1	2
Plain, w/ partially hydrogenated soybean oil, salted	1 oz	152	10	2	168	15	1	2
Plain, w/ partially hydrogenated soybean oil, unsalted	1 oz	152	10	2	2	15	1	2
Reduced fat, w/o salt	1 oz	138	6	1	2	19	2	2
Sour cream & onion	1 oz	151	10	3	177	15	1	2
POTATO FLOUR	1 cup	571	1	0	88	133	9	11
POTATO PANCAKES (2.75" dia)	1	59	3	1	168	6	1	1
POTATOES								
Au gratin, dry mix, prepared w/ water, whole milk & butter	5.5 oz pkg	764	34	21	3609	106	7	19

ITEM DESCRIPTION	Serving Size	Calories	Total Fat (g)	Saturated Fat (g)	Sodium (mg)	Carbohydrates (g)	Fiber (g)	Protein (g)
Au gratin, homemade, w/ butter	1 cup	323	19	12	1061	28	4	12
Au gratin, homemade, w/ margarine	1 cup	323	19	9	1061	28	4	12
Baked (2-1/4" x 3-1/4")	1 potato	160	0	0	17	36	4	4
Baked, flesh only	1/2 cup	57	0	0	3	13	1	1
Baked, skin only	1 skin	115	0	0	12	27	5	2
Boiled, cooked in skin, flesh only	1/2 cup	68	0	0	3	16	1	1
Boiled, cooked in skin, skin only	1 skin	27	0	0	5	6	1	1
Boiled, cooked w/o skin (2-1/4" x 3-1/4")	1 potato	144	0	0	8	33	3	3
Canned	1 cup	132	0	0	651	30	4	4
Canned, drained	1 cup	108	0	0	394	24	4	3
Canned, drained, no salt	1 cup	112	0	0	9	24	4	3
French fried, cottage cut, frozen, oven heated w/o salt	10 fries	109	4	2	22	17	2	2
French fried, frozen, oven heated, w/o salt	10 fries	166	9	3	307	20	2	2
Hashed browns, frozen, plain, prepared	1 patty	63	3	1	10	8	1	1
Hashed browns, homemade	1 cup	413	20	3	534	55	5	5
Mashed, dehydrated, prepared w/ milk, water & margarine	1 cup	244	10	3	359	34	3	5
Mashed, dehydrated, prepared w/o milk & butter	1 cup	227	10	6	540	30	5	4
Mashed, homemade, whole milk added	1 cup	174	1	1	634	37	3	4
Mashed, homemade, whole milk & butter added	1 cup	237	9	4	666	35	3	4
Microwaved, cooked in skin (2-3/4" x 4-3/4")	1 potato	212	0	0	16	49	5	5
Microwaved, cooked in skin, flesh only	1/2 cup	78	0	0	5	18	1	2
Microwaved, cooked in skin, skin only	1 skin	77	0	0	9	17	3	3
O'Brien, homemade	1 cup	157	2	2	421	30	0	5
Puffs, frozen, oven heated	1 cup	243	11	2	614	36	3	3

ITEM DESCRIPTION	Serving Size	Calories	Total Fat (g)	Saturated Fat (g)	Sodium (mg)	Carbohydrates (g)	Fiber (g)	Protein (g)
Red, baked (2-1/4" x 3-1/4")	1 potato	154	0	0	21	34	3	4
Red, fresh (2-1/4" x 3-1/4")	1 potato	149	0	0	13	34	4	4
Russet, baked (2-1/4" x 3-1/4")	1 potato	168	0	0	24	37	4	5
Russet, fresh (2-1/4" x 3-1/4")	1 potato	168	0	0	11	38	3	5
Scalloped, homemade w/ butter or margarine	1 cup	216	9	6	821	26	5	7
Scalloped, mix, prepared w/ water, whole milk, & butter	5.5 oz pkg	764	35	22	2803	105	9	17
White, baked (2-1/4" x 3-1/4")	1 potato	130	0	0	10	29	3	3
White, fresh (2-1/4" x 3-1/4")	1 potato	147	0	0	13	33	5	4
POTATO SALAD (homemade)	1 cup	358	21	4	1322	28	3	7
POTATO STICKS	1/2 cup	94	6	2	45	10	1	1
POULTRY SEASONING	1 tbsp	14	0	0	1	3	1	0
POUT (cooked in dry heat)	3 oz	87	1	0	66	0	0	18
PRETZELS								
Hard, chocolate coated	1 oz	130	5	2	161	20	0	2
Hard, plain, salted	1 oz	108	1	0	486	22	1	3
Hard, plain, unsalted	1 oz	108	1	0	82	22	1	3
Hard, whole wheat	1 oz	103	1	0	58	23	2	3
Soft, salted	1 med	389	4	1	1615	80	2	9
Soft, unsalted	1 med	389	4	1	794	82	2	9
PRICKLY PEARS (fresh)	1 fruit	42	1	0	5	10	4	1
PRUNE JUICE (canned)	1 cup	182	0	0	10	45	3	2
PRUNES								
Canned in heavy syrup	1 cup	246	0	0	7	65	9	2
Dehydrated, stewed	1 cup	316	1	0	6	83	0	3
Dehydrated, uncooked	1 cup	447	1	0	7	118	0	5
Puree	2 tbsp	93	0	0	8	23	1	1
Stewed, w/ added sugar	1 cup	308	1	0	5	82	9	3
Stewed, w/o added sugar	1 cup	265	0	0	2	70	8	2
Uncooked	1 cup	417	1	0	3	111	12	4
PUDDINGS								
Chocolate, instant, prepared w/ whole milk	1/2 cup	163	5	3	417	28	1	5

ITEM DESCRIPTION	Serving Size	Calories	Total Fat (g)	Saturated Fat (g)	Sodium (mg)	Carbohydrates (g)	Fiber (g)	Protein (g)
Chocolate, reg, prepared w/ whole milk	1/2 cup	169	4	3	136	28	1	5
Chocolate, ready to eat	1/2 cup	153	5	1	164	25	0	2
Coconut cream, instant, prepared w/ 2% milk	1/2 cup	157	3	2	362	28	0	4
Coconut cream, instant, prepared w/ whole milk	1/2 cup	172	5	3	362	28	0	4
Coconut cream, reg, prepared w/ 2% milk	1/2 cup	146	4	3	228	25	0	4
Coconut cream, reg, prepared w/ whole milk	1/2 cup	160	5	4	227	25	0	4
Lemon, instant, prepared w/ whole milk	1/2 cup	169	4	3	392	30	0	4
Rice, ready to eat	1/2 cup	133	3	2	139	22	1	4
Tapioca, ready to eat	1/2 cup	143	4	1	160	24	0	2
Tapioca, ready to eat, fat free	1/2 cup	105	0	0	209	24	0	2
Vanilla, instant, prepared w/ whole milk	1/2 cup	162	4	2	406	28	0	4
Vanilla, ready to eat	1/2 cup	143	4	1	156	25	0	2
Vanilla, ready to eat, fat free	3-1/2 oz	88	0	0	189	20	0	2
Vanilla, reg, prepared w/ whole milk	1/2 cup	157	4	2	216	26	0	4
PUFF PASTRY								
Sheet, frozen, baked	1 sheet	1367	94	13	620	112	4	18
Shell, frozen, baked	1 shell	223	15	2	101	18	1	3
PUMMELO (fresh)	1 fruit	231	0	0	6	59	6	5
PUMPKIN								
Boiled, mashed	1 cup	49	0	0	2	12	3	2
Canned, w/o salt	1 cup	83	1	0	12	20	7	3
Canned, w/ salt	1 cup	83	1	0	590	20	7	3
Fresh, cubed	1 cup	30	0	0	1	8	1	1
PUMPKIN FLOWERS (boiled)	1 cup	20	0	0	8	4	1	1
PUMPKIN FLOWERS (fresh)	1 cup	5	0	0	2	1	0	0
PUMPKIN LEAVES								
Boiled	1 cup	15	0	0	6	2	2	2

ITEM DESCRIPTION	Serving Size	Calories	Total Fat (g)	Saturated Fat (g)	Sodium (mg)	Carbohydrates (g)	Fiber (g)	Protein (g)
Fresh	1 cup	7	0	0	4	1	0	1
PUMPKIN PIE MIX (canned)	1 cup	281	0	0	562	71	22	3
PUMPKIN PIE SPICE	1 tbsp	19	1	0	3	4	1	0
PUMPKIN SEEDS								
Dried	1 oz	151	13	2	5	5	1	7
Kernels, roasted, w/o salt	1 oz	146	12	2	5	4	1	9
Kernels, roasted, w/ salt	1 oz	146	12	2	161	4	1	9
Whole, roasted, w/o salt	1 oz	125	5	1	5	15	0	5
Whole, roasted, w/ salt	1 oz	125	5	1	161	15	0	5
PURSLANE								
Boiled	1 cup	21	0	0	51	4	0	2
Fresh	1 cup	7	0	0	19	1	0	1
QUAIL EGGS (fresh)	1 egg	14	1	0	13	0	0	1
QUINCES (fresh)	1 fruit	52	0	0	4	14	2	0
QUINOA (cooked)	1 cup	222	4	0	13	39	5	8
RABBIT (domestic, composite of cuts, stewed)	3 oz	167	7	2	40	0	0	25
RADICCHIO (fresh, shredded)	1 cup	9	0	0	9	2	0	1
RADISHES								
Hawaiian style, pickled	1 cup	42	0	0	1184	8	3	2
Oriental, boiled, slices	1 cup	25	0	0	19	5	2	1
Oriental, dried	1 cup	314	1	0	322	74	0	9
Oriental, fresh (7" long)	1 radish	61	0	0	71	14	5	2
Fresh, slices	1 cup	19	0	0	45	4	2	1
White icicle, fresh, slices	1 cup	14	0	0	16	3	1	1
RADISH SEEDS (fresh)	1 cup	16	1	0	2	1	0	1
RAISINS								
Golden, seedless	1 cup	498	1	0	20	131	7	6
Purple, seedless	1 cup	493	1	0	18	131	6	5
RAMBUTAN (canned in syrup)	1 cup	123	0	0	16	31	1	1
RASPBERRIES								
Fresh	1 cup	64	1	0	1	15	8	1
Red, canned in heavy syrup	1 cup	233	0	0	8	60	8	2
Red, frozen, sweetened	1 cup	258	0	0	2	65	11	2

ITEM DESCRIPTION	Serving Size	Calories	Total Fat (g)	Saturated Fat (g)	Sodium (mg)	Carbohydrates (g)	Fiber (g)	Protein (g)
REFRIED BEANS								
Canned, fat free	1 cup	182	1	0	1012	31	11	12
Canned, frijoles rojos volteados	1 cup	336	16	2	874	36	11	12
Canned, traditional	1 cup	217	3	1	1069	36	12	13
Canned, vegetarian	1 cup	201	2	0	1041	33	11	13
Pace Salsa Refried Beans	1/2 cup	72	0	0	590	14	4	4
Pace Spicy Jalapeño Refried Beans	1/2 cup	76	0	0	590	14	5	5
Pace Traditional Refried Beans	1/2 cup	80	0	0	690	13	5	5
RHUBARB								
Fresh, diced	1 cup	26	0	0	5	6	2	1
Frozen, cooked, w/ sugar	1 cup	278	0	0	2	75	5	1
RICE								
Brown, long grain, cooked	1 cup	216	2	0	10	45	4	5
Brown, medium grain, cooked	1 cup	218	2	0	2	46	4	5
White, from Chinese restaurant, steamed	1 cup	199	0	0	7	45	1	4
White, glutinous	1 cup	169	0	0	9	37	2	4
White, long grain	1 cup	205	0	0	2	45	1	4
White, long grain, instant	1 cup	193	1	0	7	41	1	4
White, long grain, parboiled	1 cup	194	1	0	3	41	1	5
White, medium grain	1 cup	242	0	0	0	53	1	4
White, short grain	1 cup	242	0	0	0	53	0	4
White, w/ pasta	1 cup	246	6	1	1147	43	5	5
Wild, cooked	1 cup	166	1	0	5	35	3	7
RICE BRAN (crude)	1 cup	373	25	5	6	59	25	16
RICE BRAN OIL	1 tbsp	120	14	3	0	0	0	0
RICE CAKES								
Brown rice, buckwheat	1 cake	34	0	0	10	7	0	1
Brown rice, buckwheat, unsalted	1 cake	34	0	0	0	7	0	1
Brown rice, corn	1 cake	35	0	0	26	7	0	1
Brown rice, multigrain	1 cake	35	0	0	23	7	0	1
Brown rice, multigrain, unsalted	1 cake	35	0	0	0	7	0	1
Brown rice, plain	1 cake	35	0	0	29	7	0	1
Brown rice, plain, unsalted	1 cake	35	0	0	2	7	0	1

ITEM DESCRIPTION	Serving Size	Calories	Total Fat (g)	Saturated Fat (g)	Sodium (mg)	Carbohydrates (g)	Fiber (g)	Protein (g)
Brown rice, rye	1 cake	35	0	0	10	7	0	1
Brown rice, sesame seed	1 cake	35	0	0	20	7	0	1
Brown rice, sesame seed, unsalted	1 cake	35	0	0	0	7	0	1
Brown	1 cup	574	4	1	13	121	7	11
White	1 cup	578	2	1	0	127	4	9
ROAST BEEF HASH (Hormel, canned)	1 cup	385	24	10	793	23	4	21
ROCKFISH (Pacific, cooked in dry heat)	3 oz	103	2	0	65	0	0	20
ROE (cooked in dry heat)	3 oz	173	7	2	99	2	0	24
ROLLS								
Dinner, egg (2-1/2" dia)	1 roll	107	2	1	191	18	1	3
Dinner, oat bran	1 roll	78	2	0	136	13	1	3
Dinner, plain, commercial (2" sq)	1 roll	78	2	0	134	13	1	3
Dinner, plain, homemade, made w/ 2% milk (2-1/2" dia)	1 roll	111	3	1	145	19	1	3
Dinner, rye (2-3/8" dia)	1 roll	80	1	0	250	15	1	3
Dinner, wheat	1 roll	76	2	0	95	13	1	2
French	1 roll	105	2	0	231	19	1	3
Hamburger or hot dog, mixed grain	1 roll	113	3	1	197	19	2	4
Hamburger or hot dog, plain	1 roll	120	2	0	206	21	1	4
Hamburger or hot dog, reduced calorie	1 roll	84	1	0	190	18	3	4
Kaiser (3-1/2" dia)	1 roll	167	2	0	310	30	1	6
Pillsbury Cinnamon Rolls, w/ icing	1 serv	145	5	2	340	23	1	2
Pumpernickel (2-1/2" dia)	1 roll	100	1	0	205	19	2	4
Sweet, cinnamon, commercial w/raisins (2-3/4" dia)	1 roll	223	10	2	230	31	1	4
Sweet, cinnamon, refrigerated dough w/ frosting	1 roll	109	4	1	250	17	0	2
Sweet, w/ cheese	1 roll	238	12	4	236	29	1	5
Wonder Hamburger Rolls	1 roll	117	2	0	256	22	1	3
ROSEMARY								
Fresh	1 tbsp	2	0	0	0	0	0	0
Dried	1 tbsp	11	1	0	2	2	1	0
ROUGHY (orange, cooked in dry heat)	3 oz	89	1	0	59	0	0	19

ITEM DESCRIPTION	Serving Size	Calories	Total Fat (g)	Saturated Fat (g)	Sodium (mg)	Carbohydrates (g)	Fiber (g)	Protein (g)
ROWAL (fresh)	1/2 cup	127	2	0	5	27	7	3
RUM								
80 proof	1 fl oz	64	0	0	0	0	0	0
86 proof	1 fl oz	70	0	0	0	0	0	0
90 proof	1 fl oz	73	0	0	0	0	0	0
94 proof	1 fl oz	76	0	0	0	0	0	0
RUTABAGAS								
Boiled, cubed	1 cup	66	0	0	34	15	3	2
Fresh	1 large	278	2	0	154	63	19	9
RYE FLOUR								
Dark	1 cup	415	3	0	1	88	29	18
Light	1 cup	374	1	0	2	82	15	9
Medium	1 cup	361	2	0	3	79	15	10
SABLEFISH								
Cooked in dry heat	3 oz	212	17	3	61	0	0	15
Smoked	1 oz	73	6	1	209	0	0	5
SAFFLOWER								
Oil, linoleic, over 70%	1 tbsp	120	14	1	0	0	0	0
Oil, oleic, over 70%	1 tbsp	120	14	1	0	0	0	0
Seed meal, defatted	1 oz	97	1	0	1	14	0	10
Seeds, dried	1 oz	147	11	1	1	10	0	5
SAFFRON	1 tbsp	7	0	0	3	1	0	0
SAGE (ground)	1 tbsp	6	0	0	0	1	1	0
SAKE	1 fl oz	39	0	0	1	1	0	0
SALAD DRESSINGS								
1000 Island, commercial	1 tbsp	59	6	1	138	2	0	0
1000 Island, fat free	1 tbsp	21	0	0	117	5	1	0
1000 Island, reduced fat	1 tbsp	29	2	0	125	4	0	0
Bacon & tomato	1 tbsp	49	5	1	163	0	0	0
Blue or Roquefort cheese, commercial	1 tbsp	71	8	1	140	1	0	0
Blue or Roquefort cheese, fat free	1 tbsp	20	0	0	138	4	0	0
Blue or Roquefort cheese, low calorie	1 tbsp	15	1	0	180	0	0	1

ITEM DESCRIPTION	Serving Size	Calories	Total Fat (g)	Saturated Fat (g)	Sodium (mg)	Carbohydrates (g)	Fiber (g)	Protein (g)
Blue or Roquefort cheese, reduced calorie	1 tbsp	14	0	0	258	2	0	0
Buttermilk, light	1 tbsp	30	2	0	136	3	0	0
Caesar	1 tbsp	80	9	1	158	0	0	0
Caesar, low calorie	1 tbsp	16	1	0	162	3	0	0
Creamy, w/ sour cream or buttermilk & oil, reduced calorie	1 tbsp	24	2	0	153	1	0	0
Creamy, w/ sour cream or buttermilk & oil, reduced calorie, cholesterol free	1 tbsp	21	1	0	140	2	0	0
Creamy, w/ sour cream or buttermilk & oil, reduced calorie, fat free	1 tbsp	18	0	0	170	3	0	0
French, commercial	1 tbsp	73	7	1	134	2	0	0
French, commercial, w/o salt	1 tbsp	69	7	1	0	2	0	0
French, fat free	1 tbsp	21	0	0	126	5	0	0
French, homemade	1 tbsp	88	10	2	92	0	0	0
French, reduced calorie	1 tbsp	32	2	0	160	4	0	0
French, reduced fat	1 tbsp	36	2	0	126	5	0	0
French, reduced fat, w/o salt	1 tbsp	37	2	0	5	5	0	0
Green goddess	1 tbsp	64	7	1	130	1	0	0
Honey mustard, reduced calorie	1 tbsp	31	2	0	135	4	0	0
Italian, commercial	1 tbsp	43	4	1	243	2	0	0
Italian, commercial, w/o salt	1 tbsp	43	4	1	4	2	0	0
Italian, fat free	1 tbsp	7	0	0	158	1	0	0
Italian, reduced calorie	1 tbsp	28	3	0	199	1	0	0
Italian, reduced fat	1 tbsp	11	1	0	205	1	0	0
Italian, reduced fat, w/o salt	1 tbsp	11	1	0	4	1	0	0
Kraft Free Fat Free Italian Dressing	1 tbsp	10	0	0	215	2	0	0
Kraft Free Fat Free Ranch Dressing	1 tbsp	24	0	0	177	5	0	0
Kraft Light Done Right! Italian Dressing	1 tbsp	26	2	0	114	1	0	0
Kraft Light Done Right! Ranch Dressing	1 tbsp	38	3	0	151	2	0	0
Kraft Ranch Dressing	1 tbsp	74	8	1	144	1	0	0
Kraft Zesty Italian Dressing	1 tbsp	54	6	1	253	1	0	0
Peppercorn, commercial	1 tbsp	76	8	1	143	0	0	0
Ranch, commercial	1 tbsp	73	8	1	122	1	0	0

ITEM DESCRIPTION	Serving Size	Calories	Total Fat (g)	Saturated Fat (g)	Sodium (mg)	Carbohydrates (g)	Fiber (g)	Protein (g)
Ranch, fat free	1 tbsp	17	0	0	106	4	0	0
Ranch, reduced fat	1 tbsp	29	2	0	136	3	0	0
Russian	1 tbsp	53	4	0	149	5	0	0
Russian, low calorie	1 tbsp	23	1	0	139	4	0	0
Sesame seed	1 tbsp	66	7	1	150	1	0	0
Spray, assorted flavors	~10 sprays	13	1	0	88	1	0	0
Sweet & sour	1 tbsp	2	0	0	33	1	0	0
Vinegar & oil, homemade	1 tbsp	72	8	1	0	0	0	0
SALAMI								
Beef & pork, cooked	3 slices	124	10	3	535	1	0	8
Beef & pork, less sodium	3.5 oz	396	31	11	623	15	0	15
Beef, cooked	1 slice	68	6	3	296	0	0	3
Dry or hard, pork	3 slices	122	10	4	678	0	0	7
Dry or hard, pork & beef	3 slices	104	8	3	543	1	0	6
Italian pork	1 oz	119	10	4	529	0	0	6
Oscar Mayer Salami, beer	1 slice	52	4	1	283	0	0	3
Oscar Mayer Salami Cotto, beef	1 slice	47	4	2	301	0	0	3
Oscar Mayer Salami Cotto, beef, pork & chicken	1 slice	56	5	2	252	1	0	3
Oscar Mayer Salami, Genoa	1 slice	35	3	1	164	0	0	2
Oscar Mayer Salami, hard	1 slice	33	3	1	178	0	0	2
SALMON								
Atlantic, farmed, cooked in dry heat	3 oz	175	11	2	52	0	0	19
Atlantic, wild, cooked in dry heat	3 oz	155	7	1	48	0	0	22
Chinook, cooked in dry heat	3 oz	196	11	3	51	0	0	22
Chinook, smoked	1 oz	33	1	0	222	0	0	5
Chinook, smoked, lox	1 oz	33	1	0	567	0	0	5
Chum, canned	3 oz	175	5	1	414	0	0	18
Chum, canned, w/o salt	3 oz	175	5	1	64	0	0	18
Chum, cooked in dry heat	3 oz	131	4	1	54	0	0	22
Coho, farmed, cooked in dry heat	3 oz	151	7	2	44	0	0	21
Coho, wild, cooked in dry heat	3 oz	118	4	1	49	0	0	20
Coho, wild, cooked in moist heat	3 oz	156	6	1	45	0	0	23
Pink, canned	3 oz	118	5	1	471	0	0	17

ITEM DESCRIPTION	Serving Size	Calories	Total Fat (g)	Saturated Fat (g)	Sodium (mg)	Carbohydrates (g)	Fiber (g)	Protein (g)
Pink, canned, w/o salt	3 oz	118	5	1	64	0	0	17
Pink, cooked in dry heat	3 oz	127	4	1	73	0	0	22
Sockeye, canned	3 oz	141	6	1	306	0	0	20
Sockeye, canned, w/o salt	3 oz	130	6	1	64	0	0	17
Sockeye, cooked in dry heat	3 oz	184	9	2	56	0	0	23
SALMON OIL	1 tbsp	123	14	3	0	0	0	0
SALSA								
Pace Chipotle Chunky Salsa	2 tbsp	8	0	0	230	2	1	0
Pace Cilantro Chunky Salsa	2 tbsp	8	0	0	270	2	1	0
Pace Lime & Garlic Chunky Salsa	2 tbsp	12	0	0	210	3	1	0
Pace Salsa Verde	2 tbsp	15	0	0	230	2	1	0
Pace Tequila Lime Salsa	2 tbsp	15	0	0	190	3	1	0
Pace Thick & Chunky Salsa	2 tbsp	8	0	0	230	2	1	0
Pace Triple Pepper Salsa	2 tbsp	15	0	0	190	3	1	1
Ready to serve	2 tbsp	9	0	0	192	2	1	0
SALSIFY								
Boiled, slices	1 cup	92	0	0	22	21	4	4
Fresh, slices	1 cup	109	0	0	27	25	4	4
SALT (table)	1 tbsp	0	0	0	6976	0	0	0
SANDWICH SPREAD								
Meatless	1 tbsp	22	1	0	94	1	1	1
Oscar Mayer Sandwich Spread, pork, chicken, beef	1 serv	71	5	2	246	5	0	2
Pork & beef	1 tbsp	35	3	1	152	2	0	1
Poultry salad	1 tbsp	26	2	0	49	1	0	2
SARDINE OIL	1 tbsp	123	14	4	0	0	0	0
SARDINES								
Atlantic, canned in oil	1 cup	310	17	2	752	0	0	37
Pacific, canned in tomato sauce	1 cup	166	9	2	368	1	0	19
SAUERKRAUT								
Canned	1 cup	27	0	0	939	6	4	1
Canned, low sodium	1 cup	31	0	0	437	6	4	1
SAUSAGE								
Beerwurst, beer salami, pork & beef	2 oz	155	13	5	410	2	1	8

ITEM DESCRIPTION	Serving Size	Calories	Total Fat (g)	Saturated Fat (g)	Sodium (mg)	Carbohydrates (g)	Fiber (g)	Protein (g)
Beerwurst, pork (4" dia x 1/8" thick)	1 slice	55	4	1	285	0	0	3
Berliner, pork, beef	1 slice	53	4	1	298	1	0	4
Blood	1 slice	95	9	3	170	0	0	4
Bratwurst, beef & pork, smoked	2.3 oz	196	17	4	560	1	0	8
Bratwurst, chicken, cooked	3 oz	148	9	0	60	0	0	16
Bratwurst, pork, beef & turkey, light, smoked	2.3 oz	123	9	0	648	1	0	10
Bratwurst, pork, cooked	1 link	283	25	8	719	2	0	12
Bratwurst, veal, cooked	2.96 oz	286	27	13	50	0	0	12
Chicken & beef, smoked	1 cup, pcs	408	33	10	1408	0	0	26
Chorizo, pork & beef (4" 'link)	1 link	273	23	9	741	1	0	14
Honey roll, beef (4" dia x 1/8" thick)	1 slice	42	2	1	304	1	0	4
Italian, pork, cooked (1/4 lb link)	1 link	286	23	8	1002	4	0	16
Italian, sweet links	3 oz link	125	7	3	479	2	0	14
Kielbasa, pork & beef, nonfat dry milk	1 link	232	20	7	678	2	0	9
Kielbasa, turkey & beef, smoked	2 oz	127	10	3	672	2	0	7
Knockwurst, pork & beef	1 link	221	20	7	670	2	0	8
Liverwurst, pork (2-1/2" dia x 1/4" thick)	1 slice	59	5	2	155	0	0	3
Oscar Mayer Braunschweiger Liver Sausage, slices	1 slice	93	8	3	325	1	0	4
Oscar Mayer Braunschweiger Liver Sausage, tube	1 serv	191	17	6	626	1	0	8
Oscar Mayer Pork Sausage Links	1 link	82	7	3	201	0	0	4
Oscar Mayer Smokie Links	1 link	130	12	4	433	1	0	5
Oscar Mayer Smokies, beef	1 link	127	11	5	416	1	0	5
Oscar Mayer Smokies, cheese	1 link	130	12	4	450	1	0	6
Oscar Mayer Smokies Sausage Little, cheese, pork & turkey	1 link	28	3	1	93	0	0	1
Oscar Mayer Smokies Sausage Little, pork & turkey	1 link	27	2	1	92	0	0	1
Oscar Mayer Summer Sausage, beef thuringer	1 slice	71	6	3	328	0	0	3
Oscar Mayer Summer Sausage, thuringer	1 slice	70	6	2	329	0	0	3

ITEM DESCRIPTION	Serving Size	Calories	Total Fat (g)	Saturated Fat (g)	Sodium (mg)	Carbohydrates (g)	Fiber (g)	Protein (g)
Polish, beef & chicken, hot	5 pcs	142	11	4	847	2	0	10
Polish, beef & pork, smoked	2.7 oz	229	20	7	644	2	0	9
Polish, pork (10" long x 1-1/4" dia)	1 link	740	65	23	1989	4	0	32
Pork & beef, patty	1 patty	107	10	3	217	1	0	4
Pork & turkey, patty	1 patty	77	6	2	220	0	0	6
Pork sausage rice links, brown & serve	2 links	183	17	3	310	1	0	6
Smoked link, pork (4" long x 1-1/8" dia)	1 link	209	19	6	562	0	0	8
Smoked link, pork & beef	1 oz	320	29	10	911	2	0	12
Smoked link, pork & beef, w/flour & nonfat dry milk (4" long x 1-1/8" dia)	1 link	182	15	5	865	3	0	10
Smoked link, pork & beef, w/nonfat dry milk (4" long x 1-1/8" dia)	1 link	213	19	7	798	1	0	9
Turkey, pork, & beef, reduced fat, smoked	1 cup	353	25	9	1407	4	0	27
Vienna, canned, chicken, beef & pork (2" long x 7/8" dia)	1 link	37	3	1	155	0	0	2
SAUSAGE BISCUITS (Jimmy Dean, frozen)	1 sandwich	192	14	4	441	12	1	5
SAUSAGE SUBSTITUTE								
Meatless	1 link	64	5	1	222	2	1	5
Morningstar Farms Sausage Style Recipe Crumbles, frozen	2/3 cup	90	2	0	445	8	1	10
Morningstar Farms Veggie Sausage Links, frozen	1 link	72	3	0	302	3	2	9
Morningstar Farms Veggie Sausage Patties, frozen	1 patty	80	3	0	255	3	2	10
Worthington Low Fat Veja-Links, canned	1 link	38	1	0	190	1	0	5
Worthington Prosage Links, frozen	2 links	64	2	0	369	2	1	9
Worthington Saucettes, canned	1 link	83	6	0	202	2	1	6
Worthington Veja-Links, canned	1 link	48	3	0	164	1	1	5
SAVORY (ground)	1 tbsp	12	0	0	1	3	2	0
SCALLIONS (fresh, chopped)	1 tbsp	2	0	0	1	0	0	0
SCALLOPS (breaded & fried)	6 pcs	386	19	5	919	38	0	16

ITEM DESCRIPTION	Serving Size	Calories	Total Fat (g)	Saturated Fat (g)	Sodium (mg)	Carbohydrates (g)	Fiber (g)	Protein (g)
SCALLOP SQUASH								
Boiled, mashed	1 cup	38	0	0	2	8	5	2
Fresh, slices	1 cup	23	0	0	1	5	0	2
SCALLOPS SUBSTITUTE								
(imitation, made from surimi)	3 oz	84	0	0	676	9	0	11
SCUP (cooked in dry heat)	3 oz	115	3	0	46	0	0	21
SEA BASS (cooked in dry heat)	3 oz	105	2	1	74	0	0	20
SEA TROUT (cooked in dry heat)	3 oz	113	4	1	63	0	0	18
SEAWEED								
Agar, fresh	2 tbsp	3	0	0	1	1	0	0
Irish moss, fresh	2 tbsp	5	0	0	7	1	0	0
Kelp, fresh	2 tbsp	4	0	0	23	1	0	0
Laver, fresh	2 tbsp	4	0	0	5	1	0	1
Spirulina, dried	1 tbsp	20	1	0	73	2	0	4
Wakame, fresh	2 tbsp	4	0	0	87	1	0	0
SEMOLINA	1 cup	601	2	0	2	122	7	21
SESAME BUTTER								
Paste	1 tbsp	94	8	1	2	4	1	3
Tahini	1 tbsp	89	8	1	5	3	1	3
Tahini, from fresh & ground kernels	1 tbsp	86	7	1	11	4	1	3
Tahini, from roasted & toasted kernels	1 tbsp	89	8	1	17	3	1	3
Tahini, from unroasted kernels	1 tbsp	85	8	1	0	3	1	3
High fat	1 oz	149	11	1	12	8	0	9
Low fat	1 oz	94	0	0	11	10	0	14
Part defatted	1 oz	108	3	0	12	10	0	11
SESAME MEAL (part defatted)	1 oz	161	14	2	11	7	0	5
SESAME OIL	1 tbsp	120	14	2	0	0	0	0
SESAME SEEDS								
Kernels, dried	1 cup	946	92	14	70	18	17	31
Kernels, toasted, w/o salt	1 cup	726	61	9	50	33	21	22
Kernels, toasted, w/ salt	1 cup	726	61	9	753	33	22	22
Whole, dried	1 cup	825	72	10	16	34	17	26
Whole, roasted & toasted	1 cup	814	69	10	16	37	20	24

ITEM DESCRIPTION	Serving Size	Calories	Total Fat (g)	Saturated Fat (g)	Sodium (mg)	Carbohydrates (g)	Fiber (g)	Protein (g)
SESAME STICKS								
Wheat based, salted	1 oz	153	10	2	422	13	1	3
Wheat based, unsalted	1 oz	153	10	2	8	13	0	3
SESBANIA FLOWER								
Fresh	1 cup	5	0	0	3	1	0	0
Steamed	1 cup	23	0	0	11	5	0	1
SHAD (American, cooked in dry heat)	3 oz	214	15	0	55	0	0	18
SHAKES								
Fast food, chocolate	12 fl oz	358	10	7	274	58	5	10
Fast food, strawberry	12 fl oz	319	8	5	234	53	1	10
Fast food, vanilla	12 fl oz	370	16	10	202	49	2	8
SHALLOTS								
Freeze-dried	1 tbsp	3	0	0	1	1	0	0
Fresh, chopped	1 tbsp	7	0	0	1	2	0	0
SHARK (cooked, battered & fried)	3 oz	194	12	3	104	5	0	16
SHEANUT OIL	1 tbsp	120	14	6	0	0	0	0
SHELLIE BEANS (canned)	1 cup	74	0	0	818	15	8	4
SHERBET (orange)	1/2 cup	107	1	1	34	23	1	1
SHORTENING								
Baking, soybean, palm & cottonseed, hydrogenated	1 tbsp	113	13	4	0	0	0	0
Cakes & frostings, soybean, hydrogenated	1 tbsp	113	13	3	0	0	0	0
Confectionery, coconut or palm oil, hydrogenated	1 tbsp	113	13	12	0	0	0	0
Confectionery, fractionated palm	1 tbsp	120	14	9	0	0	0	0
Frying, heavy, beef tallow & cottonseed	1 tbsp	115	13	6	0	0	0	0
Frying, heavy, palm, hydrogenated	1 tbsp	113	13	6	0	0	0	0
Frying, heavy, soybean, hydrogenated	1 tbsp	113	13	3	0	0	0	0
Frying, soybean & cottonseed, hydrogenated	1 tbsp	113	13	2	0	0	0	0
Household, lard & vegetable oil	1 tbsp	115	13	5	0	0	0	0
Household, soybean & cottonseed, hydrogenated	1 tbsp	113	13	3	0	0	0	0

ITEM DESCRIPTION	Serving Size	Calories	Total Fat (g)	Saturated Fat (g)	Sodium (mg)	Carbohydrates (g)	Fiber (g)	Protein (g)
Household, soybean & palm, hydrogenated	1 tbsp	113	13	3	0	0	0	0
Household, vegetable	1 tbsp	113	13	3	1	0	0	0
Soybean & cottonseed, hydrogenated	1 tbsp	113	13	3	0	0	0	0
SHRIMP								
Breaded & fried	3 oz	206	10	2	292	10	0	18
Canned	3 oz	85	1	0	660	0	0	17
Cooked in moist heat	3 oz	84	1	0	190	0	0	18
Imitation, made from surimi	3 oz	86	1	0	599	8	0	11
SMELT (rainbow, cooked in dry heat)	3 oz	105	3	0	65	0	0	19
SNACK BARS								
Cocoavia Chocolate Almond Snack Bar	1 bar	76	3	1	57	11	1	2
Cocoavia Chocolate Blueberry Snack Bar	1 bar	72	2	1	57	13	1	1
Corn flake crust, w/ fruit	1 oz bar	107	2	0	47	21	1	1
Crisped rice bar, chocolate chip	1 oz bar	113	4	1	78	20	1	1
Kudos Whole Grain Bar, chocolate chip	1 bar	118	4	1	69	20	1	1
Kudos Whole Grain Bar, M&M's milk chocolate	1 bar	100	3	2	82	18	1	1
Kudos Whole Grain Bar, peanut butter	1 bar	130	6	3	75	18	1	2
Power Bar, chocolate	1 bar	247	2	1	99	47	4	10
Snickers Marathon Chewy Chocolate Peanut Bar	1 bar	218	7	3	254	26	1	13
Snickers Marathon Double Chocolate Nut Bar	1 bar	151	4	2	147	23	5	10
Snickers Marathon Energy Bar	1 bar	170	5	2	169	22	3	10
Snickers Marathon Honey Nut Oat Bar	1 bar	166	3	2	140	24	5	10
Snickers Marathon Multi-Grain Bar	1 bar	223	7	3	230	30	2	10
Snickers Marathon Protein Perfect Bar, caramel nut	1 bar	322	8	4	180	42	8	20
SNACK CAKES								
Crème filled, chocolate w/ frosting	1 cake	200	8	2	194	30	2	2
Crème filled, sponge	1 cake	157	5	2	168	27	0	1

ITEM DESCRIPTION	Serving Size	Calories	Total Fat (g)	Saturated Fat (g)	Sodium (mg)	Carbohydrates (g)	Fiber (g)	Protein (g)
SNAP BEANS								
Canned, all styles, seasoned	1/2 cup	18	0	0	425	4	2	1
Green, boiled	1 cup	44	0	0	1	10	4	2
Green, canned	1 cup	36	0	0	409	7	4	2
Green, canned, no salt	1 cup	36	0	0	34	8	4	2
Green, fresh	1 cup	34	0	0	7	8	4	2
Green, frozen, all styles, microwaved	1 cup	44	0	0	3	8	4	2
Green, frozen, boiled	1 cup	38	0	0	1	9	4	2
Yellow, boiled	1 cup	44	0	0	4	10	4	2
Yellow, canned	1 cup	36	0	0	622	8	4	2
Yellow, canned, no salt	1 cup	36	0	0	34	8	4	2
Yellow, fresh	1 cup	34	0	0	7	8	4	2
Yellow, frozen, boiled	1 cup	38	0	0	12	9	4	2
SNAPPER (cooked in dry heat)	3 oz	109	1	0	48	0	0	22
SODA								
Chocolate flavored	1 fl oz	13	0	0	27	3	0	0
Club soda	16 fl oz	0	0	0	100	0	0	0
Cola	16 fl oz	201	0	0	20	52	0	0
Cola or pepper, w/ aspartame, w/o caffeine	16 fl oz	5	0	0	19	1	0	1
Cola or pepper, w/ saccharine, w/ caffeine	16 fl oz	0	0	0	76	0	0	0
Cola, reduced sugar, w/ sweeteners	8 fl oz	71	0	0	14	18	0	0
Cream soda	16 fl oz	252	0	0	59	66	0	0
Ginger ale	16 fl oz	166	0	0	34	43	0	0
Grape	16 fl oz	213	0	0	74	56	0	0
Lemon-lime	16 fl oz	202	0	0	49	51	0	0
Orange	16 fl oz	238	0	0	60	61	0	0
Pepper	16 fl oz	201	0	0	49	51	0	0
Root beer	16 fl oz	202	0	0	64	52	0	0
Other than cola or pepper, low calorie	16 fl oz	0	0	0	28	0	0	0
Other than cola or pepper, low calorie, w/ aspartame	16 fl oz	0	0	0	28	0	0	0

ITEM DESCRIPTION	Serving Size	Calories	Total Fat (g)	Saturated Fat (g)	Sodium (mg)	Carbohydrates (g)	Fiber (g)	Protein (g)
Other than cola or pepper, low calorie, w/ saccharine	16 fl oz	0	0	0	76	0	0	0
SOFRITO SAUCE (homemade)	1/2 cup	244	19	0	1179	6	2	13
SORGHUM	1 cup	651	6	1	12	143	12	22
SORGHUM SYRUP	1 tbsp	61	0	0	2	16	0	0
SOUP								
Bean w/ bacon, mix, prepared w/ water	1 cup	106	2	1	928	16	9	5
Bean w/ frankfurters, canned, prepared w/ water	1 cup	188	7	2	1092	22	0	10
Bean w/ ham, canned, chunky, ready to serve	1 cup	231	9	3	972	27	11	13
Bean w/ pork, canned, prepared w/ water	1 cup	168	6	1	928	22	8	8
Beef & mushroom, canned, prepared w/ water	1 cup	73	3	1	942	6	0	6
Beef & mushroom, low sodium, chunky	1 cup	173	6	4	63	24	1	11
Beef, chunky, canned, ready to serve	1 cup	162	3	1	880	25	2	10
Beef noodle, canned, prepared w/ water	1 cup	83	3	1	930	9	1	5
Beef stroganoff, canned, chunky, ready to serve	1 cup	235	11	6	1044	22	1	12
Beef w/ country vegetable, chunky, canned, ready to serve	1 pkg	334	7	3	1978	46	0	22
Black bean, canned, prepared w/ water	1 cup	114	2	0	1203	19	8	6
Cheese, canned, prepared w/ milk	1 cup	231	15	9	1019	16	1	9
Cheese, canned, prepared w/ water	1 cup	156	10	7	958	11	1	5
Chicken, chunky, canned, ready to serve	1 cup	174	6	2	867	17	2	12
Chicken corn chowder, chunky, ready to serve	1 pkg	534	34	9	1612	40	5	17
Chicken gumbo, canned, prepared w/ water	1 cup	56	1	0	954	8	2	3
Chicken mushroom, canned, prepared w/ water	1 cup	132	9	2	942	9	0	4

ITEM DESCRIPTION	Serving Size	Calories	Total Fat (g)	Saturated Fat (g)	Sodium (mg)	Carbohydrates (g)	Fiber (g)	Protein (g)
Chicken mushroom chowder, chunky, ready to serve	1 pkg	431	24	6	1827	38	8	16
Chicken noodle, canned, prepared w/ water	1 cup	62	2	1	657	7	1	3
Chicken noodle, chunky, canned, ready to serve	1 cup	91	2	1	840	10	1	8
Chicken noodle, low sodium, canned, prepared w/ water	1 cup	62	2	1	429	7	1	3
Chicken noodle, mix, prepared w/ water	1 cup	56	1	0	561	9	0	2
Chicken rice, canned, chunky, ready to serve	1 cup	127	3	1	888	13	1	12
Chicken rice, mix, prepared w/ water	1 cup	58	1	0	931	9	1	2
Chicken vegetable, canned, prepared w/ water	1 cup	77	3	1	972	9	1	4
Chicken vegetable, chunky, canned, ready to serve	1 cup	166	5	1	833	19	0	12
Chicken vegetable, chunky, reduced fat, reduced sodium, ready to serve	1 pkg	182	2	1	872	29	0	12
Chicken w/ dumplings, canned, prepared w/ water	1 cup	96	6	1	860	6	1	6
Chicken w/ rice, canned, prepared w/ water	1 cup	58	2	0	812	7	1	4
Chili beef, canned, prepared w/ water	1 cup	149	3	2	1013	24	3	7
Clam chowder, Manhattan style, canned, chunky, ready to serve	1 cup	134	3	2	1001	19	3	7
Clam chowder, Manhattan style, canned, prepared w/ water	1 cup	75	2	0	563	12	2	2
Clam chowder, New England, canned, prepared w/ 2% milk	1 cup	154	5	2	902	19	1	8
Clam chowder, New England, canned, prepared w/ water	1 cup	87	3	1	853	13	1	4
Consomme, w/ gelatin, mix, prepared w/ water	1 cup	17	0	0	3299	2	0	2
Crab, canned, ready to serve	1 cup	76	2	0	1235	10	1	5
Cream of asparagus, canned, prepared w/ milk	1 cup	161	8	3	1042	16	1	6

ITEM DESCRIPTION	Serving Size	Calories	Total Fat (g)	Saturated Fat (g)	Sodium (mg)	Carbohydrates (g)	Fiber (g)	Protein (g)
Cream of asparagus, canned, prepared w/ water	1 cup	85	4	1	981	11	1	2
Cream of celery, canned, prepared w/ milk	1 cup	164	10	4	1009	15	1	6
Cream of celery, canned, prepared w/ water	1 cup	90	6	1	949	9	1	2
Cream of chicken, canned, prepared w/ milk	1 cup	191	11	5	1047	15	0	7
Cream of chicken, canned, prepared w/ water	1 cup	117	7	2	986	9	0	3
Cream of chicken, mix, prepared w/ water	1 cup	107	5	3	1185	13	0	2
Cream of mushroom, canned, prepared w/ 2% milk	1 cup	169	10	3	837	14	0	6
Cream of mushroom, canned, prepared w/ water	1 cup	104	7	2	789	8	0	2
Cream of mushroom, low sodium, ready to serve	1 cup	129	9	2	49	11	1	2
Cream of onion, canned, prepared w/ milk	1 cup	186	9	4	1004	18	1	7
Cream of onion, canned, prepared w/ water	1 cup	107	5	1	927	13	1	3
Cream of potato, canned, prepared w/milk	1 cup	149	6	4	1061	17	1	6
Cream of potato, canned, prepared w/ water	1 cup	73	2	1	1000	11	1	2
Cream of shrimp, canned, prepared w/ water	1 cup	88	5	3	954	8	0	3
Egg drop, Chinese restaurant	1 cup	65	1	0	892	10	0	3
Escarole, canned, ready to serve	1 cup	27	2	1	3864	2	0	2
Gazpacho, canned, ready to serve	1 cup	46	0	0	739	4	1	7
Green pea, canned, prepared w/ milk	1 cup	239	7	4	970	32	3	13
Green pea, canned, prepared w/ water	1 cup	161	3	1	891	26	5	8
Hot & sour, Chinese restaurant	1 cup	91	3	1	876	10	0	6
Lentil, w/ ham, canned, ready to serve	1 cup	139	3	1	1319	20	0	9

ITEM DESCRIPTION	Serving Size	Calories	Total Fat (g)	Saturated Fat (g)	Sodium (mg)	Carbohydrates (g)	Fiber (g)	Protein (g)
Minestrone, canned, prepared w/ water	1 cup	82	3	1	911	11	1	4
Minestrone, chunky, canned, ready to serve	1 cup	127	3	1	864	21	6	5
Mushroom barley, canned, prepared w/ water	1 cup	73	2	0	891	12	1	2
Mushroom w/ beef stock, canned, prepared w/ water	1 cup	85	4	2	969	9	1	3
Mushroom, mix, prepared w/ water	1 cup	83	5	1	1020	11	1	2
Onion, canned, prepared w/ water	1 cup	56	2	0	1028	8	1	4
Onion, mix, prepared w/ water	1 cup	28	0	0	796	6	1	1
Oxtail, mix, prepared w/ water	1 cup	68	2	1	1159	9	0	3
Oyster stew, canned, prepared w/ milk	1 cup	135	8	5	1041	10	0	6
Oyster stew, canned, prepared w/ water	1 cup	58	4	3	981	4	0	2
Pea, low sodium, prepared w/ water	1 cup	161	3	1	26	26	5	8
Pepperpot, canned, prepared w/ water	1 cup	100	5	2	948	9	1	6
Potato ham chowder, chunky, ready to serve	1 pkg	431	28	9	1962	30	3	15
Ramen noodle, beef	1 pkg	371	13	7	1702	54	2	9
Ramen noodle, chicken	1 pkg	371	13	6	1760	54	2	9
Scotch broth, canned, prepared w/ water	1 cup	80	3	1	1000	9	1	5
Shark fin, restaurant prepared	1 cup	99	4	1	1082	8	0	7
Sirloin burger w/ vegetable, ready to serve	1 pkg	415	20	7	1946	37	12	23
Split pea, canned, reduced sodium, prepared w/ water	1 cup	180	2	1	420	30	5	10
Split pea, w/ ham, canned, prepared w/ water	1 cup	190	4	2	1007	28	2	10
Split pea, w/ ham, chunky, canned, ready to serve	1 cup	185	4	2	965	27	4	11
Split pea, w/ ham, chunky, reduced fat, reduced sodium, ready to serve	1 pkg	410	6	2	1849	61	0	28
Stockpot, canned, prepared w/ water	1 cup	99	4	1	1047	11	0	5

ITEM DESCRIPTION	Serving Size	Calories	Total Fat (g)	Saturated Fat (g)	Sodium (mg)	Carbohydrates (g)	Fiber (g)	Protein (g)
Tomato beef w/ noodle, canned, prepared w/ water	1 cup	137	4	2	895	21	2	4
Tomato bisque, canned, prepared w/ milk	1 cup	198	7	3	1109	29	1	6
Tomato bisque, canned, prepared w/ water	1 cup	124	3	1	1047	24	1	2
Tomato, canned, prepared w/ 2% milk	1 cup	139	3	2	723	22	2	6
Tomato, canned, prepared w/ water	1 cup	74	1	0	675	16	2	2
Tomato, low sodium, prepared w/ water	1 cup	74	1	0	60	16	2	2
Tomato, mix, prepared w/ water	1 cup	101	2	1	943	19	1	2
Tomato rice, canned, prepared w/ water	1 cup	116	3	0	788	21	2	2
Tomato vegetable, mix, prepared w/ water	1 cup	54	1	0	323	10	1	2
Turkey, chunky, canned, ready to serve	1 cup	135	4	1	923	14	0	10
Turkey noodle, canned, prepared w/ water	1 cup	68	2	1	815	9	1	4
Turkey vegetable, canned, prepared w/ water	1 cup	72	3	1	906	9	1	3
Vegetable beef, canned, prepared w/ water	1 cup	76	2	1	773	10	2	5
Vegetable beef, microwavable	1 pkg	128	2	1	1098	10	4	18
Vegetable beef, mix, prepared w/ water	1 cup	53	1	1	789	8	1	3
Vegetable, chunky, canned, ready to serve	1 cup	125	4	1	880	19	1	4
Vegetable, condensed, low sodium, prepared w/ water	1 cup	83	1	0	491	15	3	3
Vegetable w/beef broth, canned, prepared w/ water	1 cup	80	2	0	800	13	2	3
Vegetable w/chicken, canned, prepared w/ water, low sodium	1 cup	166	5	1	84	21	1	12
Vegetarian vegetable, canned, prepared w/ water	1 cup	67	2	0	815	12	1	2

ITEM DESCRIPTION	Serving Size	Calories	Total Fat (g)	Saturated Fat (g)	Sodium (mg)	Carbohydrates (g)	Fiber (g)	Protein (g)
Wonton, Chinese restaurant	1 cup	71	1	0	905	12	0	5
SOUP, BRAND NAME								
Campbell's Chunky, baked potato w/ cheddar & bacon bits	1 cup	159	6	1	870	23	2	4
Campbell's Chunky, baked potato w/ steak & cheese	1 cup	211	10	2	941	21	3	9
Campbell's Chunky, beef rib roast w/ potatoes & herbs	1 cup	108	1	1	889	17	3	8
Campbell's Chunky, beef w/ country vegetable	1 cup	147	3	1	889	21	4	10
Campbell's Chunky, beef w/ white & wild rice	1 cup	159	3	1	990	24	3	8
Campbell's Chunky, chicken & dumplings	1 cup	181	7	2	889	19	4	9
Campbell's Chunky, chicken, broccoli, cheese, & potato	1 cup	201	11	4	909	14	1	7
Campbell's Chunky, chicken corn chowder	1 cup	194	9	1	850	20	3	8
Campbell's Chunky, classic chicken noodle	1 cup	115	3	1	889	15	2	8
Campbell's Chunky, fajita chicken w/ rice & beans	1 cup	142	1	0	850	23	4	9
Campbell's Chunky, grilled chicken sausage gumbo	1 cup	140	3	1	850	21	3	8
Campbell's Chunky, grilled chicken, vegetable, & pasta	1 cup	100	2	1	880	15	2	8
Campbell's Chunky, grilled sirloin steak, hearty vegetable	1 cup	125	2	1	889	19	4	8
Campbell's Chunky, Healthy Request, chicken noodle	1 cup	120	3	1	480	15	1	7
Campbell's Chunky, Healthy Request, vegetable	1 cup	118	0	0	480	24	4	4
Campbell's Chunky, hearty bean & ham	1 cup	181	2	1	779	30	8	11
Campbell's Chunky, hearty chicken w/ vegetable	1 cup	93	1	1	789	13	2	7
Campbell's Chunky, herb roasted chicken, potatoes, garlic	1 cup	113	1	1	870	17	3	8

ITEM DESCRIPTION	Serving Size	Calories	Total Fat (g)	Saturated Fat (g)	Sodium (mg)	Carbohydrates (g)	Fiber (g)	Protein (g)
Campbell's Chunky, Manhattan clam chowder	1 cup	127	4	1	831	19	3	5
Campbell's Chunky, microwavable, beef w/ country vegetables	1 cup	149	3	1	899	21	5	10
Campbell's Chunky, microwavable, chicken & dumplings	1 cup	191	9	2	889	18	3	8
Campbell's Chunky, microwavable, classic chicken noodle	1 cup	110	2	1	840	14	2	8
Campbell's Chunky, microwavable, grilled chicken & sausage gumbo	1 cup	120	3	1	779	18	3	7
Campbell's Chunky, microwavable, Healthy Request, chicken noodle	1 cup	110	3	1	480	15	1	7
Campbell's Chunky, microwavable, New England clam chowder	1 cup	201	12	2	870	18	3	6
Campbell's Chunky, microwavable, old fashioned vegetable beef	1 cup	110	1	0	880	13	3	9
Campbell's Chunky, microwavable, sirloin burger w/ country vegetables	1 cup	159	4	2	870	18	4	10
Campbell's Chunky, New England clam chowder	1 cup	211	9	1	889	25	5	7
Campbell's Chunky, old fashioned potato & ham chowder	1 cup	191	11	4	801	17	2	6
Campbell's Chunky, old fashioned vegetable beef	1 cup	130	3	1	889	18	4	9
Campbell's Chunky, roadhouse beef bean chili	1 cup	233	8	4	870	25	8	15
Campbell's Chunky, Salisbury steak w/ mushrooms & onions	1 cup	152	5	2	889	19	5	9
Campbell's Chunky, savory chicken w/ white & wild rice	1 cup	118	2	1	811	18	2	7
Campbell's Chunky, savory pot roast	1 cup	118	1	1	880	18	3	8
Campbell's Chunky, savory vegetable	1 cup	108	1	1	769	22	4	3
Campbell's Chunky, slow roasted beef w/ mushrooms	1 cup	118	1	1	831	18	3	8
Campbell's Chunky, split pea & ham	1 cup	169	3	1	779	27	4	12

ITEM DESCRIPTION	Serving Size	Calories	Total Fat (g)	Saturated Fat (g)	Sodium (mg)	Carbohydrates (g)	Fiber (g)	Protein (g)
Campbell's Chunky, steak & potato	1 cup	130	2	1	921	18	2	10
Campbell's Healthy Request, chicken w/ rice, condensed	1/2 cup	73	2	1	480	9	1	2
Campbell's Healthy Request, cream of celery, condensed	1/2 cup	67	2	0	480	12	1	1
Campbell's Healthy Request, cream of chicken, condensed	1/2 cup	81	3	1	460	12	1	2
Campbell's Healthy Request, cream of mushroom, condensed	1/2 cup	69	2	1	470	10	1	2
Campbell's Healthy Request, homestyle chicken noodle, condensed	1/2 cup	60	2	1	480	8	1	3
Campbell's Healthy Request, minestrone, condensed	1/2 cup	80	1	0	460	15	3	3
Campbell's Healthy Request, tomato, condensed	1/2 cup	91	2	1	470	17	1	2
Campbell's Healthy Request, vegetable, condensed	1/2 cup	100	1	0	480	19	3	4
Campbell's Red & White, 25% less sodium, chicken noodle, condensed	1/2 cup	60	2	1	660	8	1	3
Campbell's Red & White, 25% less sodium, cream of mushroom, condensed	1/2 cup	110	8	1	650	9	2	1
Campbell's Red & White, 25% less sodium, tomato, condensed	1/2 cup	91	0	0	529	20	1	2
Campbell's Red & White, 98% fat free, broccoli cheese, condensed	1/2 cup	71	2	1	790	12	1	3
Campbell's Red & White, 98% fat free, cream of broccoli, condensed	1/2 cup	69	2	1	701	10	2	2
Campbell's Red & White, 98% fat free, cream of celery, condensed	1/2 cup	60	3	1	580	8	1	1
Campbell's Red & White, 98% fat free, cream of chicken, condensed	1/2 cup	69	3	1	590	10	1	2
Campbell's Red & White, 98% fat free, cream of mushroom, condensed	1/2 cup	69	3	1	630	9	1	2
Campbell's Red & White, bean w/ bacon, condensed	1/2 cup	170	4	2	860	25	8	8

ITEM DESCRIPTION	Serving Size	Calories	Total Fat (g)	Saturated Fat (g)	Sodium (mg)	Carbohydrates (g)	Fiber (g)	Protein (g)
Campbells Red & White, beef consomme, condensed	1/2 cup	20	0	0	810	1	0	4
Campbell's Red & White, beef noodle, condensed	1/2 cup	71	2	1	820	8	1	4
Campbell's Red & White, beef w/ vegetable & barley, condensed	1/2 cup	89	2	1	890	15	3	5
Campbell's Red & White, beefy mushroom, condensed	1/2 cup	50	2	1	890	6	0	3
Campbell's Red & White, broccoli cheese, condensed	1/2 cup	100	5	2	820	12	0	2
Campbell's Red & White, cheddar cheese, condensed	1/2 cup	110	5	2	890	12	1	2
Campbell's Red & White, chicken alphabet, condensed	1/2 cup	71	2	1	660	11	1	4
Campbell's Red & White, chicken & dumplings, condensed	1/2 cup	71	2	1	760	10	1	3
Campbell's Red & White, chicken & stars, condensed	1/2 cup	71	2	1	640	10	1	3
Campbell's Red & White, chicken gumbo, condensed	1/2 cup	60	1	1	869	10	1	2
Campbell's Red & White, chicken noodle, condensed	1/2 cup	60	2	1	890	8	1	3
Campbell's Red & White, chicken noodle, Noodleo's, condensed	1/2 cup	79	2	1	620	12	1	4
Campbell's Red & White, chicken vegetable, condensed	1/2 cup	79	1	1	890	15	2	3
Campbell's Red & White, chicken w/ rice, condensed	1/2 cup	71	2	1	820	13	1	2
Campbell's Red & White, chicken wonton, condensed	1/2 cup	60	1	1	869	8	0	4
Campbell's Red & White, cream of asparagus, condensed	1/2 cup	110	7	2	830	9	3	2
Campbell's Red & White, cream of broccoli, condensed	1/2 cup	91	4	1	750	12	1	2
Campbell's Red & White, cream of celery, condensed	1/2 cup	91	6	1	861	9	3	1

ITEM DESCRIPTION	Serving Size	Calories	Total Fat (g)	Saturated Fat (g)	Sodium (mg)	Carbohydrates (g)	Fiber (g)	Protein (g)
Campbell's Red & White, cream of chicken, condensed	1/2 cup	120	8	3	870	10	2	3
Campbell's Red & White, cream of chicken w/ herbs, condensed	1/2 cup	81	4	1	810	9	2	2
Campbell's Red & White, cream of mushroom, condensed	1/2 cup	100	6	2	870	9	2	1
Campbell's Red & White, cream of mushroom w/ roasted garlic, condensed	1/2 cup	69	3	1	711	11	2	2
Campbell's Red & White, cream of onion, condensed	1/2 cup	100	6	2	800	10	3	1
Campbell's Red & White, cream of potato, condensed	1/2 cup	91	2	1	800	15	2	2
Campbell's Red & White, cream of shrimp, condensed	1/ 2 cup	91	5	1	861	8	1	2
Campbell's Red & White, creamy chicken noodle, condensed	1/2 cup	120	7	2	870	11	4	4
Campbell's Red & White, curly noodle, condensed	1/2 cup	79	2	0	630	11	1	4
Campbell's Red & White, Dora the Explorer, condensed	1/2 cup	71	2	1	580	10	1	3
Campbell's Red & White, double noodle in chicken broth, condensed	1/ 2 cup	100	2	1	620	17	2	4
Campbell's Red & White, fiesta nacho cheese, condensed	1/2 cup	120	8	3	790	10	1	3
Campbell's Red & White, French onion, condensed	1/2 cup	45	2	1	900	6	1	2
Campbell's Red & White, golden mushroom, condensed	1/2 cup	81	4	1	890	10	1	2
Campbell's Red & White, Goldfish pasta w/ chicken	1/2 cup	71	2	1	600	11	1	3
Campbell's Red & White, Goldfish pasta w/ meatballs	1/2 cup	79	2	1	559	11	2	4
Campbell's Red & White, green pea, condensed	1/2 cup	180	3	1	870	28	4	9
Campbell's Red & White, homestyle chicken noodle, condensed	1/2 cup	71	2	1	706	8	1	4

ITEM DESCRIPTION	Serving Size	Calories	Total Fat (g)	Saturated Fat (g)	Sodium (mg)	Carbohydrates (g)	Fiber (g)	Protein (g)
Campbell's Red & White, Italian style wedding, condensed	1/2 cup	89	2	1	810	12	3	4
Campbell's Red & White, lentil, condensed	1/2 cup	140	1	1	800	24	6	9
Campbell's Red & White, Manhattan clam chowder, condensed	1/2 cup	71	1	1	879	12	2	2
Campbell's Red & White, mega noodle, condensed	1/2 cup	89	2	1	600	14	2	4
Campbell's Red & White, microwavable bowls, chicken noodle	1 cup	74	2	1	870	10	1	4
Campbell's Red & White, microwavable bowls, creamy tomato	1 cup	157	5	1	750	25	3	3
Campbell's Red & White, microwavable bowls, tomato	1 cup	108	0	0	789	24	3	3
Campbell's Red & White, microwavable bowls, vegetable beef	1 cup	83	0	0	880	15	3	5
Campbell's Red & White, minestrone, condensed	1/2 cup	89	1	1	960	17	3	4
Campbell's Red & White, New England clam chowder, condensed	1/2 cup	89	2	1	879	13	1	4
Campbell's Red & White, old fashioned tomato rice, condensed	1/2 cup	110	2	1	770	23	1	1
Campbell's Red & White, pepper pot, condensed	1/2 cup	89	4	1	980	9	1	5
Campbell's Red & White, Scotch broth, condensed	1/2 cup	69	2	1	880	9	2	3
Campbell's Red & White, Shrek shaped pasta	1/2 cup	71	2	1	580	11	3	4
Campbell's Red & White, Southwest-style chicken vegetable, condensed	1/2 cup	110	1	1	830	21	4	5
Campbell's Red & White, split pea w/ ham & bacon, condensed	1/2 cup	180	3	2	850	27	5	10
Campbell's Red & White, tomato bisque, condensed	1/2 cup	130	4	1	879	23	1	2

ITEM DESCRIPTION	Serving Size	Calories	Total Fat (g)	Saturated Fat (g)	Sodium (mg)	Carbohydrates (g)	Fiber (g)	Protein (g)
Campbell's Red & White, tomato, condensed	1/2 cup	91	0	0	711	20	1	2
Campbell's Red & White, vegetable beef, condensed	1/2 cup	79	1	1	890	15	3	5
Campbell's Red & White, vegetable, condensed	1/2 cup	100	1	1	890	20	3	4
Campbell's Red & White, vegetarian vegetable, condensed	1/2 cup	89	1	0	790	18	2	3
Campbell's Select, 98% fat free, New England clam chowder	1 cup	105	2	0	870	16	3	6
Campbell's Select, chicken w/ egg noodles	1 cup	100	3	1	480	13	2	7
Campbell's Select, Italian-style wedding	1 cup	110	3	1	789	15	2	7
Campbell's Select, Mexican style chicken tortilla	1 cup	127	3	1	921	18	3	8
Campbell's Select, minestrone	1 cup	96	0	0	899	19	4	4
Campbell's Select, savory chicken & long grain rice	1 cup	93	0	0	970	15	1	7
Campbell's Soup at Hand, chicken & stars	1 serv	64	1	1	891	10	2	3
Campbell's Soup at Hand, chicken w/ mini noodles	1 serv	79	2	1	979	11	2	4
Campbell's Soup at Hand, cream of broccoli	1 serv	143	7	2	891	17	7	3
Campbell's Soup at Hand, creamy chicken	1 serv	131	9	2	891	13	4	4
Campbell's Soup at Hand, creamy tomato	1 serv	189	4	1	939	34	4	4
Campbell's Soup at Hand, New England clam chowder	1 serv	122	6	1	891	13	4	4
Campbell's Soup at Hand, vegetable beef	1 serv	61	1	1	930	10	1	3
Healthy Choice, chicken & rice, canned	1 cup	89	1	0	434	14	2	6
Healthy Choice, chicken noodle, canned	1 cup	100	2	1	474	13	2	9

ITEM DESCRIPTION	Serving Size	Calories	Total Fat (g)	Saturated Fat (g)	Sodium (mg)	Carbohydrates (g)	Fiber (g)	Protein (g)
Healthy Choice, garden vegetable, canned	1 cup	125	1	0	480	25	5	5
SOUR CREAM								
Cultured	1 tbsp	23	2	1	10	0	0	0
Imitation, cultured	2 tbsp	60	6	5	29	2	0	1
Kraft Breakstone's, fat free	2 tbsp	29	0	0	23	5	0	2
Kraft Breakstone's, reduced fat	2 tbsp	47	4	2	18	2	0	1
Reduced fat, cultured	1 tbsp	20	2	1	6	1	0	0
SOYBEAN OIL								
Hydrogenated, w/ cottonseed	1 tbsp	120	14	2	0	0	0	0
Lecithin	1 tbsp	104	14	2	0	0	0	0
Partially hydrogenated	1 tbsp	120	14	2	0	0	0	0
Regular	1 tbsp	120	14	2	0	0	0	0
SOYBEANS								
Boiled	1 cup	298	15	2	2	17	10	29
Curd cheese	1 cup	340	18	3	45	16	0	28
Dry roasted	1 cup	776	37	5	3	56	14	68
Fresh	1 cup	830	37	5	4	56	17	68
Green, boiled	1 cup	254	12	1	25	20	8	22
Green, fresh	1 cup	376	17	2	38	28	11	33
Roasted	1 cup	810	44	6	7	58	30	61
Sprouted, fresh	1 cup	85	5	1	10	7	1	9
Sprouted, steamed	1 cup	76	4	1	9	6	1	8
Sprouted, steamed, w/ salt	1 cup	76	4	1	231	6	1	8
SOY CHIPS (or crisps, salted)	1 oz	107	2	0	239	15	1	8
SOY CREAMER								
Silk French Vanilla Creamer	1 tbsp	20	1	0	10	3	0	0
Silk Hazelnut Creamer	1 tbsp	20	1	0	10	3	0	0
Silk Original Creamer	1 tbsp	15	1	0	10	1	0	0
SOY FLOUR								
Defatted	1 cup	346	1	0	21	40	18	49
Defatted, crude protein, stirred	1 cup	372	9	1	9	31	16	50
Full fat, fresh, crude protein, stirred	1 cup	369	18	3	11	27	8	32
Full fat, fresh, stirred	1 cup	366	17	3	11	30	8	29

ITEM DESCRIPTION	Serving Size	Calories	Total Fat (g)	Saturated Fat (g)	Sodium (mg)	Carbohydrates (g)	Fiber (g)	Protein (g)
Full fat, roasted, crude protein, stirred	1 cup	373	19	3	10	26	0	32
Full fat, roasted, stirred	1 cup	375	19	3	10	29	8	30
Low fat, crude protein, stirred	1 cup	325	6	1	16	30	9	45
Low fat, stirred	1 cup	330	8	1	8	31	14	40
SOY MEAL (defatted, fresh)	1 cup	414	3	0	4	49	0	55
SOYMILK								
All flavors, enhanced	1 cup	109	5	1	122	8	1	7
All flavors, lowfat	1 cup	100	2	0	90	18	2	4
All flavors, nonfat	1 cup	66	0	0	139	10	1	6
All flavors, unsweetened	1 cup	80	4	1	90	4	1	7
Chocolate	1 cup	153	4	1	129	24	1	5
Chocolate & other flavors, light	1 cup	114	2	0	112	20	2	5
Original & vanilla	1 cup	104	4	0	114	12	1	6
Original & vanilla, light	1 cup	73	2	0	117	9	1	6
Original & vanilla, light, unsweetened	1 cup	83	2	0	153	9	2	6
Silk, chai	1 cup	129	4	1	100	19	0	6
Silk, chocolate	1 cup	141	4	1	100	23	2	5
Silk, coffee	1 cup	151	4	1	100	25	0	5
Silk, light, chocolate	1 cup	119	2	0	100	22	2	5
Silk, light, plain	1 cup	70	2	0	119	8	1	6
Silk, light, vanilla	1 cup	80	2	0	95	10	1	6
Silk, mocha	1 cup	141	4	1	100	22	0	5
Silk, nog	1/2 cup	90	2	0	74	15	0	3
Silk, plain	1 cup	100	4	1	119	8	1	7
Silk Plus Fiber	1 cup	100	4	1	95	14	5	6
Silk Plus, for bone health	1 cup	100	4	1	95	11	2	6
Silk Plus Omega-3 DHA	1 cup	109	5	1	119	8	1	7
Silk, unsweetened	1 cup	80	4	1	85	4	1	7
Silk, vanilla	1 cup	100	4	1	95	10	1	6
Silk, very vanilla	1 cup	129	4	1	141	19	1	6
Vitasoy, light, vanilla	1 cup	73	2	0	119	10	0	4
Vitasoy Organic Classic Original Soymilk	1 cup	114	4	1	160	11	1	8

ITEM DESCRIPTION	Serving Size	Calories	Total Fat (g)	Saturated Fat (g)	Sodium (mg)	Carbohydrates (g)	Fiber (g)	Protein (g)
Vitasoy Organic Creamy Original Soymilk	1 cup	107	4	0	160	11	1	7
SOY PROTEIN								
Concentrate, acid wash	1 oz	94	0	0	255	9	2	16
Concentrate, alcohol extraction	1 oz	94	0	0	1	9	2	16
Isolate	1 oz	96	1	0	285	2	2	23
Isolate, potassium type	1 oz	92	0	0	14	3	2	23
SOY SAUCE								
Made from hydrolyzed vegetable protein	1 tbsp	7	0	0	1024	1	0	0
Made from soy & wheat (shoyu)	1 tbsp	8	0	0	902	1	0	1
Made from soy & wheat (shoyu), low sodium	1 tbsp	8	0	0	533	1	0	1
Made from soy (tamari)	1 tbsp	11	0	0	1005	1	0	2
SOY YOGURT								
Silk, banana strawberry	1 container	150	2	0	26	29	1	4
Silk, black cherry	1 container	150	2	0	20	29	1	4
Silk, blueberry	1 container	150	2	0	26	29	1	4
Silk, key lime	1 container	150	2	0	26	30	1	4
Silk, peach	1 container	160	2	0	26	32	1	4
Silk, plain	1 container	150	4	0	30	22	1	6
Silk, raspberry	1 container	150	2	0	26	30	1	4
Silk, strawberry	1 container	160	2	0	26	31	1	4
Silk, vanilla, family size	1 container	179	4	0	30	31	1	6
Silk, vanilla, single serving	1 container	150	3	0	20	25	1	5
SPAGHETTI SAUCE								
(marinara, ready to serve)	1 cup	224	7	2	1054	35	7	5
SPAGHETTI SQUASH								
Boiled or baked	1 cup	42	0	0	28	10	2	1
Fresh, cubed	1 cup	31	1	0	17	7	0	1
SPAM								
Hormel luncheon meat, pork & chicken, canned, light	2 oz	107	8	3	578	1	0	9
Hormel luncheon meat, pork w/ ham, canned	2 oz	174	15	6	767	2	0	7

ITEM DESCRIPTION	Serving Size	Calories	Total Fat (g)	Saturated Fat (g)	Sodium (mg)	Carbohydrates (g)	Fiber (g)	Protein (g)
SPEARMINT								
Dried	1 tbsp	5	0	0	6	1	0	0
Fresh	2 tbsp	5	0	0	3	1	1	0
SPELT (cooked)	1 cup	246	2	0	10	51	8	11
SPICES								
Oregano, dried	1 tsp	3	0	0	0	1	0	0
Tarragon, dried	1 tsp	2	0	0	0	0	0	0
Thyme, dried	1 tsp	3	0	0	1	1	0	0
SPINACH								
Boiled	1 cup	41	0	0	126	7	4	5
Canned	1 cup	44	1	0	746	7	4	5
Canned, drained	1 cup	49	1	0	58	7	5	6
Canned, no salt	1 cup	44	1	0	176	7	5	5
Fresh	1 cup	7	0	0	24	1	1	1
Frozen, chopped or leaf	1 cup	45	1	0	115	7	5	6
Frozen, chopped or leaf, boiled	10 oz pkg	75	2	0	213	11	8	9
New Zealand, boiled, chopped	1 cup	22	0	0	193	4	0	2
New Zealand, fresh, chopped	1 cup	8	0	0	73	1	0	1
SPINACH SOUFFLÉ	1 cup	233	18	8	770	8	1	11
SPLIT PEAS								
Boiled	1 cup	231	1	0	4	41	16	16
Fresh	1 cup	672	2	0	30	119	50	48
SPORTS DRINKS								
Fluid replacement, electrolyte solution	8 fl oz	25	0	0	252	6	0	0
Fruit flavored, low calorie	8 fl oz	26	0	0	84	7	0	0
Gatorade, fruit flavored	8 fl oz	63	0	0	95	16	0	0
Powerade, lemon-lime	8 fl oz	78	0	0	54	19	0	0
Propel Fitness Water, fruit flavored	8 fl oz	12	0	0	31	3	0	0
SPOT (cooked in dry heat)	3 oz	134	5	2	31	0	0	20
SPRING ONIONS (fresh, chopped)	1 tbsp	2	0	0	1	0	0	0
SQUID (fried)	3 oz	149	6	2	260	7	0	15
STRAWBERRIES								
Canned in heavy syrup	1 cup	234	1	0	10	60	4	1

ITEM DESCRIPTION	Serving Size	Calories	Total Fat (g)	Saturated Fat (g)	Sodium (mg)	Carbohydrates (g)	Fiber (g)	Protein (g)
Fresh, halved	1 cup	49	0	0	2	12	3	1
Frozen, sweetened, whole	1 cup	199	0	0	3	54	5	1
Frozen, sweetened, slices	1 cup	245	0	0	8	66	5	1
Frozen, unsweetened	1 cup	77	0	0	4	20	5	1
STRAWBERRY-FLAVOR DRINK								
(mix, powder, prepared w/ whole milk)	8 fl oz	234	8	5	128	33	0	8
STRAWBERRY TOPPING	2 tbsp	107	0	0	9	28	0	0
STRIPED BASS (cooked in dry heat)	3 oz	105	3	1	75	0	0	19
STUFFING								
Brownberry, sage & onion mix	1 serv	261	3	1	1126	49	4	9
Stove Top, chicken flavor, prepared	1/2 cup	107	1	0	429	20	1	4
STURGEON								
Cooked in dry heat	3 oz	115	4	1	59	0	0	18
Smoked	1 oz	49	1	0	210	0	0	9
SUCCOTASH								
Boiled	1 cup	221	2	0	33	47	9	10
Canned, w/ cream style corn	1 cup	205	1	0	652	47	8	7
Canned, w/ whole kernel corn	1 cup	161	1	0	564	36	7	7
Frozen, boiled	1 cup	158	2	0	76	34	7	7
SUCKER (white, cooked in dry heat)	3 oz	101	3	0	43	0	0	18
SUGAR								
Brown	1 cup	836	0	0	62	216	0	0
Granulated	1 tsp	16	0	0	0	4	0	0
Maple	1 tsp	11	0	0	0	3	0	0
Powdered, sifted	1 cup	389	0	0	1	100	0	0
Powdered, unsifted	1 cup	467	0	0	1	120	0	0
SUMMER SQUASH								
All varieties, boiled, slices	1 cup	36	1	0	2	8	3	2
All varieties, fresh, slices	1 cup	18	0	0	2	4	1	1
SUNFISH								
(pumpkin seed, cooked in dry heat)	3 oz	97	1	0	88	0	0	21
SUNFLOWER OIL								
High oleic, 70% & over	1 tbsp	124	14	1	0	0	0	0
Linoleic, 65%	1 tbsp	120	14	1	0	0	0	0

ITEM DESCRIPTION	Serving Size	Calories	Total Fat (g)	Saturated Fat (g)	Sodium (mg)	Carbohydrates (g)	Fiber (g)	Protein (g)
Linoleic, hydrogenated	1 tbsp	120	14	2	0	0	0	0
Linoleic, less than 60%	1 tbsp	120	14	1	0	0	0	0
SUNFLOWER SEED BUTTER								
w/o salt	1 tbsp	93	8	1	0	4	0	3
w/ salt	1 tbsp	93	8	1	83	4	0	3
SUNFLOWER SEED FLOUR								
(part defatted)	1 cup	209	1	0	2	23	3	31
SUNFLOWER SEEDS								
Dry roasted, w/ salt	1 cup	745	64	7	525	31	12	25
Oil roasted, w/o salt	1 cup	799	69	10	4	31	14	27
Oil roasted, w/ salt	1 cup	799	69	10	554	31	14	27
Toasted, w/o salt	1 cup	829	76	8	4	28	15	23
Toasted, w/ salt	1 cup	829	76	8	821	28	15	23
SURIMI	3 oz	84	1	0	122	6	0	13
SWAMP CABBAGE								
Boiled, chopped	1 cup	20	0	0	120	4	2	2
Fresh, chopped	1 cup	11	0	0	63	2	1	1
SWEETENERS								
Aspartame, Equal	1 tsp	13	0	0	0	3	0	0
Fructose, dry, powder	1 tsp	15	0	0	1	4	0	0
Saccharine	1 pckt	4	0	0	4	1	0	0
Sucralose, Splenda	1 pckt	3	0	0	0	1	0	0
SWEET POTATO CHIPS	1 oz	141	7	1	10	18	1	1
SWEET POTATOES								
Canned in syrup	1 cup	203	0	0	100	48	6	2
Canned in syrup, drained	1 cup	212	1	0	76	50	6	3
Canned, mashed	1 cup	258	1	0	191	59	4	5
Canned, vacuum packed, mashed	1 cup	232	1	0	135	54	5	4
Cooked, baked in skin (5" long x 2" dia)	1 potato	103	0	0	41	24	4	2
Cooked, boiled, w/o skin, mashed	1 cup	249	0	0	89	58	8	4
Cooked, candied, homemade (2-1/1" x 2" dia)	1 pc	151	3	1	74	29	3	1
Fresh, cubed	1 cup	114	0	0	73	27	4	2

ITEM DESCRIPTION	Serving Size	Calories	Total Fat (g)	Saturated Fat (g)	Sodium (mg)	Carbohydrates (g)	Fiber (g)	Protein (g)
Frozen, baked, cubed	1 cup	176	0	0	14	41	3	3
Leaves, fresh, chopped	1 cup	12	0	0	3	2	1	1
Leaves, steamed	1 cup	22	0	0	8	5	1	1
SWISS CHARD								
Boiled, chopped	1 cup	35	0	0	313	7	4	3
Fresh	1 cup	7	0	0	77	1	1	1
SWORDFISH (cooked in dry heat)	3 oz	132	4	1	98	0	0	22
TABASCO SAUCE	1 tsp	1	0	0	30	0	0	0
TACO SAUCE								
Pace Green	2 tbsp	4	0	0	100	1	0	0
Pace Red	1 tbsp	8	0	0	130	2	0	0
TACO SEASONING MIX (Pace)	2 tbsp	10	0	0	428	3	1	0
TACO SHELLS baked (5" dia)	1	59	3	1	49	8	1	1
TAMARIND								
Nectar, canned	1 cup	143	0	0	18	37	1	0
Fresh	1 fruit	5	0	0	1	1	0	0
TANGERINE JUICE								
Canned, sweetened	1 cup	124	1	0	2	30	1	1
Fresh	1 cup	106	0	0	2	25	1	1
Frozen concentrate, sweetened	1 cup	111	0	0	2	27	0	1
TANGERINES								
Canned in juice	1 cup	92	0	0	12	24	2	2
Canned in juice, drained	1 cup	72	0	0	9	18	2	1
Canned in light syrup	1 cup	154	0	0	15	41	2	1
Fresh (2-1/4" dia)	1 fruit	40	0	0	2	10	1	1
TAPIOCA (pearl, dry)	1 cup	544	0	0	2	135	1	0
TARO								
Cooked, slices	1 cup	187	0	0	20	46	7	1
Fresh, slices	1 cup	116	0	0	11	28	4	2
Leaves, fresh	1 cup	12	0	0	1	2	1	1
Leaves, steamed	1 cup	35	1	0	3	6	3	4
Shoots, cooked, slices	1 cup	20	0	0	3	4	0	1
Shoots, fresh, slices	1 cup	9	0	0	1	2	0	1
Tahitian, cooked, slices	1 cup	60	1	0	74	9	0	6

ITEM DESCRIPTION	Serving Size	Calories	Total Fat (g)	Saturated Fat (g)	Sodium (mg)	Carbohydrates (g)	Fiber (g)	Protein (g)
Tahitian, fresh, slices	1 cup	55	1	0	62	9	0	3
Tomatoes, green, fresh	1 cup	41	0	0	23	9	2	2
TARO CHIPS	1 oz	141	7	2	97	19	2	1
TEA								
Brewed w/ distilled water	6 fl oz	2	0	0	0	1	0	0
Brewed w/ tap water	8 fl oz	2	0	0	7	1	0	0
Chamomile	6 fl oz	2	0	0	2	0	0	0
Herbal, other than chamomile	6 fl oz	2	0	0	2	0	0	0
Instant, sweetened w/ saccharine, lemon	8 fl oz	5	0	0	14	1	0	0
Instant, sweetened w/ sugar, lemon	8 fl oz	91	0	0	5	22	0	0
Instant, unsweetened	8 fl oz	2	0	0	10	0	0	0
TEA SEED OIL	1 tbsp	120	14	3	0	0	0	0
TEMPEH	1 cup	320	18	4	15	16	0	31
TEQUILA SUNRISE (canned)	1 fl oz	34	0	0	18	4	0	0
TERIYAKI SAUCE	1 tbsp	16	0	0	690	3	0	1
THYME (fresh)	1 tsp	1	0	0	0	0	0	0
TILAPIA (Beacon Light)	3 oz	85	1	0	35	1	0	15
TILEFISH (cooked in dry heat)	3 oz	125	4	1	50	0	0	21
TOASTER PASTRIES								
Brown sugar cinnamon	1 pastry	206	7	2	212	34	1	3
Fruit	1 pastry	211	6	1	180	37	1	3
Fruit, frosted	1 pastry	215	6	1	172	39	0	2
Kellogg's Low Fat Pop Tarts, frosted brown sugar cinnamon	1 pastry	188	3	1	210	39	1	2
Kellogg's Low Fat Pop Tarts, frosted chocolate fudge	1 pastry	190	3	1	249	40	1	3
Kellogg's Low Fat Pop Tarts, frosted strawberry	1 pastry	191	3	1	201	40	1	2
Kellogg's Low Fat Pop Tarts, strawberry	1 pastry	192	3	1	220	40	1	2
Kellogg's Pop Tarts, apple cinnamon	1 pastry	205	5	1	174	37	1	2
Kellogg's Pop Tarts, blueberry	1 pastry	212	7	1	207	36	1	2
Kellogg's Pop Tarts, brown sugar cinnamon	1 pastry	219	9	1	214	32	1	3

ITEM DESCRIPTION	Serving Size	Calories	Total Fat (g)	Saturated Fat (g)	Sodium (mg)	Carbohydrates (g)	Fiber (g)	Protein (g)
Kellogg's Pop Tarts, cherry	1 pastry	204	5	1	220	37	1	2
Kellogg's Pop Tarts, frosted blueberry	1 pastry	203	5	1	207	37	1	2
Kellogg's Pop Tarts, frosted brown sugar cinnamon	1 pastry	211	7	1	184	34	1	3
Kellogg's Pop Tarts, frosted cherry	1 pastry	204	5	1	220	37	1	2
Kellogg's Pop Tarts, frosted chocolate fudge	1 pastry	201	5	1	203	37	1	3
Kellogg's Pop Tarts, frosted chocolate vanilla cream	1 pastry	203	5	1	229	37	1	3
Kellogg's Pop Tarts, frosted grape	1 pastry	203	5	1	198	38	1	2
Kellogg's Pop Tarts, frosted raspberry	1 pastry	205	6	1	211	37	1	2
Kellogg's Pop Tarts, frosted strawberry	1 pastry	203	5	1	169	38	1	2
Kellogg's Pop Tarts, frosted wild berry	1 pastry	210	5	1	168	39	1	2
Kellogg's Pop Tarts, s'mores	1 pastry	204	5	1	199	36	1	3
Kellogg's Pop Tarts, strawberry	1 pastry	205	5	2	185	37	1	2
TOFU								
Dried, frozen (koyadofu)	1 pc	82	5	1	1	2	1	8
Ex firm, prepared w/ nigari	1/5 block	83	5	0	7	2	0	9
Firm, prepared w/ nigari	1/5 block	64	4	1	11	2	1	7
Fried	1 pc	35	3	0	2	1	1	2
Hard, prepared w/ nigari	1/4 block	178	12	2	2	5	1	15
Okara	1 cup	94	2	0	11	15	0	4
Salted & fermented (fuyu)	1 block	13	1	0	316	1	0	1
Soft, prepared w/ nigari	1/5 block	55	3	0	7	2	0	6
Mori-Nu, silken, ex firm	1 slice	46	2	0	53	2	0	6
Mori-Nu, silken, firm	1 slice	52	2	0	30	2	0	6
Mori-Nu, silken, lite, ex firm	1 slice	32	1	0	82	1	0	6
Mori-Nu, silken, lite, firm	1 slice	31	1	0	71	1	0	5
Mori-Nu, silken, soft	1 slice	46	2	0	4	2	0	4
Nasoya Lite, firm	1/4 pkg	43	1	0	27	1	1	7
Nasoya Organic, ex firm	1/5 pkg	77	4	1	3	2	1	8

ITEM DESCRIPTION	Serving Size	Calories	Total Fat (g)	Saturated Fat (g)	Sodium (mg)	Carbohydrates (g)	Fiber (g)	Protein (g)
Nasoya Organic, firm	1/5 pkg	66	3	0	3	2	1	7
Nasoya Organic, super firm, cubed	1/5 pkg	96	5	1	5	3	2	10
TOFU YOGURT	1 cup	246	5	1	92	42	1	9
TOMATILLOS (fresh)	1 med	11	0	0	0	2	1	0
TOMATO CHILI SAUCE								
Bottled, w/o salt	1 tbsp	18	0	0	3	5	0	0
Bottled, w/ salt	1 tbsp	18	0	0	228	3	1	0
TOMATO JUICE								
Canned, w/o salt	1 cup	41	0	0	24	10	1	2
Canned, w/ salt	1 cup	41	0	0	654	10	1	2
Campbell's	8 oz	49	0	0	680	10	2	2
Campbell's Healthy Request	8 oz	51	0	0	481	10	2	2
Campbell's, low sodium	8 oz	49	0	0	141	10	2	2
Campbell's Organic	8 oz	49	0	0	680	10	2	2
Tomato & vegetable, low sodium	1 cup	53	0	0	169	11	2	1
TOMATO PASTE								
Canned, w/o added salt	1/2 cup	107	1	0	128	25	5	6
Canned, w/ salt	1/2 cup	107	1	0	1035	25	5	6
TOMATO PUREE								
Canned, w/o salt	1 cup	95	1	0	70	22	5	4
Canned, w/ salt	1 cup	95	1	0	998	22	5	4
TOMATOES								
Cherry	1 cup	27	0	0	7	6	2	1
Orange, fresh	1 tomato	18	0	0	47	4	1	1
Red, canned, packed in tomato juice	1 cup	41	0	0	343	10	2	2
Red, canned, packed in tomato juice, no salt added	1 cup	41	0	0	24	10	2	2
Red, canned, stewed	1 cup	66	0	0	564	16	3	2
Red, canned, w/ green chilies	1 cup	36	0	0	966	9	0	2
Red, cooked	1 cup	43	0	0	26	10	2	2
Red, stewed	1 cup	80	3	1	460	13	2	2
Red, w/ salt	1 cup	43	0	0	593	10	2	2
Sun-dried	1 cup	139	2	0	1131	30	7	8

ITEM DESCRIPTION	Serving Size	Calories	Total Fat (g)	Saturated Fat (g)	Sodium (mg)	Carbohydrates (g)	Fiber (g)	Protein (g)
Sun-dried, packed in oil, drained	1 cup	234	15	2	293	26	6	6
Yellow, fresh, chopped	1 cup	21	0	0	32	4	1	1
TOMATO SAUCE								
Canned	1 cup	59	0	0	1284	13	4	3
Canned, Spanish style	1 cup	81	1	0	1152	18	3	4
Canned, w/ herbs & cheese	1 cup	144	5	2	1325	25	5	5
Canned, w/ mushrooms	1 cup	86	0	0	1107	21	4	4
Canned, w/ onions	1 cup	103	0	0	1350	24	4	4
Canned, w/ onions, greens peppers & celery	1 cup	102	2	0	1365	22	4	2
Canned, w/ tomato tidbits	1 cup	78	1	0	37	17	3	3
No salt	1 cup	102	0	0	27	21	4	3
TOMATO SEED OIL	1 tbsp	120	14	3	0	0	0	0
TONIC WATER	1 fl oz	10	0	0	4	3	0	0
TORTILLA CHIPS								
Low fat, baked w/o fat	1 oz	118	2	0	119	23	2	3
Low fat, made w/ Olestra, nacho cheese	1 oz	90	1	0	171	18	2	2
Low fat, unsalted	1 oz	118	2	0	4	23	2	3
Nacho cheese	1 oz	146	7	1	174	18	1	2
Nacho, made w/ masa flour	1 oz	141	7	1	201	18	2	2
Nacho, reduced fat	1 oz	126	4	1	284	20	1	2
Plain	1 oz	139	7	1	119	19	2	2
Plain, yellow corn	1 oz	139	6	1	80	19	1	2
Ranch flavor	1 oz	142	7	1	147	18	1	2
Taco flavor	1 oz	136	7	1	223	18	2	2
Unsalted, white corn	1 cup	131	6	1	4	17	1	2
TORTILLAS								
Corn (6" dia)	1 tortilla	58	1	0	3	12	1	1
Flour (6" dia)	1 tortilla	94	2	1	191	15	1	2
Mission Foods Four Tortillas, soft taco (8")	1 serv	146	3	0	249	25	0	4
TOWEL GOURD								
Boiled (1" pcs)	1 cup	100	1	0	37	26	0	1
Fresh (1" pcs)	1 cup	19	0	0	3	4	0	1

ITEM DESCRIPTION	Serving Size	Calories	Total Fat (g)	Saturated Fat (g)	Sodium (mg)	Carbohydrates (g)	Fiber (g)	Protein (g)
TRAIL MIX								
Regular	1 cup	693	44	8	344	67	0	21
Reg, unsalted	1 cup	693	44	8	15	67	0	21
Reg, w/ chocolate chips, salted nuts & seeds	1 cup	707	47	9	177	66	0	21
Reg, w/ chocolate chips, unsalted nuts & seeds	1 cup	707	47	9	39	66	0	21
Tropical	1 cup	570	24	12	14	92	0	9
TREE FERN (cooked, chopped)	1/2 cup	28	0	0	4	8	3	0
TROUT								
Cooked in dry heat	3 oz	162	7	1	57	0	0	23
Rainbow, farmed, cooked in dry heat	3 oz	144	6	2	36	0	0	21
Rainbow, wild, cooked in dry heat	3 oz	128	5	1	48	0	0	19
TUNA								
Bluefin, fresh, cooked in dry heat	3 oz	156	5	1	42	0	0	25
Canned in oil, drained	3 oz	158	7	1	337	0	0	23
Canned in oil, w/o salt, drained	3 oz	168	7	1	42	0	0	25
Canned in water, drained	3 oz	99	1	0	287	0	0	22
Canned in water, w/o salt, drained	3 oz	99	1	0	42	0	0	22
Skipjack, fresh, cooked in dry heat	3 oz	112	1	0	40	0	0	24
White, canned in oil, drained	3 oz	158	7	1	337	0	0	23
White, canned in oil, w/o salt, drained	3 oz	158	7	1	42	0	0	23
White, canned in water, drained	3 oz	109	3	1	320	0	0	20
White, canned in water, w/o salt, drained	3 oz	109	3	1	42	0	0	20
Yellowfin, fresh	3 oz	92	1	0	31	0	0	20
Yellowfin, fresh, cooked in dry heat	3 oz	118	1	0	40	0	0	25
TUNA SALAD	3 oz	159	8	1	342	8	0	14
TURBOT (European, cooked in dry heat)	3 oz	104	3	0	163	0	0	17
TURKEY								
Back, w/ skin, roasted, chopped	1 cup	340	20	6	102	0	0	37
Breast meat (3-1/2" sq)	1 slice	22	0	0	213	1	0	4
Breast, pre-basted, w/ skin, roasted	1/2 breast	1089	30	8	3430	0	0	191

ITEM DESCRIPTION	Serving Size	Calories	Total Fat (g)	Saturated Fat (g)	Sodium (mg)	Carbohydrates (g)	Fiber (g)	Protein (g)
Breast, smoked, lemon pepper flavor, 97% fat free	1 slice	27	0	0	325	0	0	6
Breast, w/ skin, roasted	1/2 breast	1633	64	18	544	0	0	248
Canned, meat only, broth drained	1 cup	220	9	3	630	0	0	32
Dark meat, roasted, chopped	1 cup	262	10	3	111	0	0	40
Dark meat, w/ skin, roasted, chopped	1 cup	309	16	5	106	0	0	38
Fryer-roasters, back, meat only, roasted	1/2 back	168	6	2	72	0	0	28
Fryer-roasters, back, w/ skin, roasted	1/2 back	265	13	4	91	0	0	34
Fryer-roasters, breast, meat only, roasted	1/2 breast	413	2	1	159	0	0	92
Fryer-roasters, breast, w/ skin, roasted	1/2 breast	526	11	3	182	0	0	100
Fryer-roasters, dark meat, meat only, roasted, chopped	1 cup	227	6	2	111	0	0	40
Fryer-roasters, leg, meat only, roasted	1 leg	356	8	3	181	0	0	65
Fryer-roasters, leg, w/ skin, roasted	1 leg	416	13	4	196	0	0	70
Fryer-roasters, light meat, meat only, roasted, chopped	1 cup	196	2	1	78	0	0	42
Fryer-roasters, meat only, roasted, chopped	1 cup	210	4	1	94	0	0	41
Fryer-roasters, wing, meat only, roasted	1 wing	98	2	1	47	0	0	19
Fryer-roasters, wing, w/ skin, roasted	1 wing	186	9	2	66	0	0	25
Giblets, simmered, some giblet fat, chopped	1 cup	289	17	6	93	1	0	30
Gizzards, simmered	1 gizzard	108	3	1	56	0	0	18
Ground, cooked (4 oz)	1 patty	193	11	3	88	0	0	22
Heart, simmered	1 heart	29	1	0	19	0	0	5
Leg, w/ skin, roasted	1 leg	1136	54	17	420	0	0	152
Light & dark meat, seasoned, diced	3 oz	117	5	1	723	1	0	16
Light meat, roasted, chopped	1 cup	220	5	1	90	0	0	42
Light meat, w/ skin, roasted, chopped	1 cup	276	12	3	88	0	0	40

ITEM DESCRIPTION	Serving Size	Calories	Total Fat (g)	Saturated Fat (g)	Sodium (mg)	Carbohydrates (g)	Fiber (g)	Protein (g)
Liver, simmered	1 liver	227	17	6	46	1	0	17
Meat & skin, roasted, chopped	1 cup	291	14	4	95	0	0	39
Meat only, roasted, chopped	1 cup	238	7	2	98	0	0	41
Neck, meat only, simmered	1 neck	274	11	4	85	0	0	41
Patties, breaded, battered, fried (2-1/4 oz)	1 patty	181	12	3	512	10	0	9
Roast, boneless, frozen, seasoned, light & dark meat, roasted, chopped	1 cup	209	8	3	918	4	0	29
Skin only, roasted	1/2 turkey	1096	98	26	131	0	0	49
Sticks, breaded, battered, fried (2-1/4 oz)	1 stick	179	11	3	536	11	0	9
Thigh, pre-basted, w/ skin, roasted	1 thigh	493	27	8	1372	0	0	59
Wing, w/ skin, roasted	1 wing	426	23	6	113	0	0	51
Cooked	1 cup, pcs	313	23	7	1874	3	0	24
Louis Rich	1 serv	35	3	1	170	0	0	2
TURKEY BOLOGNA (Louis Rich)	1 serv	52	4	1	302	1	0	3
TURKEY BREAST								
Carl Buddig, light & dark meat, smoked	2 oz	91	5	2	625	1	0	10
Louis Rich, Carving Board, smoked	1 serv	42	0	0	540	1	0	9
Louis Rich, fat free, oven roasted	1 serv	24	0	0	334	1	0	4
Louis Rich, honey roasted, fat free	1 serv	57	0	0	661	3	0	11
Louis Rich, oven roasted	1 serv	28	1	0	270	1	0	5
Louis Rich, portion fat free, oven roasted	1 serv	50	0	0	659	1	0	11
Louis Rich, portion fat free, smoked	1 serv	52	0	0	721	1	0	11
Louis Rich, smoked	1 serv	28	1	0	257	1	0	5
Oscar Mayer, fat free, smoked	1 slice	10	0	0	142	0	0	2
TURKEY FAT	1 tbsp	115	13	4	0	0	0	0
TURKEY HAM								
Cured, thigh meat	1 oz	35	1	0	312	1	0	5
Dark meat, smoked, frozen	1 oz	33	1	0	258	1	0	5
Ex lean, prepackaged or deli slices	1 cup, pcs	171	5	2	1432	4	0	27

ITEM DESCRIPTION	Serving Size	Calories	Total Fat (g)	Saturated Fat (g)	Sodium (mg)	Carbohydrates (g)	Fiber (g)	Protein (g)
Louis Rich Turkey Ham	1 serv	32	1	0	316	0	0	5
TURKEY NUGGETS (Louis Rich, breaded)	1 pc	77	5	1	190	4	0	4
TURKEY PASTRAMI	2 slices	76	4	1	559	1	0	9
TURKEY PEPPERONI (Hormel, slices)	1 serv	73	3	1	557	1	0	9
TURKEY POT PIE (frozen)	1 serv	699	35	11	1390	70	4	26
TURKEY ROLL								
Light meat	1 slice, oval	25	0	0	271	1	0	4
Light & dark meat	2 slices	85	4	1	334	1	0	10
TURKEY SALAMI								
Cooked	1 serv	47	3	1	281	0	0	5
Louis Rich Turkey Salami	1 serv	41	3	1	281	0	0	4
Louis Rich Turkey Salami Cotto	1 serv	42	3	1	285	0	0	4
TURKEY SAUSAGE								
Breakfast links, mild	1 oz link	65	5	1	164	0	0	4
Hot, smoked	1 oz link	44	2	1	260	1	0	4
Italian, smoked	1 oz link	44	2	0	260	1	0	4
Louis Rich Turkey Smoked Sausage	2 oz	90	6	1	530	2	0	8
Reduced fat, brown & serve	1 oz link	32	2	0	99	2	0	3
TURKEY TACO MEAT (frozen, cooked)	1 cup	271	14	3	1157	6	0	31
TURMERIC (ground)	1 tbsp	24	1	0	3	4	1	1
TURNIP GREENS								
Boiled, chopped	1 cup	29	0	0	42	6	5	2
Canned, no salt added	1 cup	27	0	0	42	4	2	2
Fresh, chopped	1 cup	18	0	0	22	4	2	1
Frozen, boiled	1 cup	48	1	0	25	8	6	5
TURNIPS								
Boiled, mashed	1 cup	51	0	0	37	12	5	2
Fresh	1 large	51	0	0	123	12	3	2
Frozen, boiled	1 cup	36	0	0	56	7	3	2
UCUHUBA BUTTER	1 tbsp	120	14	12	0	0	0	0
VANILLA EXTRACT								
Imitation, no alcohol	1 tbsp	7	0	0	0	2	0	0
Imitation, w/ alcohol	1 tbsp	31	0	0	1	0	0	0
Real	1 tbsp	37	0	0	1	2	0	0

ITEM DESCRIPTION	Serving Size	Calories	Total Fat (g)	Saturated Fat (g)	Sodium (mg)	Carbohydrates (g)	Fiber (g)	Protein (g)
VEAL								
Breast, fat, cooked	3 oz	443	45	18	42	0	0	8
Breast, plate half, boneless, braised	3 oz	240	16	6	54	0	0	22
Breast, point half, boneless, braised	3 oz	211	12	5	56	0	0	24
Breast, whole, boneless, braised	3 oz	226	14	6	55	0	0	23
Breast, whole, boneless, lean, braised	3 oz	185	8	3	58	0	0	26
Composite of retail cuts, fat, cooked	3 oz	546	57	28	48	0	0	8
Composite of retail cuts, lean & fat, cooked	3 oz	196	10	4	74	0	0	26
Composite of retail cuts, lean, cooked	3 oz	167	6	2	76	0	0	27
Cubed for stew, leg & shoulder, braised	3 oz	160	4	1	79	0	0	30
Ground, broiled	3 oz	146	6	3	71	0	0	21
Leg, top round, braised	3 oz	179	5	2	57	0	0	31
Leg, top round, pan fried, breaded	3 oz	202	8	3	386	8	0	23
Leg, top round, pan fried, not breaded	3 oz	179	7	3	65	0	0	27
Leg, top round, roasted	3 oz	136	4	2	58	0	0	24
Loin, braised	3 oz	241	15	6	68	0	0	26
Loin, lean, braised	3 oz	192	8	2	71	0	0	29
Loin, lean, roasted	3 oz	149	6	2	82	0	0	22
Loin, roasted	3 oz	184	10	4	79	0	0	21
Rib, braised	3 oz	213	11	4	81	0	0	28
Rib, roasted	3 oz	194	12	5	78	0	0	20
Shank, fore & hind, braised	3 oz	162	5	2	79	0	0	27
Shoulder, arm, braised	3 oz	201	9	3	74	0	0	29
Shoulder, arm, roasted	3 oz	156	7	3	76	0	0	22
Shoulder, blade, braised	3 oz	191	9	3	83	0	0	27
Shoulder, blade, roasted	3 oz	158	7	3	85	0	0	21
Sirloin, braised	3 oz	214	11	4	67	0	0	27
Sirloin, lean, braised	3 oz	173	6	2	69	0	0	29
Sirloin, lean, roasted	3 oz	143	5	2	72	0	0	22
Sirloin, roasted	3 oz	172	9	4	71	0	0	21
VEGETABLE BROTH								
Swanson	1 cup	12	0	0	940	3	0	0

ITEM DESCRIPTION	Serving Size	Calories	Total Fat (g)	Saturated Fat (g)	Sodium (mg)	Carbohydrates (g)	Fiber (g)	Protein (g)
Vegetable broth, Swanson Certified Organic	1 cup	12	0	0	550	3	0	0
VEGETABLE JUICE COCKTAIL (canned)	1 cup	46	0	0	653	11	2	2
VEGETABLE OIL (Enova)	1 tbsp	124	14	1	0	0	0	0
VEGETARIAN MEAT LOAF	1 slice	110	5	1	308	4	3	12
VEGETARIAN STEW	1 cup	304	7	1	988	17	3	42
VEGGIE BURGER								
Green Giant Harvest Burger, original, frozen	1 patty	138	4	1	411	7	6	18
Loma Linda Vege-Burger, canned	1/4 cup	63	1	0	122	2	1	12
Morningstar Farms Cheddar Burger, frozen	1 patty	142	7	2	458	10	3	13
Morningstar Farms Grillers, original, frozen	1 patty	136	6	1	270	5	3	15
Morningstar Farms Grillers, prime, frozen	1 patty	169	9	1	356	4	2	17
Morningstar Farms Grillers, recipe crumbles, frozen	.67 cup	72	2	0	235	4	3	10
Morningstar Farms Grillers, vegan, frozen	1 patty	94	2	0	280	6	4	12
Morningstar Farms Mushroom Lover's Burger, frozen	1 patty	108	6	1	221	8	1	7
Morningstar Farms Spicy Black Bean Burger, frozen	1 patty	115	4	1	348	13	5	11
Morningstar Farms Tomato & Basil Pizza Burger, frozen	1 patty	121	6	1	261	7	3	10
Worthington Vegetarian Burger, canned	1/4 cup	69	2	0	248	3	2	10
Veggie fillets	1 fillet	246	15	2	416	8	5	20
Veggie or soy burgers	1 patty	124	4	1	398	10	3	11
VEGGIE PATTIES								
Morningstar Farms Asian Veggie Patties, frozen	1 patty	104	4	1	486	10	2	7
Morningstar Farms Breakfast Patties, frozen	1 patty	78	3	0	240	4	2	8
Morningstar Farms Garden Veggie Patties, frozen	1 patty	118	4	1	352	9	3	12

ITEM DESCRIPTION	Serving Size	Calories	Total Fat (g)	Saturated Fat (g)	Sodium (mg)	Carbohydrates (g)	Fiber (g)	Protein (g)
Morningstar Farms Veggie Medley, frozen	1 patty	119	4	0	264	11	2	11
Worthington Fripats, frozen	1 patty	134	6	1	331	5	2	15
VENISON								
Ground, pan fried	1 patty	174	8	4	73	0	0	25
Loin, steak, lean, broiled	1 serv	81	1	0	31	0	0	16
VINEGAR								
Balsamic	1 tbsp	14	0	0	4	3	0	0
Cider	1 tbsp	3	0	0	1	0	0	0
Distilled	1 tbsp	3	0	0	0	0	0	0
Red wine	1 tbsp	3	0	0	1	0	0	0
VODKA								
80 proof	1 fl oz	64	0	0	0	0	0	0
86 proof	1 fl oz	70	0	0	0	0	0	0
90 proof	1 fl oz	73	0	0	0	0	0	0
94 proof	1 fl oz	76	0	0	0	0	0	0
WAFFLES								
Buttermilk, frozen, microwaved (4" dia)	1	101	3	1	232	15	1	2
Buttermilk, frozen, toasted (4" dia)	1	102	3	1	234	16	1	2
Plain, frozen, microwaved (4" dia)	1	95	3	1	218	15	1	2
Plain, frozen, toasted (4" dia)	1	103	3	1	241	16	1	2
Plain, homemade (7" dia)	1	218	11	2	383	25	0	6
Kellogg's Eggo Banana Bread Waffles	1	90	6	1	270	32	2	5
Kellogg's Eggo Golden Oat Waffles (4" dia)	1	69	1	0	135	13	1	2
Kellogg's Eggo Low Fat Blueberry Nutri-Grain Waffles (4" dia)	1	73	1	0	207	15	1	2
Kellogg's Eggo Low Fat Homestyle Waffles (4" dia)	1	83	1	0	155	15	0	2
Kellogg's Eggo Low Fat Nutri-Grain Waffles (4" dia)	1	71	1	0	215	14	1	2
WALLEYE POLLOCK (cooked in dry heat)	3 oz	96	1	0	99	0	0	20
WALNUT OIL	1 tbsp	120	14	1	0	0	0	0

ITEM DESCRIPTION	Serving Size	Calories	Total Fat (g)	Saturated Fat (g)	Sodium (mg)	Carbohydrates (g)	Fiber (g)	Protein (g)
WALNUTS								
Black, dried, chopped	1 cup	772	74	4	2	12	9	30
English, chopped	1 cup	765	76	7	2	16	8	18
WASABI ROOT (fresh, slices)	1 cup	142	1	0	22	31	10	6
WATER								
Aquafina	1 fl oz	0	0	0	0	0	0	0
Calistoga	1 fl oz	0	0	0	0	0	0	0
Crystal Geyser	1 fl oz	0	0	0	0	0	0	0
Dannon	1 fl oz	0	0	0	0	0	0	0
Dannon Fluoride to Go	1 fl oz	0	0	0	0	0	0	0
Dasani	1 fl oz	0	0	0	0	0	0	0
Evian	1 fl oz	0	0	0	0	0	0	0
Fruit flavored, sweetened, w/ added vits & minerals	1 fl oz	0	0	0	0	2	0	0
Fruit flavored, sweetened, w/ low calorie sweetener	1 fl oz	0	0	0	1	0	0	0
Generic, bottled	1 fl oz	0	0	0	1	0	0	0
Naya	1 fl oz	0	0	0	0	0	0	0
Perrier	1 fl oz	0	0	0	0	0	0	0
Poland Spring	1 fl oz	0	0	0	0	0	0	0
Tap, municipal	1 fl oz	0	0	0	1	0	0	0
Tap, well	1 fl oz	0	0	0	1	0	0	0
WATER CHESTNUTS								
Canned, slices	1/2 cup	35	0	0	6	9	2	1
Fresh, slices	1/2 cup	60	0	0	9	15	2	1
WATERCRESS (fresh, chopped)	1 cup	4	0	0	14	0	0	1
WATERMELON								
Fresh, diced	1 cup	46	0	0	2	12	1	1
Seeds, dried	1 cup	602	51	11	107	17	0	31
WAXGOURD								
Boiled, cubed	1 cup	24	0	0	187	5	2	1
Fresh, cubed	1 cup	17	0	0	147	4	4	1
WHEAT								
Durum	1 cup	651	5	1	4	137	0	26

ITEM DESCRIPTION	Serving Size	Calories	Total Fat (g)	Saturated Fat (g)	Sodium (mg)	Carbohydrates (g)	Fiber (g)	Protein (g)
Hard red spring	1 cup	632	4	1	4	131	23	30
Hard red winter	1 cup	628	3	1	4	137	23	24
Hard white	1 cup	657	3	1	4	146	23	22
Soft red winter	1 cup	556	3	0	3	125	21	17
Soft white	1 cup	571	3	1	3	127	21	18
Sprouted	1 cup	214	1	0	17	46	1	8
WHEAT BRAN (crude)	1 cup	125	2	0	1	37	25	9
WHEAT FLOUR								
White, all purpose, enriched, bleached	1 cup	455	1	0	2	95	3	13
White, all purpose, enriched, self rising	1 cup	442	1	0	1588	93	3	12
White, all purpose, enriched, unbleached	1 cup	455	1	0	2	95	3	13
White, all purpose, unenriched	1 cup	455	1	0	2	95	3	13
White, bread, enriched	1 cup	495	2	0	3	99	3	16
White, cake, enriched	1 cup	496	1	0	3	107	2	11
White, tortilla mix, enriched	1 cup	450	12	5	751	75	0	11
Whole grain	1 cup	407	2	0	6	87	15	16
WHEAT GERM	1 cup	414	11	2	14	60	15	27
WHEAT GERM OIL	1 tbsp	120	14	3	0	0	0	0
WHELK (cooked in moist heat)	3 oz	234	1	0	350	13	0	41
WHIPPED CREAM (topping, pressurized)	1 tbsp	8	1	0	4	0	0	0
WHIPPED TOPPING (frozen, low fat)	1 cup	168	10	8	54	18	0	2
WHISKEY								
80 proof	1 fl oz	64	0	0	0	0	0	0
86 proof	1 fl oz	70	0	0	0	0	0	0
90 proof	1 fl oz	73	0	0	0	0	0	0
94 proof	1 fl oz	76	0	0	0	0	0	0
WHISKEY SOUR								
Canned	1 fl oz	37	0	0	14	4	0	0
Prepared from bottled mix	1 fl oz	47	0	0	19	4	0	0
Prepared from bottled mix, w/sodium	1 fl oz	45	0	0	6	4	0	0

ITEM DESCRIPTION	Serving Size	Calories	Total Fat (g)	Saturated Fat (g)	Sodium (mg)	Carbohydrates (g)	Fiber (g)	Protein (g)
WHITE BEANS								
Boiled	1 cup	249	1	0	11	45	11	17
Canned	1 cup	299	1	0	13	56	13	19
Fresh	1 cup	673	1	0	32	122	31	47
Small, boiled	1 cup	254	1	0	4	46	19	16
Small, fresh	1 cup	722	3	1	26	134	54	45
WHITEFISH								
Cooked in dry heat	3 oz	146	6	1	55	0	0	21
Smoked	1 oz	30	0	0	285	0	0	7
WHITE SAUCE								
Homemade, med thick	1 cup	368	27	7	885	23	1	10
Homemade, thick	1 cup	465	35	9	932	29	1	10
Homemade, thin	1 cup	262	17	5	820	19	0	9
WHITING (cooked in dry heat)	3 oz	146	1	0	112	0	0	20
WINE								
All	1 fl oz	24	0	0	1	1	0	0
Cooking	1 fl oz	14	0	0	182	2	0	0
Dessert, dry	1 fl oz	45	0	0	3	3	0	0
Dessert, sweet	1 fl oz	47	0	0	3	4	0	0
Light	1 fl oz	14	0	0	2	0	0	0
Non-alcoholic	1 fl oz	2	0	0	2	0	0	0
Red	1 fl oz	25	0	0	1	1	0	0
Red, Barbera	1 fl oz	25	0	0	0	1	0	0
Red, Burgundy	1 fl oz	25	0	0	0	1	0	0
Red, Cabernet Franc	1 fl oz	24	0	0	0	1	0	0
Red, Cabernet Sauvignon	1 fl oz	24	0	0	0	1	0	0
Red, Carignane	1 fl oz	22	0	0	0	1	0	0
Red, Claret	1 fl oz	24	0	0	0	1	0	0
Red, Gamay	1 fl oz	23	0	0	0	1	0	0
Red, Lemberger	1 fl oz	24	0	0	0	1	0	0
Red, Merlot	1 fl oz	24	0	0	1	1	0	0
Red, Mouvedre	1 fl oz	26	0	0	0	1	0	0
Red, Petite Sirah	1 fl oz	25	0	0	0	1	0	0
Red, Pinot Noir	1 fl oz	24	0	0	0	1	0	0

ITEM DESCRIPTION	Serving Size	Calories	Total Fat (g)	Saturated Fat (g)	Sodium (mg)	Carbohydrates (g)	Fiber (g)	Protein (g)
Red, Sangiovese	1 fl oz	25	0	0	0	1	0	0
Red, Syrah	1 fl oz	24	0	0	0	1	0	0
Red, Zinfandel	1 fl oz	26	0	0	0	1	0	0
White	1 fl oz	24	0	0	1	1	0	0
White, Chenin Blanc	1 fl oz	24	0	0	0	1	0	0
White, Fume Blanc	1 fl oz	24	0	0	0	1	0	0
White, Gewurztraminer	1 fl oz	24	0	0	0	1	0	0
White, late harvest	1 fl oz	34	0	0	0	4	0	0
White, Muller Thurgau	1 fl oz	22	0	0	0	1	0	0
White, Muscat	1 fl oz	25	0	0	0	2	0	0
White, Pinot Blanc	1 fl oz	24	0	0	0	1	0	0
White, Pinot Gris (Grigio)	1 fl oz	24	0	0	0	1	0	0
White, Riesling	1 fl oz	24	0	0	0	1	0	0
White, Sauvignon Blanc	1 fl oz	24	0	0	0	1	0	0
White, Semillon	1 fl oz	24	0	0	0	1	0	0
WINGED BEANS								
Boiled	1 cup	253	10	1	22	26	0	18
Immature seeds, boiled	1 cup	24	0	0	2	2	0	3
Immature seeds, fresh, slices	1 cup	22	0	0	2	2	0	3
WINTER SQUASH								
All varieties, baked, cubed	1 cup	76	1	0	2	18	6	2
All varieties, fresh, cubed	1 cup	39	0	0	5	10	2	1
WOLFFISH								
(Atlantic, cooked in dry heat)	3 oz	105	3	0	93	0	0	19
WONTON WRAPPERS	1 wrapper	93	0	0	183	19	1	3
WORCESTERSHIRE SAUCE	1 tbsp	13	0	0	167	3	0	0
YAMS								
Boiled or baked, cubed	1 cup	158	0	0	11	37	5	2
Fresh, cubed	1 cup	177	0	0	14	42	6	2
Mountain, fresh, cubed	1 cup	91	0	0	18	22	0	2
Mountain, steamed, cubed	1 cup	119	0	0	17	29	0	3
YARD LONG BEANS								
Boiled, slices	1 cup	49	0	0	4	10	0	3
Fresh, slices	1 cup	43	0	0	4	8	0	3

ITEM DESCRIPTION	Serving Size	Calories	Total Fat (g)	Saturated Fat (g)	Sodium (mg)	Carbohydrates (g)	Fiber (g)	Protein (g)
Mature seeds, boiled	1 cup	202	1	0	9	36	6	14
Mature seeds, fresh	1 cup	579	2	1	28	103	18	41
YEAST								
Baker's, active dry	1 tsp	12	0	0	2	2	1	2
Baker's, compressed	0.6 oz cake	18	0	0	5	3	1	1
YEAST EXTRACT SPREAD	1 tsp	9	0	0	216	1	0	2
YELLOW BEANS								
Boiled	1 cup	255	2	0	9	45	18	16
Fresh	1 cup	676	5	1	24	119	49	43
YELLOWTAIL								
Cooked in dry heat	3 oz	159	6	0	43	0	0	25
Raw	3 oz	124	4	1	33	0	0	20
YOGURT								
Breyers Light n' Lively, strawberry	4.4 oz	135	1	1	56	27	0	4
Breyers Light, nonfat strawberry, w/aspartame & fructose	8 oz	125	0	0	102	22	0	8
Breyers, low fat strawberry	8 oz	218	2	1	118	41	0	9
Breyers Smooth & Creamy, low fat strawberry	8 oz	232	2	1	125	45	1	9
Dannon Fruit on the Bottom, Blueberry	6 oz	140	1.5	1	130	26	1	6
Dannon Light & Fit, Blueberry	1 serv	80	0	0	75	16	0	5
Fruit, low fat, 10 grams protein	8 fl oz	250	3	2	142	47	0	10
Fruit, low fat, 11 grams protein	8 fl oz	250	3	2	159	46	0	11
Fruit, low fat, 9 grams protein	8 fl oz	243	3	2	130	46	0	9
Fruit, low fat, w/ low calorie sweetener	8 fl oz	257	3	2	142	46	0	12
Fruit varieties, nonfat	8 fl oz	233	0	0	142	47	0	11
Plain, low fat	8 fl oz	154	4	2	172	17	0	13
Plain, skim milk	8 fl oz	137	0	0	189	19	0	14
Plain, whole milk	8 fl oz	149	8	5	113	11	0	9
Vanilla, low fat	8 fl oz	208	3	2	162	34	0	12
Yoplait Light, Harvest Peach	6 oz	100	0	0	85	19	0	5
Yoplait Original, Strawberry	6 oz	170	0	1	80	33	0	5

ITEM DESCRIPTION	Serving Size	Calories	Total Fat (g)	Saturated Fat (g)	Sodium (mg)	Carbohydrates (g)	Fiber (g)	Protein (g)
ZUCCHINI								
Baby, fresh	1 med	2	0	0	0	0	0	0
Boiled, w/ skin, slices	1 cup	29	0	0	5	7	3	1
Fresh, w/ skin	1 cup	18	0	0	11	4	1	1
Frozen, boiled, w/ skin	1 cup	38	0	0	4	8	3	3
Italian style, canned	1 cup	66	0	0	849	16	0	2

popular restaurants

ARBY'S

ITEM DESCRIPTION	Serving Size	Calories	Total Fat (g)	Saturated Fat (g)	Sodium (mg)	Carbohydrates (g)	Fiber (g)	Protein (g)
BEVERAGES								
Capri Sun Fruit Juice	1	100	0	0	30	24	0	0
Coffee	1 oz	5	0	0	0	0	0	2
Diet Pepsi®	22 oz	0	0	0	50	0	0	0
Dr Pepper®	22 oz	225	0	0	75	65	0	0
Iced FruiTea, Diet Blackberry	1	0	0	0	0	4	0	0
Iced FruiTea, Diet Peach	1	0	0	0	0	4	0	0
Iced FruiTea, Mandarin Peach	1	90	0	0	0	23	0	0
Iced FruiTea, Passion Fruit	1	100	0	0	0	25	0	0
Milk, 1% Low Fat Chocolate	1	180	3	2	19	32	1	8
Milk, 2% Reduced Fat White	1	118	5	3	116	12	0	8
Mountain Dew®	22 oz	230	0	0	70	60	0	0
Pepsi®	22 oz	210	0	0	50	58	0	0
Sierra Mist	22 oz	210	0	0	40	56	0	0
Tea, Sweet	16 oz	120	0	0	15	32	0	0
BREAKFAST ITEMS								
Biscuit	1	273	15	4	786	28	1	5
Biscuit w/ Bacon	1	340	21	6	1028	29	1	9
Biscuit w/ Bacon, Egg & Cheese	1	461	30	10	1446	30	1	17
Biscuit w/ Chicken	1	417	23	5	1240	39	1	15
Biscuit w/ Ham	1	323	17	4	1315	29	1	14
Biscuit w/ Ham, Egg & Cheese	1	444	26	8	1734	31	1	21
Biscuit w/ Sausage	1	436	31	9	1160	28	1	10
Biscuit w/ Sausage Gravy	1	1040	60	22	4700	107	1	7
Biscuit w/ Sausage, Egg & Cheese	1	557	40	13	1579	30	1	18
Croissant	1	190	10	6	190	21	1	3
Croissant w/ Bacon & Egg	1	337	22	10	651	23	1	11
Croissant w/ Bacon, Egg & Cheese	1	378	25	12	850	23	1	14
Croissant w/ Ham & Cheese	1	281	15	9	918	22	1	14
Croissant w/ Ham, Egg & Cheese	1	361	21	10	1138	23	1	19
Croissant w/ Sausage & Egg	1	433	32	13	784	23	1	12
Croissant w/ Sausage, Egg & Cheese	1	475	35	15	982	23	1	15

ITEM DESCRIPTION	Serving Size	Calories	Total Fat (g)	Saturated Fat (g)	Sodium (mg)	Carbohydrates (g)	Fiber (g)	Protein (g)
French Toastix	1	312	13	2	492	44	1	6
Muffin, Blueberry	1	320	12	2	490	49	1	4
Sausage Patty	1	210	20	7	480	0	0	6
Sourdough w/ Bacon, Egg & Cheese	1	437	21	8	1220	40	2	20
Sourdough w/ Egg & Cheese	1	392	17	7	1058	40	2	17
Sourdough w/ Ham, Egg & Cheese	1	442	19	7	1586	41	2	26
Sourdough w/ Sausage, Egg & Cheese	1	556	33	12	1431	40	2	22
Wrap w/ Bacon, Egg & Cheese	1	515	29	8	1367	50	2	16
Wrap w/ Ham, Egg, & Cheese	1	575	31	10	2005	51	2	25
Wrap w/ Sausage, Egg & Cheese	1	689	45	15	1849	50	2	21
DESSERTS								
Apple Turnover w/ Icing	1	380	14	7	287	58	3	4
Cherry Turnover w/ Icing	1	364	13	7	269	58	1	4
Chocolate Twist	1	250	12	4	110	34	2	4
Cinnamon Roll	1	330	15	5	540	42	2	6
Cinnamon Twist	1	260	13	7	210	32	2	4
Cookies, Chocolate Chunk	1	209	10	5	163	27	0	2
Shake, Chocolate Malt Swirl	1	620	17	10	454	101	1	16
Shake, Chocolate Swirl	1	620	17	10	449	101	1	16
Shake, Jamocha Swirl	1	611	17	10	485	99	1	16
Shake, Vanilla	1	572	18	11	458	86	0	17
Sticky Bun, Pecan	1	511	27	7	587	60	3	7
TJ Cinnamons Mocha Chill®	1	306	7	4	214	48	1	11
TJ Icing	1	119	5	3	58	18	0	0
DRESSINGS AND SPREADS								
Arby's Sauce	1 serv	15	0	0	177	4	0	0
Cheese Sauce, Cheddar	1 serv	25	2	0	182	2	0	0
Dipping Sauce, Barbecue	1 pkg	44	0	0	343	11	0	0
Dipping Sauce, Bronco Berry®	1 pkg	92	0	0	27	23	0	0
Dipping Sauce, Buffalo	1 pkg	10	0	0	790	2	0	0
Dipping Sauce, Honey Mustard	1 pkg	129	12	2	151	6	0	0
Dipping Sauce, Ranch	1 pkg	158	16	4	277	2	0	1
Dressing, Balsamic Vinaigrette	1 pkg	130	12	2	460	5	0	0
Dressing, Buttermilk Ranch	1 pkg	230	24	4	390	2	0	1

ITEM DESCRIPTION	Serving Size	Calories	Total Fat (g)	Saturated Fat (g)	Sodium (mg)	Carbohydrates (g)	Fiber (g)	Protein (g)
Dressing, Dijon Honey Mustard	1 pkg	180	17	3	240	0	0	1
Horsey Sauce®	1 serv	62	5	1	173	3	0	0
Ketchup	1 pkg	13	0	0	158	3	0	0
Mayonnaise	1 pkg	105	11	2	74	0	0	0
Sauce, Marinara	1 pkg	30	2	0	0	4	1	1
Spicy Three Pepper Sauce®	1 serv	22	1	0	140	3	0	0
Syrup	1 serv	78	0	0	25	20	0	0
Tangy Southwest Sauce®	1 serv	249	26	4	278	3	0	0
KIDS MENU								
Applesauce	1	90	0	0	10	22	2	0
Curly Fries Meal	1	234	14	3	548	27	3	3
Popcorn Chicken Meal	1	272	12	2	698	20	1	18
Roast Beef Sandwich Meal	1	272	10	4	740	34	2	16
SALADS								
Chopped Farmhouse Chicken Salad, Crispy	1	395	19	7	857	25	4	25
Chopped Farmhouse Chicken Salad, Grilled	1	229	11	6	579	9	3	20
Chopped Italian Salad	1	386	28	12	1420	11	3	21
Chopped Turkey Club Salad	1	230	11	6	801	9	3	22
SANDWICHES								
Arby-Q	1	340	11	4	1089	48	2	17
Arby's Melt	1	298	12	4	922	36	2	16
Beef 'n Cheddar	reg	440	21	6	1275	43	2	22
Chicken Fillet, Crispy	1	488	23	4	1210	47	2	26
Chicken Fillet, Roast	1	383	16	3	921	37	2	23
Chicken Salad w/ Pecans	1	769	39	10	1240	79	9	30
Chicken, Bacon & Swiss, Crispy	1	544	25	7	1632	50	2	32
Chicken, Bacon & Swiss, Roast	1	439	18	6	1343	40	2	30
Chicken, Cordon Bleu Sandwich, Crispy	1	577	28	7	1936	47	2	37
Chicken, Cordon Bleu Sandwich, Roast	1	472	20	6	1646	37	2	34
Corned Beef Reuben	1	590	32	9	1685	55	3	32
Ham & Swiss Melt	1	268	8	3	1042	35	1	17
Roast Beef	reg	320	14	5	953	34	2	21
Roast Beef Super	1	398	19	6	1060	40	2	21

ITEM DESCRIPTION	Serving Size	Calories	Total Fat (g)	Saturated Fat (g)	Sodium (mg)	Carbohydrates (g)	Fiber (g)	Protein (g)
Roast Chicken Club	1	498	20	7	1540	46	2	30
Roast Ham & Swiss	1	691	31	8	1952	75	5	33
Roast Turkey & Swiss	1	708	30	8	1677	74	5	41
Roast Turkey, Ranch & Bacon	1	818	38	11	2146	75	5	46
Roastburger, All American	1	408	18	7	1122	44	2	18
Roastburger, Bacon & Bleu	1	466	23	9	1375	44	2	21
Roastburger, Bacon Cheddar	1	443	18	8	1427	44	2	23
Sourdough Ham Melt	1	380	16	5	1280	39	2	19
Sourdough Roast Beef Melt	1	351	14	4	1048	40	2	17
Swiss Melt	1	303	12	4	919	37	2	16
Toasted Sub, Classic Italian	1	596	27	7	1831	65	3	25
Toasted Sub, French Dip & Swiss	1	533	19	8	2169	67	3	29
Toasted Sub, Philly Beef	1	610	30	9	1549	62	3	29
Toasted Sub, Turkey Bacon Club	1	605	24	6	1701	65	3	35
Ultimate BLT	1	779	45	11	1571	75	6	23
SIDES AND SNACKS								
Bacon	4 pcs	77	6	2	301	1	0	5
Cheddar Fries	med	546	33	5	1525	62	6	7
Curly Fries	med	496	29	5	1160	58	6	7
Double Meat for Roastburger	1 serv	119	9	4	532	0	0	13
Jalapeño Bites®	5 pcs	305	21	9	526	29	2	5
Loaded Potato Bites®	5 pcs	353	22	7	800	27	2	11
Mozzarella Sticks	4 pcs	426	28	13	1370	38	2	18
Onion Petals	reg	248	17	3	249	26	2	3
Popcorn Chicken	reg	363	16	3	930	27	2	24
Potato Cakes	3 pcs	369	28	5	587	39	3	3

AU BON PAIN

BAKED ITEMS

Bagel, Asiago Cheese	1	340	6	4	600	55	0	15
Bagel, Cinnamon Crisp	1	410	7	3	390	76	2	10
Bagel, Cinnamon Raisin	1	310	1	0	440	66	1	11
Bagel, Everything	1	340	5	0	980	62	1	13
Bagel, Honey 9 Grain	1	340	4	0	480	67	4	12

ITEM DESCRIPTION	Serving Size	Calories	Total Fat (g)	Saturated Fat (g)	Sodium (mg)	Carbohydrates (g)	Fiber (g)	Protein (g)
Bagel, Jalapeño Double Cheddar	1	340	10	5	630	52	0	17
Bagel, Onion Dill	1	290	1	0	440	58	1	11
Bagel, Plain	1	280	1	0	430	57	0	11
Bagel, Poppy	1	320	4	0	430	58	1	12
Bagel, Sesame Seed	1	320	5	1	430	58	1	12
Baguette, Artisan	sm	240	2	1	570	46	2	8
Baguette, Artisan	lg	310	3	1	760	62	3	10
Baguette, Artisan Honey Multigrain	sm	250	3	0	500	49	5	8
Baguette, Artisan Honey Multigrain	lg	340	4	0	670	66	6	11
Blondie	1	330	19	6	350	61	3	7
Bread Bowl	1	620	3	1	1690	121	1	26
Bread, Artisan Sundried Tomato	1	270	1	0	760	55	3	9
Bread, Country White	1	270	1	0	660	56	2	9
Bread, Whole Wheat Multigrain	1	260	3	0	630	53	9	11
Breadstick, Asiago	1	180	4	3	340	28	0	8
Breadstick, Cheddar Jalapeño	1	130	2	1	250	25	0	6
Breadstick, Cinnamon Raisin	1	180	0	0	220	40	1	6
Breadstick, Everything	1	170	3	0	490	31	0	7
Breadstick, Rosemary Garlic	1	180	5	1	710	30	1	6
Breadstick, Sesame	1	180	4	1	220	30	1	7
Brownie, Chocolate Cheesecake	1	370	14	4	260	58	1	5
Brownie, Chocolate Chip	1	380	17	5	390	62	1	5
Brownie, Hazelnut Mocha	1	430	21	5	360	58	3	6
Brownie, Rocky Road	1	410	17	5	430	62	2	6
Ciabatta	lg	300	1	0	780	61	3	10
Ciabatta	sm	180	1	0	470	37	2	6
Cinnamon Roll w/ Icing	1	400	15	8	270	60	2	8
Cookie, Chocolate Chip	1	260	12	6	220	37	1	2
Cookie, Confetti w/ M&M's	1	260	12	6	200	36	0	3
Cookie, English Toffee	1	230	13	5	170	26	1	2
Cookie, Mini Chocolate Chip	1	70	3	2	55	9	0	1
Cookie, Mini Oatmeal Raisin	1	60	2	1	50	9	1	1
Cookie, Oatmeal Raisin	1	230	8	4	190	36	2	3
Cookie, Shortbread	1	310	18	9	270	34	1	3

ITEM DESCRIPTION	Serving Size	Calories	Total Fat (g)	Saturated Fat (g)	Sodium (mg)	Carbohydrates (g)	Fiber (g)	Protein (g)
Cookie, White Chocolate Chunk Macadamia Nut	1	280	15	7	240	34	1	3
Crème de Fleur	1	490	25	14	410	57	2	11
Croissant, Almond	1	600	38	14	300	55	4	13
Croissant, Apple	1	270	11	6	160	44	3	5
Croissant, Chocolate	1	430	22	13	210	58	3	7
Croissant, Ham & Cheese	1	390	20	11	650	38	2	15
Croissant, Plain	1	300	17	9	220	31	1	6
Croissant, Raspberry Cheese	1	360	17	9	280	46	2	8
Croissant, Spinach & Cheese	1	290	16	9	300	28	2	10
Croissant, Sweet Cheese	1	390	19	10	310	48	2	9
Crumb Cake	1	470	25	13	780	56	1	5
Danish, Cherry	1	420	20	10	340	54	1	7
Danish, Lemon	1	440	20	10	360	57	1	7
Danish, Sweet Cheese	1	470	24	13	390	54	1	9
Farm House Roll	1	320	6	1	670	57	3	10
Focaccia	1	350	7	1	680	61	1	12
Lahvash	1	280	4	1	660	56	4	9
Macaroon, Chocolate Dipped Cranberry Almond	1	300	15	11	190	36	3	4
Muffin, Blueberry	1	490	17	2	500	74	2	9
Muffin, Carrot Walnut	1	520	25	6	800	66	4	8
Muffin, Chocolate Chip	1	580	23	6	480	83	3	9
Muffin, Corn	1	460	16	3	550	69	2	9
Muffin, Cranberry Walnut	1	500	23	2	450	61	4	9
Muffin, Double Chocolate Chunk	1	570	23	7	450	80	4	10
Muffin, Low-fat Triple Berry	1	290	2	0	490	67	2	3
Muffin, Raisin Bran	1	480	11	2	600	85	10	12
Muffin, Southwest Jalapeño	1	560	30	6	610	64	1	8
Palmier	1	440	23	15	330	53	1	1
Pecan Roll	1	630	32	11	330	80	3	10
Pound Cake, Banana Nut	1	520	28	5	470	60	1	7
Pound Cake, Lemon	1 pc	520	27	6	460	64	0	5
Pound Cake, Marble	1 pc	490	27	5	520	59	1	6

ITEM DESCRIPTION	Serving Size	Calories	Total Fat (g)	Saturated Fat (g)	Sodium (mg)	Carbohydrates (g)	Fiber (g)	Protein (g)
Pound Cake, Mint Chocolate	1	530	28	6	590	65	3	7
Scone, Chocolate Orange Pecan	1	580	28	13	360	74	3	10
Scone, Cinnamon	1	530	27	16	400	60	2	9
Scone, Orange	1	470	23	13	420	57	1	10
Shortbread, Chocolate Dipped	1	380	22	12	310	42	1	4
Strudel, Apple	1	430	24	13	270	48	1	5
Strudel, Cherry	1	460	26	16	270	49	2	5
Tulip, Chocolate Cherry	1	410	21	5	370	54	2	5
Tulip, Lemon Drop	1	410	19	5	330	55	1	5
BEVERAGES								
Caffe Americano	med (16 oz)	10	0	0	25	2	0	0
Caffe Latte	med (16 oz)	260	14	9	220	21	0	14
Cappuccino	med (16 oz)	150	8	5	110	13	0	8
Caramel Macchiato	med (16 oz)	430	12	8	190	68	0	12
Chai Latte	med (16 oz)	380	14	8	170	51	0	14
Chocolate Milk	sm (12 oz)	320	9	5	100	54	3	10
Diet Pepsi	med (22 oz)	0	0	0	70	0	0	0
Diet Sierra Mist	med (22 oz)	0	0	0	70	0	0	0
Hot Chocolate	med (16 oz)	460	15	9	170	74	4	16
Iced Caffe Latte	med (16 oz)	150	8	5	110	13	0	8
Iced Caramel Macchiato	med (16 oz)	390	10	6	160	65	0	10
Iced Chai Latte	med (16 oz)	260	7	5	90	42	0	7
Iced Coffee, Decaf French Roast	med (22 oz)	10	0	0	20	2	0	0
Iced Coffee, French Roast	med (22 oz)	10	0	0	20	2	0	0
Iced Coffee, French Vanilla	med (22 oz)	10	0	0	20	2	0	1
Iced Latte, Mocha	med (16 oz)	300	15	9	100	40	2	9
Iced Latte, Vanilla	med (16 oz)	330	7	5	95	59	0	7
Iced Latte, White Chocolate	med (16 oz)	330	13	8	190	51	0	6
Iced Tea, Peach	med (22 oz)	240	0	0	0	61	0	0
Latte, Mocha	med (16 oz)	390	20	12	200	48	2	13
Latte, Vanilla	med (16 oz)	410	12	7	150	66	0	12
Latte, White Chocolate	med (16 oz)	410	17	11	240	58	0	11
Lemonade	med (22 oz)	310	0	0	0	82	0	0
Mountain Dew	med (22 oz)	300	0	0	110	85	0	0

ITEM DESCRIPTION	Serving Size	Calories	Total Fat (g)	Saturated Fat (g)	Sodium (mg)	Carbohydrates (g)	Fiber (g)	Protein (g)
Orange Juice	sm (8 oz)	110	0	0	0	26	0	2
Orange Soda	med (22 oz)	360	0	0	70	96	0	0
Pepsi	med (22 oz)	280	0	0	55	77	0	0
Pepsi, Caffeine Free	med (22 oz)	280	0	0	55	77	0	0
Root Beer	med (22 oz)	280	0	0	110	80	0	0
Sierra Mist	med (22 oz)	280	0	0	70	72	0	0
Smoothie, Caramel Blast	med (16 oz)	540	17	12	105	104	0	6
Smoothie, Coffee Blast	med (16 oz)	440	21	15	115	71	0	8
Smoothie, Mocha Blast	med (16 oz)	440	17	12	95	80	2	7
Smoothie, Peach	med (16 oz)	310	1	0	115	69	4	4
Smoothie, Strawberry	med (16 oz)	310	1	0	110	66	3	4
Smoothie, Vanilla Blast	med (16 oz)	540	17	12	100	104	0	6
BREAKFAST ITEMS								
Apple Croissants Tart	1	80	4	2	55	12	1	1
Bagel w/ Bacon	1	340	6	2	640	57	0	16
Bagel w/ Bacon & Egg	1	420	8	3	990	60	0	25
Bagel w/ Bacon, Egg & Cheese	1	500	15	6	1120	59	0	30
Bagel w/ Egg	1	360	4	1	780	59	0	21
Bagel w/ Egg & Cheese	1	430	10	5	900	58	0	25
Bagel, Asiago w/ Prosciutto & Egg	1	520	16	7	1690	60	1	34
Bagel, Asiago w/ Sausage, Egg & Cheddar	1	810	47	23	1540	58	1	38
Bagel, Onion Dill w/ Smoked Salmon & Wasabi	1	430	11	5	1090	64	1	23
Ciabatta Melt w/ Bacon & Egg	1	500	26	14	1250	40	2	26
Eggs, Scrambled	1 serv	35	3	1	90	1	0	3
French Pecan Toast	1	70	4	2	45	8	0	2
Oatmeal	med (12 oz)	210	4	1	10	38	5	8
Pineapple Blueberry Cobbler	1	45	2	0	35	8	1	1
Portobello, Egg & Cheddar	1	490	26	13	1140	41	3	22
Potatoes, Roasted	1 serv	35	1	0	110	6	1	1
Quinoa, Cinnamon Walnut	1 serv	45	3	0	0	4	1	2
Salsa Verde Sandwich w/ Egg & Cheddar	1	450	22	12	1080	41	2	21
Sausage w/ Peppers & Onions	1 serv	50	5	2	90	1	0	2

ITEM DESCRIPTION	Serving Size	Calories	Total Fat (g)	Saturated Fat (g)	Sodium (mg)	Carbohydrates (g)	Fiber (g)	Protein (g)
Southwest Corn Casserole	1 serv	60	4	2	85	4	0	3
DRESSINGS AND SPREADS								
Artichoke Aioli	1 serv	70	6	1	230	2	0	1
Basil Pesto	1 serv	120	12	2	220	1	0	2
Chili Dijon	1 serv	120	12	2	130	3	1	1
Cream Cheese, Honey Pecan	1 serv	200	16	10	135	10	0	2
Cream Cheese, Lite	1 serv	120	9	6	280	5	0	4
Cream Cheese, Sundried Tomato	1 serv	140	11	7	170	5	1	4
Cream Cheese, Vegetable	1 serv	170	16	10	270	3	0	3
Dressing, Balsamic Vinaigrette	1 serv	120	9	2	360	8	0	0
Dressing, Blue Cheese	1 serv	310	33	6	460	2	0	2
Dressing, Caesar	1 serv	270	28	5	370	4	0	1
Dressing, Fat Free Raspberry Vinaigrette	1 serv	50	0	0	190	12	0	0
Dressing, Hazelnut Vinaigrette	1 serv	270	25	4	300	11	0	1
Dressing, Light Ranch	1 serv	120	11	2	410	3	0	2
Dressing, Lite Honey Mustard	1 serv	170	9	2	380	20	0	1
Dressing, Lite Olive Oil Vinaigrette	1 serv	110	10	2	420	6	0	0
Dressing, Pomegranate Vinaigrette	1 serv	250	22	4	160	12	0	0
Dressing, Sesame Ginger	1 serv	230	20	3	680	12	0	1
Dressing, Thai Peanut	1 serv	160	8	1	740	20	0	2
Honey Mustard Sauce	1 serv	200	3	0	240	41	1	2
Mayonnaise	1 serv	70	7	1	220	2	0	0
Mayonnaise, Herb	1 serv	110	11	2	160	1	0	0
Mayonnaise, Jalapeño	1 serv	50	5	1	310	1	0	2
Mustard	1 serv	0	0	0	70	0	0	0
Spread, Herb Bagel	1 serv	140	12	8	340	4	0	5
Spread, Mediterranean	1 serv	120	11	3	430	2	1	2
Spread, Sun-Dried Tomato	1 serv	45	4	0	70	1	0	0
KIDS MENU								
Chicken Nuggets	1 serv	250	10	2	840	24	1	18
Chicken Sandwich, Grilled	1 serv	480	12	3	1030	60	2	24
Grilled Cheese	1	670	41	25	1060	55	2	20
Macaroni & Cheese	1	250	14	9	690	18	0	10

ITEM DESCRIPTION	Serving Size	Calories	Total Fat (g)	Saturated Fat (g)	Sodium (mg)	Carbohydrates (g)	Fiber (g)	Protein (g)
Pasta, Buttered Penne	1	260	12	7	95	31	1	6
Turkey Sandwich, Smoked	1	430	11	3	1400	60	2	19
MAIN MENU								
Apple Cranberry Orzo, Roasted	1 oz	45	1	0	25	9	1	1
Beef Stroganoff	1 oz	35	3	1	105	2	0	2
Carrots, Roasted	1 oz	15	0	0	60	3	1	0
Cheese Tortellini Primavera (salad bar)	1 oz	45	2	1	115	4	0	2
Cheese Tortellini Primavera	12 oz	530	26	13	1370	53	4	19
Chicken Marsala	1 oz	30	2	1	100	2	0	2
Chicken w/ Burgundy Wine Sauce	1 oz	25	1	0	110	1	0	3
Chicken w/ Penne Broccoli Alfredo (salad bar)	1 oz	40	2	1	90	3	0	3
Chicken w/ Penne Broccoli Alfredo	12 oz	470	19	10	1100	38	2	33
Fire Roasted Exotic Grains & Vegetables	1 oz	40	1	0	85	7	1	1
Green Beans w/ Almonds, Roasted	1 oz	20	1	0	60	2	1	1
Italian Sausage & Peppers	1 oz	40	3	1	105	3	0	3
Lasagna, Meat (salad bar)	1 oz	45	3	1	150	3	0	2
Lasagna, Meat	11 oz	480	28	13	1640	29	2	28
Lasagna, Spinach & Artichoke	1 oz	35	2	1	130	4	0	2
Mayan Chicken Harvest Rice Bowl	1 serv	490	14	3	1430	67	4	25
Mayan Chicken Harvest Rice Bowl w/ Brown Rice	1 serv	540	16	3	1430	71	7	23
Mediterranean Spinach & Chickpea Ragout	1 oz	20	0	0	75	4	1	1
Moroccan Bulgur Wheat Pilaf	1 oz	50	3	0	55	8	1	1
Orecchiette & Chicken Apple Sausage	1 oz	40	2	0	70	3	0	2
Penne w/ Chicken & Fire-Roasted Pepper Sauce	1 oz	35	1	0	95	4	0	2
Polenta	1 oz	45	2	1	110	5	1	1
Quinoa	1 oz	25	0	0	50	4	1	1
Rice, Brown	1 oz	35	1	0	60	6	0	0
Rice, White	1 oz	30	0	0	55	6	0	0
Salmon Curry Harvest Rice Bowl	1 serv	560	17	8	1300	69	2	32
Salmon Curry Harvest Rice Bowl w/ Brown Rice	1 serv	610	20	8	1350	73	5	31

ITEM DESCRIPTION	Serving Size	Calories	Total Fat (g)	Saturated Fat (g)	Sodium (mg)	Carbohydrates (g)	Fiber (g)	Protein (g)
Salmon Provencal	1 oz	25	1	0	85	1	0	3
Steak Churrasco Harvest Rice Bowl	1 serv	510	15	4	1430	69	2	29
Steak Churrasco Harvest Rice Bowl w/ Brown Rice	1 serv	560	18	4	1490	73	5	28
Tsaziki	1 oz	15	0	0	40	2	0	1
White Bean Cacciatore	1 oz	20	1	0	85	3	1	1
SALADS								
Barbecue Beef	1 oz	35	1	0	90	4	0	2
Black Bean & Corn	1	130	0	0	310	25	5	5
Brown Rice & Hazelnut Waldorf	1	180	10	2	240	22	2	1
Brown Rice Waldorf	1 oz	45	3	0	60	5	0	0
Caesar Asiago	side	130	6	3	270	12	2	6
Caesar Asiago	1	220	12	6	480	18	3	11
Chef's Salad	1	240	15	7	1120	8	3	22
Chicken Caesar Asiago, Grilled	1	300	13	6	740	18	3	28
Chicken Pesto	1	160	8	3	420	1	1	20
Chicken, Mediterranean	1	290	16	6	1230	12	3	23
Chicken, Thai Peanut	1	240	8	0	280	19	4	22
Chickpea & Tomato	1	100	1	0	200	19	6	5
Chickpea & Tomato Cucumber	1	230	12	5	810	23	7	11
Egg & Cucumber	1 oz	40	3	1	90	1	0	2
Garden	1	70	2	0	85	13	3	4
Garden	side	50	2	0	65	8	2	2
Green Bean & Almond	1	100	6	1	85	7	3	3
Orzo Toscano	1 oz	35	1	0	90	6	1	1
Panzanella, Southwest	1 oz	50	3	0	55	7	0	1
Pasta, Southwest Fusilli	1 oz	45	3	0	65	4	0	1
Potato Bacon	1 oz	40	2	0	125	5	1	1
Radicchio	1	410	28	8	410	30	6	11
Salmon Niçoise	1	390	17	3	710	25	4	32
Sesame Brown Rice & Orange	1 oz	45	3	0	70	6	0	1
Sesame Chicken, Mandarin	1	310	17	1	410	29	3	20
Tomato Cucumber	1 oz	10	0	0	40	2	0	0
Tomato, Green Bean & Almond	1 oz	20	2	0	50	2	0	0

ITEM DESCRIPTION	Serving Size	Calories	Total Fat (g)	Saturated Fat (g)	Sodium (mg)	Carbohydrates (g)	Fiber (g)	Protein (g)
Tuna	1 oz	40	3	0	100	1	0	4
Tuna Garden	1	240	12	2	480	15	4	20
Tuna, Mediterranean	1	120	8	2	290	4	1	9
Turkey & Strawberry	1	110	4	0	410	11	4	10
Turkey Cobb, Smoked	1	330	19	8	1060	15	4	25
Watermelon & Feta	1 oz	15	1	0	25	3	0	0
SANDWICHES								
Caprese	1	680	32	15	1200	65	4	30
Chicken & Mozzarella	1	680	24	8	1440	66	2	48
Chicken Pesto	1	650	23	5	1540	65	2	43
Chicken, Arizona	1	690	28	11	1600	60	4	47
Chicken, Barbecue on Farmhouse Roll	1	790	29	11	1820	81	4	49
Eggplant & Mozzarella	1	660	30	12	1520	70	6	26
Mediterranean Wrap	1	610	29	7	1770	73	8	18
Pork, Maui Baked	1	640	21	10	1250	72	4	43
Portobello & Goat Cheese	1	550	25	9	1340	62	6	19
Prosciutto Mozzarella	1	780	40	16	2270	67	4	40
Roast Beef Caesar	1	670	27	8	1520	64	3	40
Salmon Salsa Verde	1	550	15	5	1000	66	3	36
Steakhouse Ciabatta	1	710	30	11	1810	73	4	44
Tuna Melt	1	670	29	10	1120	68	5	41
Tuna, Spicy	1	470	16	3	1180	60	11	29
Turkey Club, Smoked	1	690	31	13	2290	59	3	41
Turkey Melt	1	780	32	13	2340	77	3	42
Turkey, Apple & Radicchio	1	480	16	3	1870	61	10	28
Turkey, Baja	1	650	24	9	1860	68	5	41
Wrap, Chicken Caesar Asiago	1	610	28	9	1440	61	5	34
Wrap, Hot Mayan Chicken	1	590	14	3	1420	92	6	24
Wrap, Hot Pork Carnitas	1	690	13	3	1480	106	7	36
Wrap, Hot Steak Churrasco	1	560	15	3	1460	84	5	25
Wrap, Southwest Tuna	1	750	40	13	1470	66	7	39
Wrap, Thai Peanut Chicken	1	530	15	2	1340	79	6	30
SIDES AND SNACKS								
Almonds, Chocolate Covered	1 serv	220	6	6	35	19	1	4

ITEM DESCRIPTION	Serving Size	Calories	Total Fat (g)	Saturated Fat (g)	Sodium (mg)	Carbohydrates (g)	Fiber (g)	Protein (g)
Almonds, Tamari	1 serv	180	14	1	160	5	3	9
Apples, Blue Cheese & Cranberries	1 serv	200	10	4	270	27	3	4
Beef, Thai Peanut	1 serv	120	5	1	290	5	1	12
Brie, Fruit & Crackers	1 serv	200	11	6	280	18	0	6
Cheddar, Fruit & Crackers	1 serv	200	12	6	280	18	0	8
Cheese, Herb w/ Fruit & Crackers	1 serv	190	11	6	450	20	1	4
Chicken, Thai Peanut & Snow Peas	1 serv	140	4	1	480	9	1	17
Chocolate Duo	1 serv	160	9	5	40	18	0	3
Chocolate Nonpareils	1 serv	190	9	5	0	29	0	1
Cranberries, Dark Chocolate	1 serv	170	9	5	0	27	3	1
Fruit Cup	sm	70	0	0	15	18	1	1
Fruit Romanoff w/ Almonds	1 serv	200	7	2	15	34	3	3
Gelatin, Lemon	1 serv	120	0	0	210	29	0	2
Gelatin, Lime	1 serv	120	0	0	190	29	0	2
Gelatin, Orange	1 serv	130	0	0	160	30	0	2
Granola	1 serv	230	8	1	75	37	3	5
Grapes	1 serv	160	0	0	0	41	2	2
Hummus & Cucumber	1 serv	130	8	0	460	10	3	3
Licorice, Red	1 serv	140	1	1	20	30	0	1
Majuka Fruit Trail Mix	1 serv	140	7	2	0	17	2	2
Mango Coconut Mousse	1 serv	170	10	6	45	18	0	3
Mozzarella & Tomato	1 serv	180	14	7	290	5	1	10
Muesli	1 serv	390	8	2	50	76	7	11
Nuts, Mixed	1 serv	180	16	3	60	7	1	5
Pineapple	1 serv	110	0	0	0	30	3	1
Raspberry Mousse	1 serv	150	6	4	45	20	0	3
Snack Mix, The 19th Hole	1 serv	160	9	1	200	15	1	4
Soy Mix	1 serv	110	7	1	0	13	3	7
Strawberry, Chocolate Covered	1	35	2	2	5	5	1	0
Tiramisu	1 serv	170	11	6	45	15	0	3
Trail Mix, New	1 serv	120	5	1	5	20	2	2
Turkey, Smoked w/ Asparagus, Cranberry Chutney & Gorgonzola	1 serv	140	5	4	730	10	1	13
Turkish Apricots	1 serv	120	0	0	10	29	4	1

ITEM DESCRIPTION	Serving Size	Calories	Total Fat (g)	Saturated Fat (g)	Sodium (mg)	Carbohydrates (g)	Fiber (g)	Protein (g)
Watermelon	1 serv	70	0	0	0	17	1	1
Yogurt Blueberry w/ Blueberries	sm	250	3	2	135	50	0	8
Yogurt Strawberry w/ Blueberries	sm	250	2	2	135	50	0	7
Yogurt Vanilla w/ Blueberries	sm	220	3	2	180	41	0	9
SOUPS								
Baked Stuffed Potato	med	350	20	10	990	29	2	9
Bisque, Corn & Green Chili	med	260	15	7	1540	27	3	6
Bisque, Wild Mushroom	med	190	9	2	1020	22	2	5
Black Bean	med	260	1	0	1100	46	26	15
Black-Eyed Pea, Southern	med	170	2	0	980	29	9	11
Broccoli Cheddar	med	300	21	10	990	20	2	11
Carrot Ginger	med	140	5	0	960	22	3	1
Chicken & Dumpling	med	210	7	3	1280	28	2	11
Chicken Florentine	med	250	13	6	1050	25	1	8
Chicken Gumbo	med	180	8	1	880	21	2	6
Chicken Noodle	med	130	3	1	1050	19	2	8
Clam Chowder	med	320	18	7	1020	27	1	9
Corn Chowder	med	350	18	8	1120	40	3	9
Cream of Chicken & Wild Rice	med	240	14	5	970	22	1	6
Curried Rice & Lentil	med	170	2	0	1260	30	8	8
French Moroccan Tomato Lentil	med	190	2	0	1060	32	10	10
French Onion	med	130	5	3	1310	19	2	3
Garden Vegetable	med	80	2	0	1070	13	3	3
Gazpacho	med	90	5	0	1520	11	3	2
Hearty Cabbage	reg	110	5	2	1030	14	3	5
Italian Wedding	med	170	7	3	1300	19	3	8
Jamaican Black Bean	med	250	1	0	440	43	23	16
Mediterranean Pepper	med	170	5	1	590	26	8	7
Pasta E Fagioli	med	260	8	2	1010	35	9	12
Portuguese Kale	med	130	5	1	1220	15	4	5
Potato Cheese	med	260	14	9	1250	24	2	7
Potato Leek	med	300	19	10	1000	28	2	5
Red Beans, Italian Sausage & Rice	med	270	6	2	1080	40	17	14
Split Pea w/ Ham	med	250	2	0	1220	41	15	18

ITEM DESCRIPTION	Serving Size	Calories	Total Fat (g)	Saturated Fat (g)	Sodium (mg)	Carbohydrates (g)	Fiber (g)	Protein (g)
Stew, Beef & Vegetable	med	310	16	3	1070	25	3	18
Stew, Brunswick	med	300	10	4	1150	35	3	19
Stew, Chicken & Vegetable	med	290	17	5	940	26	3	11
Thai Coconut Curry	med	160	7	2	1050	21	2	4
Tomato	med	200	7	3	1150	27	3	6
Tomato Basil Bisque	med	210	9	5	500	27	4	7
Tomato Cheddar	reg	240	16	6	1070	17	2	8
Tomato Florentine	med	130	3	1	1020	18	2	6
Tomato Rice	med	120	1	0	280	24	2	4
Tortilla, Southwest	med	190	10	3	1160	23	4	4
Vegetable, Beef Barley	med	140	3	2	1010	21	4	9
Vegetable, Southwest	med	170	5	1	400	28	6	6
Vegetable, Tuscan	med	170	5	2	1190	23	3	7
Vegetarian Chili	med	220	2	0	970	39	20	12
Vegetarian Lentil	med	170	2	0	1200	31	11	9
Vegetarian Minestrone	med	120	2	0	1130	20	4	5
Vegetarian, Black Bean	med	260	1	0	1100	46	26	15
TOPPINGS AND EXTRAS								
Bacon	1 serv	60	5	2	210	0	0	5
Cheese, Brie	1 serv	160	14	9	330	0	1	7
Cheese, Cheddar	2 pcs	160	13	7	270	1	0	10
Cheese, Feta	1 serv	80	6	4	320	1	0	5
Cheese, Goat	1 serv	100	8	6	150	1	0	6
Cheese, Gorgonzola	1 serv	200	16	12	770	2	0	12
Cheese, Mozzarella	1 serv	120	9	6	105	0	0	9
Cheese, Swiss	1 serv	150	12	8	90	2	0	12
Chicken Breast	1 serv	120	2	0	420	0	0	26
Croutons	1 pkg	190	6	1	310	29	1	5
Granola	1 serv	230	8	1	75	37	3	5
Guacamole	1 serv	50	5	1	115	2	2	0
Ham	1 serv	100	4	2	1190	0	0	18
Hummus, Roasted Red Pepper	1 serv	80	5	0	250	6	2	2
Peppers, Roasted Red	1 serv	10	0	0	105	2	0	0
Prosciutto	1 serv	110	6	3	940	2	0	14

ITEM DESCRIPTION	Serving Size	Calories	Total Fat (g)	Saturated Fat (g)	Sodium (mg)	Carbohydrates (g)	Fiber (g)	Protein (g)
Roast Beef	1 serv	150	6	2	300	0	0	23
Sausage Patty	1 serv	210	20	7	360	0	0	8
Tuna Salad Mix	1 serv	160	10	2	400	3	1	17
Turkey Breast	1 serv	80	1	0	980	2	0	16

BLIMPIE

BREAKFAST ITEMS

ITEM DESCRIPTION	Serving Size	Calories	Total Fat (g)	Saturated Fat (g)	Sodium (mg)	Carbohydrates (g)	Fiber (g)	Protein (g)
Biscuit w/ Bacon, Egg & Cheese	1	432	24	17	1579	37	1	17
Biscuit w/ Egg & Cheese	1	385	21	15	1377	37	1	14
Biscuit w/ Ham, Egg & Cheese	1	420	21	16	1655	39	1	19
Biscuit w/ Sausage, Egg & Cheese	1	535	35	20	1687	37	1	20
Biscuit, Plain	1	263	11	10	830	34	1	6
Bluffin w/ Bacon, Egg & Cheese	1	293	14	7	973	27	2	16
Bluffin w/ Egg & Cheese	1	245	10	5	771	27	2	13
Bluffin w/ Ham, Egg & Cheese	1	280	11	6	1049	29	2	18
Bluffin w/ Sausage, Egg & Cheese	1	395	24	10	1081	27	2	19
Bluffin, Plain	1	129	1	0	242	25	2	5
Burrito w/ Bacon, Egg & Cheese	1	553	24	12	2095	56	5	31
Burrito w/ Egg & Cheese	1	506	20	11	1892	56	5	28
Burrito w/ Ham, Egg & Cheese	1	559	21	11	2310	58	5	36
Burrito w/ Sausage, Egg & Cheese	1	656	34	16	2202	56	5	34
Cinnamon Roll	1	449	20	9	729	60	2	9
Croissant w/ Bacon, Egg & Cheese	1	396	115	12	1026	30	1	16
Croissant w/ Egg & Cheese	1	349	111	11	823	30	1	12
Croissant w/ Ham, Egg & Cheese	1	384	112	11	1102	31	1	17
Croissant w/ Sausage, Egg & Cheese	1	499	125	16	1133	30	1	18
Croissant, Plain	1	233	102	6	295	28	1	5
Panini Breakfast	4 in	494	14	5	1408	67	2	26

DESSERTS

ITEM DESCRIPTION	Serving Size	Calories	Total Fat (g)	Saturated Fat (g)	Sodium (mg)	Carbohydrates (g)	Fiber (g)	Protein (g)
Brownie	1	182	7	3	115	28	1	2
Cookie, Chocolate Chunk	1	196	10	4	153	25	0	2
Cookie, Oatmeal Raisin	1	170	7	3	142	26	1	2
Cookie, Peanut Butter	1	198	12	5	161	20	1	3
Cookie, Sugar	1	327	17	6	286	41	1	3

ITEM DESCRIPTION	Serving Size	Calories	Total Fat (g)	Saturated Fat (g)	Sodium (mg)	Carbohydrates (g)	Fiber (g)	Protein (g)
Cookie, White Chocolate Macadamia Nut	1	198	12	5	161	20	1	3
Turnover, Apple	1	340	21	10	190	35	1	4
Turnover, Cherry	1	350	21	10	190	35	1	4
DRESSINGS AND SPREADS								
Dressing, Blue Cheese	1 serv	230	24	5	440	2	n/a	2
Dressing, Buttermilk Ranch	1 serv	230	24	4	380	2	n/a	1
Dressing, Creamy Caesar	1 serv	210	21	4	520	2	n/a	1
Dressing, Creamy Italian	1 serv	180	18	3	420	4	0	0
Dressing, Dijon Honey Mustard	1 serv	180	17	3	240	8	n/a	1
Dressing, Fat-Free Italian	1 serv	25	0	n/a	390	5	0	0
Dressing, Light Buttermilk Ranch	1 serv	70	4	1	310	8	n/a	1
Dressing, Light Italian	1 serv	20	1	0	770	2	n/a	0
Dressing, Peppercorn	1 serv	240	26	4	453	1	0	1
Dressing, Special	1 serv	70	7	1	0	0	n/a	0
Dressing, Thousand Island	1 serv	210	20	3	350	6	0	0
Honey Mustard	1 serv	43	1	0	168	7	1	1
Mayonnaise	1 serv	202	22	3	202	0	0	0
Mustard, Deli Style	1 serv	5	0	0	60	0	0	0
Mustard, Spicy Brown	1 serv	5	0	0	60	0	n/a	0
Oil Blend	1 serv	130	14	2	0	0	0	0
Red Wine Vinegar	1 serv	5	0	0	0	1	0	0
Sauce, Red Hot Original	1 serv	10	0	0	760	2	0	0
KIDS MENU								
Ham & American Cheese	3 in	262	9	5	901	32	2	15
Tuna	3 in	277	11	2	457	30	2	14
Turkey	3 in	187	2	0	598	31	2	10
SALADS								
Antipasto	1	245	14	6	1627	12	4	20
Buffalo Chicken	1	222	9	5	842	10	4	25
Chef	1	176	7	4	805	10	2	18
Chicken Caesar	1	192	8	4	463	6	3	25
Coleslaw	side	160	9	2	240	20	2	1
Garden	1	29	0	0	16	6	3	2
Macaroni	side	330	22	5	790	28	2	5

ITEM DESCRIPTION	Serving Size	Calories	Total Fat (g)	Saturated Fat (g)	Sodium (mg)	Carbohydrates (g)	Fiber (g)	Protein (g)
Northwest Potato	side	260	17	4	390	22	3	3
Potato	side	230	12	3	490	28	3	3
Seafood	reg	122	4	1	582	17	3	6
Tuna	reg	272	18	3	517	7	2	18
Ultimate Club	1	287	16	9	1196	10	3	25
SANDWICHES								
Blimpie Best	6 in	420	14	6	1371	49	3	25
Blimpie Best, Super Stacked	6 in	523	19	8	2128	52	3	37
Blimpie Trio, Super Stacked	6 in	488	12	5	1773	52	3	41
BLT	6 in	447	22	5	933	46	3	15
BLT, Super Stacked	6 in	639	41	9	1438	43	2	22
Chicken Teriyaki	6 in	428	9	4	1315	50	1	35
Chicken Teriyaki on Wheat	6 in	416	10	5	1255	47	5	36
Chicken w/ Cheddar, Bacon & Ranch	6 in	642	34	10	1648	48	3	36
Ciabatta, Buffalo Chicken	1	583	27	7	2050	50	3	32
Ciabatta, Grilled Chicken Caesar	1	617	24	6	1584	63	3	34
Ciabatta, Mediterranean	1	447	8	2	1719	65	3	26
Ciabatta, Roast Beef, Turkey & Cheddar	1	588	30	9	1941	51	3	28
Ciabatta, Sicilian	1	637	25	7	2520	68	3	33
Ciabatta, Turkey Italiano	1	502	11	4	2164	64	3	30
Ciabatta, Tuscan	1	600	23	7	2150	65	3	29
Ciabatta, Ultimate Club	1	480	21	6	1538	47	2	27
Club	6 in	386	10	4	1063	49	3	25
Cuban	6 in	413	11	5	1628	43	1	29
French Dip	6 in	413	11	5	1652	46	1	30
Ham & Swiss	6 in	391	10	5	1026	50	3	25
Ham & Swiss on Wheat	6 in	368	11	5	965	44	6	26
Ham, Salami & Cheese	6 in	443	16	7	1306	49	3	25
Meatball	6 in	607	32	14	2072	51	4	28
Pastrami, Hot	6 in	435	16	7	1354	42	1	30
Pastrami, Hot, Super Stacked	6 in	571	23	10	2113	43	1	46
Philly Steak & Onion	6 in	499	24	10	1233	45	1	26
Reuben	6 in	571	24	7	1221	54	3	34
Roast Beef & Provolone	6 in	408	11	5	1051	47	3	31

ITEM DESCRIPTION	Serving Size	Calories	Total Fat (g)	Saturated Fat (g)	Sodium (mg)	Carbohydrates (g)	Fiber (g)	Protein (g)
Roast Beef, Turkey & Cheddar	6 in	571	30	9	1769	48	3	27
Seafood	6 in	333	7	1	840	56	4	13
Tuna	6 in	483	21	3	776	46	3	25
Turkey & Avocado	6 in	381	9	1	1406	52	4	21
Turkey & Bacon, Super Stacked	6 in	582	24	11	2622	48	2	40
Turkey & Cranberry	6 in	350	4	1	1219	58	3	20
Turkey & Provolone	6 in	393	10	4	1405	49	3	26
Vegetarian Special	6 in	593	30	10	1766	66	4	17
Veggie Supreme	6 in	553	28	16	1415	48	3	29
VegiMax	6 in	522	20	6	1272	56	5	28
Wrap, Chicken Caesar	reg	607	29	9	1586	56	4	30
Wrap, Roast Beef & Cheddar	reg	684	36	12	1928	59	6	32
Wrap, Southwestern	reg	530	22	6	1771	61	4	23
Wrap, Steak & Onion	reg	774	47	15	1795	62	6	28
Wrap, Zesty	reg	569	26	10	1979	59	6	28
SIDES AND SNACKS								
Cheetos, Crunchy	1 pkg	160	10	3	290	15	1	2
Chips, Baked Potato	1 pkg	124	2	0	169	26	2	2
Chips, Cheddar Sour Cream	1 pkg	240	15	5	285	21	2	3
Chips, KC Master Barbecue	1 pkg	240	15	5	300	23	2	3
Chips, KC Master Barbecue, Baked	1 pkg	135	3	0	236	25	2	2
Chips, Multigrain Harvest Cheddar	1 pkg	210	9	2	285	29	3	3
Chips, Multigrain Original	1 pkg	209	9	1	139	29	4	3
Chips, Potato	1 pkg	225	15	5	270	23	2	3
Doritos, Cooler Ranch	1 pkg	245	12	3	297	32	2	4
Doritos, Nacho Cheese	1 pkg	245	12	3	332	30	2	4
Fritos	1 pkg	320	20	2	210	30	2	4
Pretzels, Classic Thin Style	1 pkg	223	2	0	n/a	47	2	4
SOUPS								
Bean w/ Ham	1	140	1	0	1070	23	11	8
Beef Steak & Noodle	1	120	3	2	780	14	0	8
Beef Stew	1	170	4	2	890	18	2	17
Captain's Corn Chowder	1	210	7	3	890	29	4	6
Chicken & Dumpling	1	170	5	3	970	19	3	11

ITEM DESCRIPTION	Serving Size	Calories	Total Fat (g)	Saturated Fat (g)	Sodium (mg)	Carbohydrates (g)	Fiber (g)	Protein (g)
Chicken Gumbo	1	90	2	0	1280	13	2	6
Chicken Noodle	1	130	4	1	1040	18	2	7
Chicken w/ White & Wild Rice	1	250	10	3	1030	15	4	14
Cream of Broccoli w/ Cheese	1	190	8	5	940	15	3	6
Cream of Potato	1	190	9	3	860	24	3	5
French Onion	1	80	4	1	1020	11	1	2
Grande Chili w/ Bean & Beef	1	250	9	5	1230	30	18	18
Harvest Vegetable	1	100	1	0	920	19	3	4
Italian Style Wedding	1	130	4	2	900	17	0	7
Minestrone	1	90	3	0	1150	14	4	4
New England Clam Chowder	1	170	3	2	1060	28	2	7
Pasta Fagioli w/ Sausage	1	150	5	2	910	22	4	7
Pilgrim Turkey Vegetables w/ Rice	1	110	2	1	800	19	2	4
Seafood Gumbo	1	100	2	1	850	16	2	4
Split Pea w/ Ham	1	130	2	0	1090	21	6	8
Tomato Basil w/ Raviolini	1	110	1	0	720	22	0	4
Yankee Pot Roast	1	80	2	1	750	12	2	5
TOPPINGS AND EXTRAS								
Bacon	1 serv	105	8	3	447	0	0	7
Bread, Cheddar Jalapeño	6 in	213	4	2	434	36	1	8
Bread, Ciabatta	1 serv	230	3	0	590	43	2	8
Bread, Honey Oat	6 in	259	8	1	405	41	5	10
Bread, Marble Rye	6 in	242	2	1	n/a	46	2	9
Bread, Wheat	6 in	190	4	1	357	34	4	9
Bread, White	6 in	213	3	1	418	40	1	7
Bread, Zesty Parmesan	6 in	236	4	2	488	39	2	9
Cappacola	1 serv	18	1	0	164	0	n/a	3
Cheese, Cheddar	1 serv	75	6	4	382	1	n/a	4
Cheese, Mild Cheddar Shredded	1 serv	114	9	6	176	0	0	7
Cheese, Parmesan Shredded	1 serv	52	4	2	145	1	0	4
Cheese, Pepper Jack	1 serv	77	7	4	135	0	0	6
Cheese, Provolone	1 serv	76	6	4	190	0	n/a	5
Cheese, Swiss	1 serv	79	6	4	44	0	0	6
Cheese, Yellow & White American	1 serv	104	9	6	507	1	n/a	6

ITEM DESCRIPTION	Serving Size	Calories	Total Fat (g)	Saturated Fat (g)	Sodium (mg)	Carbohydrates (g)	Fiber (g)	Protein (g)
Chicken Strips	1 serv	93	3	1	253	0	0	16
Corned Beef	1 serv	106	2	1	759	2	0	18
Egg	1 serv	45	3	1	188	2	0	4
Guacamole	1 serv	45	4	1	135	2	1	0
Ham	1 serv	35	1	0	278	2	n/a	5
Lettuce	1 serv	6	0	0	4	1	0	0
Meatballs	1 serv	292	21	8	1342	11	3	15
Olives	1 serv	16	2	0	124	1	0	0
Onion	3 pcs	11	0	0	1	3	0	0
Pastrami	1 serv	114	6	3	633	1	0	14
Pepperoni	1 serv	66	6	3	233	1	n/a	3
Peppers, Hot Ring	12 pcs	0	0	0	450	1	0	0
Peppers, Jalapeño	18 pcs	10	0	0	486	1	0	0
Peppers, Red Roasted	1 serv	11	0	0	112	2	0	0
Peppers, Sweet Strips	6 pcs	20	0	0	116	5	0	0
Philly Steak & Onion	1 serv	210	15	6	630	5	n/a	13
Prosciuttini	1 serv	13	0	0	177	1	0	2
Roast Beef	1 serv	46	1	0	220	0	0	8
Salami	1 serv	36	3	1	137	0	0	2
Seafood Salad	1 serv	92	4	1	415	10	1	4
Tomato	2 pcs	7	0	0	2	2	0	0
Tuna	1 serv	241	18	2	350	0	0	16
Turkey	1 serv	30	0	0	316	1	n/a	5
Wrap, Spinach Herb	12 in	310	8	3	840	52	3	9
Wrap, Traditional	12 in	310	8	3	670	52	5	9

The Nutritional Information Blimpie has provided is based on standard product formulations. Product variations may occur based on regional differences, ingredient substitutions, seasonal conditions, differences in product production at the store, and suppliers. Some items listed may not be available in all stores. This list may not include test products, limited time offers, and regional menu variations.

BOSTON MARKET

DESSERTS

Apple Gallette	1	420	22	12	280	54	3	3
Brownie, Chocolate Chip Fudge	1	320	13	3	220	49	3	5
Cookie, Chocolate Chip	1	370	19	9	340	49	2	4
Cornbread	1	180	5	1.5	320	31	0	2

ITEM DESCRIPTION	Serving Size	Calories	Total Fat (g)	Saturated Fat (g)	Sodium (mg)	Carbohydrates (g)	Fiber (g)	Protein (g)
Cupcake, Chocolate	1	350	17	6	210	48	2	3
Pie, Pecan	1	640	36	11	340	74	2	7
DRESSINGS AND SPREADS								
Dressing, Caesar Salad	1 serv	360	38	6	910	4	1	2
Dressing, Lite Ranch	1 serv	70	4	0.5	310	8	0	1
Dressing, Market Chopped Salad	1 serv	360	39	6	1710	2	0	0
MAIN MENU								
Beef Brisket	indiv	280	20	1.5	260	1	0	26
Beef Brisket	family	280	20	1.5	260	1	0	26
Beef, Shepherd's Pie	1	480	25	9	1490	40	5	25
Chicken Pot Pie, Pastry Top	1	800	48	18	1090	59	4	32
Chicken, 1/2 Rotisserie	1	610	29	9	1860	1	0	89
Chicken, 1/4 White Rotisserie	1	320	12	4	900	0	0	52
Chicken, 1/4 White Rotisserie, Skinless	1	240	4	1	890	1	0	50
Chicken, Crispy Country w/ Country Gravy	1	480	23	4.5	1150	36	1	33
Chicken, Dark (2 Thighs & Drumstick)	3 pcs	490	29	8	1600	0	0	60
Chicken, Dark Individual Meal	3 pcs	390	22	6	1270	1	0	51
Chicken, Dark Skinless (2 Thighs & Drumstick)	3 pcs	350	15	4.5	1210	0	0	52
Chicken, Dark Skinless (Thigh & 2 Drumsticks)	3 pcs	290	11	3.5	1010	0	0	45
Chicken, Rotisserie	family	310	15	4.5	930	0	0	44
Chicken, Thigh & Drumstick	2 pcs	290	17	5	950	0	0	37
Meatloaf	family	480	36	16	1030	21	0	29
Meatloaf	indiv	520	36	16	1030	21	0	29
Sirloin	family	290	15	6	440	0	0	39
Sirloin, Roasted	indiv	290	15	6	440	0	0	39
Turkey, Roasted	family	180	3	1	635	0	0	38
Turkey, Roasted	indiv	150	2.5	1	500	0	0	31
SALADS								
Caesar	entrée	420	38	10	930	9	2	12
Caesar	side	180	17	3.5	410	4	1	4
Caesar, no Dressing	lg	140	8	5	270	7	2	10
Caesar, no Dressing	sm	40	2	1.5	75	3	1	3

ITEM DESCRIPTION	Serving Size	Calories	Total Fat (g)	Saturated Fat (g)	Sodium (mg)	Carbohydrates (g)	Fiber (g)	Protein (g)
Chicken, Crispy	1	220	11	2	480	16	1	16
Chicken, Rotisserie	1	160	1	0	520	3	0	35
Market Chopped	1	480	40	8	1640	24	7	9
Sirloin, Roasted	1	160	6	2	170	0	0	26
Turkey, Roasted	1	110	2	0.5	370	0	0	23
SANDWICHES								
Beef Au Jus	1	20	0.5	0	760	3	0	1
Brisket Dip Carver	1	890	51	9	1350	63	3	43
Chicken Carver, Crispy	1	1020	42	7	2210	114	4	45
Chicken Salad	1	800	41	7	1900	65	4	40
Chicken, Boston Carver	1	750	29	8	1960	64	3	57
Chicken, Open-faced Rotisserie	1	320	8	2.5	1630	34	1	27
Chicken, Smokehouse Barbecue	1	850	29	9	2810	101	4	44
Meatloaf, Boston Carver	1	980	46	21	2350	92	4	47
Meatloaf, Open-faced	1	670	38	17	1760	48	1	34
Sirloin Dip, Boston Carver	1	900	46	13	1610	62	3	57
Sirloin, Open-faced Roasted	1	410	15	6	1640	32	1	35
Turkey, Boston Carver	1	700	26	8	1710	65	3	50
Turkey, Open-faced Roasted	1	330	6	1.5	1480	43	1	26
SIDES AND SNACKS								
Apples w/ Cinnamon	1	210	3	0	15	47	3	0
Broccoli w/ Garlic Butter	1	80	6	2	230	6	3	3
Coleslaw	1	170	9	2	270	21	2	2
Creamed Spinach	1	280	23	15	580	12	4	9
Fruit Salad	1	60	0	0	20	15	1	1
Gravy, Beef	3 oz	35	1.5	0.5	500	4	0	1
Gravy, Poultry	4 oz	50	2	0.5	690	7	0	0
Green Beans	1	60	3.5	1.5	180	7	3	2
Macaroni & Cheese	1	300	11	7	1100	35	2	11
Potatoes, Garlic Dill New	1	140	3	1	120	24	3	3
Potatoes, Mashed	1	270	11	5	820	36	4	5
Soup, Chicken Noodle	1	170	6	1.5	990	16	1	15
Soup, Chicken Tortilla w/ Toppings	1	340	22	6	1350	24	1	13
Soup, Chicken Tortilla w/o Toppings	1	90	4.5	1	940	7	1	6

ITEM DESCRIPTION	Serving Size	Calories	Total Fat (g)	Saturated Fat (g)	Sodium (mg)	Carbohydrates (g)	Fiber (g)	Protein (g)
Spinach, Garlic	1	130	9	6	200	9	5	5
Squash Casserole	1	300	19	7	1390	23	3	10
Sweet Corn	1	170	4	1	95	37	2	6
Sweet Potato Casserole	1	460	16	4.5	270	77	3	4
Vegetable Stuffing	1	190	8	1	580	25	2	3
Vegetables, Steamed	1	60	2	0	40	8	3	2

Nutrition information and ingredients are current as of the date this resource was printed. Nutrition calculations and ingredients are based on standard product formulations and recipes. Variations can be expected due to slight differences in product assembly by employees, local vendors, and other factors. This information is provided as a reference only. The allergen information provided refers to only the big 8 required allergens for labeling.

BURGER KING

BEVERAGES

ITEM DESCRIPTION	Serving Size	Calories	Total Fat (g)	Saturated Fat (g)	Sodium (mg)	Carbohydrates (g)	Fiber (g)	Protein (g)
Apple Juice, Minute Maid	1	100	0	0	15	23	0	0
Chocolate Milk, Hershey®'s 1% Low Fat	8 oz	180	2.5	1.5	140	31	1	9
Coca Cola Classic‡	sm (22 oz)	210	0	0	5	56	0	0
Coffee, Iced Mocha BK JOE®	1	360	10	6	290	66	1	6
Coffee‡ , Decaf BK JOE®	sm (16 oz)	5	0	0	10	1	0	1
Coffee‡ , Regular BK JOE®	sm (16 oz)	10	0	0	20	1	0	1
Coffee‡ , Turbo BK JOE®	sm (16 oz)	10	0	0	30	2	0	1
Diet Coke‡	sm (22 oz)	0	0	0	20	0	0	0
Dr Pepper‡	sm (22 oz)	200	0	0	50	56	0	0
Icee Coca Cola/Frozen Coke	16 oz	110	0	0	10	31	0	0
Icee Minute Maid, Cherry	16 oz	110	0	0	5	31	0	0
Milk Shake, Chocolate	med (22 oz)	670	21	13	510	119	2	11
Milk Shake, Strawberry	med (22 oz)	650	20	13	350	116	0	11
Milk Shake, Vanilla	med (22 oz)	480	20	13	320	76	0	11
Milk, Hershey®'s Fat Free	1	100	0	0	150	14	0	9
Orange Juice, Minute Maid	10 oz	140	0	0	20	33	0	2
Shake, Chocolate OREO® BK® Sundae	sm (16 oz)	700	26	16	530	116	2	11
Shake, Strawberry OREO® BK® Sundae	sm (16 oz)	680	25	16	430	114	1	10
Sprite‡	sm (22 oz)	210	0	0	45	56	0	0

BREAKFAST ITEMS

ITEM DESCRIPTION	Serving Size	Calories	Total Fat (g)	Saturated Fat (g)	Sodium (mg)	Carbohydrates (g)	Fiber (g)	Protein (g)
Biscuit w/ Bacon, Egg & Cheese	1	430	25	16	1400	34	1	17

ITEM DESCRIPTION	Serving Size	Calories	Total Fat (g)	Saturated Fat (g)	Sodium (mg)	Carbohydrates (g)	Fiber (g)	Protein (g)
Biscuit w/ Ham, Egg, & Cheese	1	410	23	15	1490	34	1	17
Biscuit w/ Sausage	1	420	27	15	1090	32	1	13
Biscuit w/ Sausage, Egg, & Cheese	1	560	37	19	1560	35	1	21
BK Wrapper™ w/ Cheesy Bacon	1	390	24	8	1060	29	2	14
Breakfast Shots™, Bacon & Cheese	2 pcs	310	20	7	800	18	1	14
Breakfast Shots™, Ham & Cheese	2 pcs	270	16	5	840	18	1	13
Breakfast Shots™, Sausage & Cheese	2 pcs	420	31	10	910	18	1	18
Cini-Minis	4 pcs	400	18	7	380	52	2	7
Croissan'wich® w/ Bacon, Egg & Cheese	1	350	19	8	870	27	0	15
Croissan'wich® w/ Egg & Cheese	1	310	16	7	730	27	0	12
Croissan'wich® w/ Ham, Egg & Cheese	1	340	17	7	1200	28	0	18
Croissan'wich® w/ Sausage & Cheese	1	380	24	10	780	26	0	14
Croissan'wich® w/ Sausage, Egg & Cheese	1	470	31	11	1030	28	0	20
Double Croissan'wich™ w/ Bacon, Egg, & Cheese	1	430	26	11	1240	29	0	20
Double Croissan'wich™ w/ Ham, Bacon, Egg, & Cheese	1	430	24	11	1570	29	0	23
Double Croissan'wich™ w/ Ham, Egg, & Cheese	1	420	21	10	1890	30	0	26
Double Croissan'wich™ w/ Ham, Sausage, Egg, & Cheese	1	550	36	14	1730	30	0	28
Double Croissan'wich™ w/ Sausage, Bacon, Egg, & Cheese	1	560	38	15	1400	29	0	25
Double Croissan'wich™ w/ Sausage, Egg, & Cheese	1	690	50	19	1560	30	0	30
French Toast Sticks	3 pcs	230	11	2	260	29	1	3
French Toast Sticks	5 pcs	380	18	3	430	49	2	5
Ham Omelet Sandwich	1	290	12	4.5	870	33	1	13
Hash Browns	sm	420	27	6	680	40	6	3
Hershey's® Sundae Pie	1	310	19	12	220	32	1	3
Pie, Dutch Apple	1	320	13	5	290	47	1	2
Vanilla Icing	1 pkg	90	0	0	25	22	0	0

ITEM DESCRIPTION

ITEM DESCRIPTION	Serving Size	Calories	Total Fat (g)	Saturated Fat (g)	Sodium (mg)	Carbohydrates (g)	Fiber (g)	Protein (g)
DRESSINGS AND SPREADS								
Caramel Sauce	1 pkg	45	0.5	0	35	10	0	0
Dipping Sauce, Barbecue	1 pkg	40	0	0	310	11	0	0
Dipping Sauce, Buffalo	1 pkg	80	8	1.5	360	2	0	0
Dipping Sauce, Honey Mustard	1 pkg	90	6	1	180	8	0	0
Dipping Sauce, Ranch	1 pkg	140	15	2.5	95	1	0	1
Dipping Sauce, Sweet & Sour	1 pkg	45	0	0	55	11	0	0
Dipping Sauce, Zesty Onion Ring	1 pkg	150	15	2.5	210	3	1	0
Dressing, Ken's® Creamy Caesar	1 pkg	210	21	4	610	4	0	3
Dressing, Ken's® Honey Mustard	1 pkg	270	23	3	510	15	0	1
Dressing, Ken's® Light Italian	1 pkg	120	11	1.5	440	5	0	0
Dressing, Ken's® Ranch	1 pkg	190	20	3	550	2	0	1
Jam, Strawberry or Grape	1 pkg	30	0	0	0	7	0	0
Ketchup	1 pkg	10	0	0	125	3	0	0
Mayonnaise	1 pkg	80	9	0.5	75	1	0	0
Syrup	1 pkg	80	0	0	20	21	0	0
MAIN MENU								
Big Fish® Sandwich	1	640	32	5	1540	66	3	23
Big Fish® Sandwich, no Tartar Sauce	1	460	13	2.5	1320	64	3	23
Burger Shots®	2 pcs	220	10	4	420	18	1	14
Cheeseburger	1	340	16	7	770	31	1	18
Chicken Fries	6 pcs	250	15	2.5	820	16	1	14
Chicken Fries	9 pcs	380	22	4	1220	24	2	21
Chicken Sandwich, Original	1	630	39	7	1390	46	3	24
Chicken Sandwich, Original, no Mayo	1	420	16	3.5	1210	46	3	24
Chicken Sandwich, Tendercrisp®	1	800	46	8	1640	68	3	32
Chicken Sandwich, Tendercrisp®, no Mayo	1	590	22	4	1450	68	3	31
Chicken Sandwich, Tendergrill®	1	490	21	4	1220	51	3	26
Chicken Sandwich, Tendergrill®, no Mayo	1	380	9	2	1130	51	3	25
Chicken Tenders®	4 pcs	180	11	2	310	13	0	9
Chicken Tenders®	6 pcs	270	16	3	460	19	0	14
Chick'n Crisp® Sandwich, Spicy	1	450	30	5	810	34	2	12
Chick'n Crisp® Sandwich, Spicy, no Mayo	1	290	12	2.5	670	34	2	12
Double Cheeseburger	1	510	29	14	1020	31	1	30

ITEM DESCRIPTION	Serving Size	Calories	Total Fat (g)	Saturated Fat (g)	Sodium (mg)	Carbohydrates (g)	Fiber (g)	Protein (g)
Double Hamburger	1	420	22	9	590	30	1	26
Double Stacker	1	620	39	16	1100	32	1	34
Double Whopper® Sandwich	1	920	58	19	1090	51	3	48
Double Whopper® Sandwich w/ Cheese	1	1010	66	24	1530	53	3	53
Double Whopper® Sandwich w/ Cheese, no Mayo	1	850	48	21	1390	52	3	53
Double Whopper® Sandwich, no Mayo	1	760	41	16	950	51	3	48
Hamburger	1	290	12	4.5	550	30	1	15
Macaroni & Cheese, Kraft®	1	160	5	1.5	340	22	1	7
Quad Stacker	1	1010	70	30	1800	34	1	64
Steakhouse Burger	1	950	59	21	1950	55	4	40
Steakhouse XT™	1	970	61	23	1930	55	4	42
Steakhouse XT™, 3 Cheese	1	1050	71	29	2150	52	3	51
Steakhouse XT™, Mushroom & Swiss	1	870	49	20	1890	54	4	43
Triple Stacker	1	820	55	23	1450	33	1	49
Triple Whopper® Sandwich	1	1160	76	27	1170	51	3	68
Triple Whopper® Sandwich w/ Cheese	1	1250	84	32	1600	52	3	73
Triple Whopper® Sandwich w/ Cheese, no Mayo	1	1090	66	29	1460	52	3	73
Triple Whopper® Sandwich, no Mayo	1	1000	59	24	1030	51	3	68
Veggie® Burger**	1	420	16	2.5	1090	46	7	23
Veggie® Burger** w/ Cheese	1	470	20	5	1300	47	7	25
Veggie® Burger**, no Mayo	1	340	8	1	1030	46	7	23
Whopper Jr.® Sandwich	1	370	21	6	560	31	2	16
Whopper Jr.® Sandwich w/ Cheese	1	420	25	8	780	31	2	18
Whopper Jr.® Sandwich w/ Cheese, no Mayo	1	340	16	7	710	31	2	18
Whopper Jr.® Sandwich, no Mayo	1	290	12	4.5	500	31	2	16
Whopper® Sandwich	1	670	40	11	1020	51	3	29
Whopper® Sandwich w/ Cheese	1	770	48	16	1450	52	3	33
Whopper® Sandwich w/ Cheese, no Mayo	1	610	30	14	1310	52	3	33
Whopper® Sandwich, no Mayo	1	520	23	9	880	51	3	28
SALADS								
Chicken Garden, Tendercrisp®	1	410	23	6	1060	27	4	27

ITEM DESCRIPTION	Serving Size	Calories	Total Fat (g)	Saturated Fat (g)	Sodium (mg)	Carbohydrates (g)	Fiber (g)	Protein (g)
Chicken Garden, Tendergrill™	1	210	7	3	780	8	3	29
Garden	1	70	4	2.5	100	7	3	4
Side	1	40	2	1	45	2	1	3
SIDES AND SNACKS								
BK™ Fresh Apple Fries	1 serv	25	0	0	0	6	1	0
Cheesy Tots® Potatoes	6 pcs	220	12	4	630	21	2	7
Cheesy Tots® Potatoes	9 pcs	330	18	6	950	31	3	11
French Fries, no Salt Added•	med	480	23	5	530	61	5	5
French Fries, Salted	med	480	23	5	820	61	5	5
Onion Rings	med	450	24	4	700	52	5	6
TOPPINGS AND EXTRAS								
Bacon	1 pc	15	1	0	50	0	0	1
Cheese, American	1 pc	45	4	2.5	220	1	0	2
Croutons, Garlic Parmesan	1 serv	60	2	0	120	9	0	1
Pickles	1 serv	1	0	0	100	0	0	0

™ & © 2009 Burger King Brands, Inc. All Rights Reserved. © 2009 The Coca-Cola Company. "Coca-Cola," "Coca-Cola Classic," "Diet Coke," "Sprite" "ICEE" and "Minute Maid" are registered trademarks of the Coca-Cola Company. All Rights Reserved. DR PEPPER is a registered trademark of Dr Pepper/Seven Up, Inc. © 2009. CHEESY TOTS® is a trademark of H.J. Heinz Company and used under license by Burger King Corporation. The HERSHEY®S trademark and trade dress are used under license. A.1.® Thick & Hearty Steak Sauce, KRAFT® Macaroni and Cheese, and OREO® are registered trademarks of Kraft Foods Holdings, Inc.

** Burger King Corporation makes no claim that the BK VEGGIE® Burger or any other of its products meets the requirements of a vegan or vegetarian diet. The patty is cooked in the microwave.

• To reduce sodium, you can order french fries without added salt.

"‡": These values represent Sodium derived from ingredients other than water. The actual amount of Sodium in the beverages will vary depending on the quantity contained in the water supply where the finished beverages are produced.

CARL'S JR.

BREAKFAST ITEMS

ITEM								
Breakfast Burger™	1	780	41	15	1460	64	3	38
Burrito w/ Bacon & Egg	1	550	32	10	990	37	1	29
Burrito w/ Steak & Eggs	1	650	36	14	1750	43	1	41
Burrito, Loaded	1	780	49	16	1480	51	3	36
French Toast Dips®, no Syrup	5 pcs	460	21	4	570	60	3	9
Hash Brown Nuggets	1 serv	350	23	4	440	32	3	3
Sourdough Breakfast Sandwich	1	450	21	8	1470	38	1	29
Sunrise Croissant™ Sandwich	1	590	44	17	810	27	1	20
DESSERTS								
Cake, Chocolate	1 pc	300	12	3	350	48	1	3
Cheesecake, Strawberry Swirl	1 pc	290	16	9	230	32	0	6

ITEM DESCRIPTION	Serving Size	Calories	Total Fat (g)	Saturated Fat (g)	Sodium (mg)	Carbohydrates (g)	Fiber (g)	Protein (g)
Cookie, Chocolate Chip	1	370	19	10	350	48	2	3
Malt, Chocolate	1	780	34	24	370	100	1	15
Malt, Oreo® Cookie	1	790	38	25	440	95	1	17
Malt, Strawberry	1	770	34	24	320	99	0	15
Malt, Vanilla	1	780	34	24	320	101	0	15
Shake, Chocolate	1	710	33	23	300	86	1	14
Shake, Oreo® Cookie	1	730	38	25	360	81	1	15
Shake, Strawberry	1	700	33	23	250	85	0	14
Shake, Vanilla	1	710	33	23	240	86	0	14
DRESSINGS AND SPREADS								
Blue Cheese Dressing	1 serv	320	34	7	410	1	0	2
House Dressing	1 serv	220	22	3.5	440	3	0	1
Low Fat Balsamic Dressing	1 serv	35	1.5	0	480	5	0	0
Thousand Island Dressing	1 serv	240	23	3.5	460	7	0	0
KIDS MENU								
Cheeseburger	kid	290	15	7	830	24	1	12
Hamburger	kid	230	10	3.5	550	24	1	9
MAIN MENU								
Burger, Bacon Cheese Six Dollar Burger™	1	950	62	23	1980	49	3	51
Burger, Big Hamburger	1	460	17	8	1090	54	3	24
Burger, Guacamole Bacon Six Dollar Burger™	1	1040	70	25	2240	53	4	49
Burger, Jalapeño Six Dollar Burger™	1	930	61	22	2190	52	3	45
Burger, Low Carb Six Dollar Burger™	1	570	43	18	1480	7	1	38
Burger, Original Six Dollar Burger™	1	890	54	20	2040	58	3	45
Burger, Super Star® w/ Cheese	1	920	58	23	1640	54	3	47
Burger, Western Bacon Six Dollar Burger®	1	1020	53	22	2520	81	3	53
Cheeseburger, Double Western Bacon™	1	960	52	23	1750	70	3	52
Cheeseburger, Western Bacon Cheeseburger®	1	710	33	13	1410	69	3	32
Chicken Club™ Sandwich, Charbroiled	1	560	27	7	1280	44	2	39
Chicken Salad, Charbroiled	1	250	9	3.5	590	14	4	29
Chicken Sandwich, Charbroiled Barbecue	1	380	7	1.5	1010	49	2	34

ITEM DESCRIPTION	Serving Size	Calories	Total Fat (g)	Saturated Fat (g)	Sodium (mg)	Carbohydrates (g)	Fiber (g)	Protein (g)
Chicken Sandwich, Charbroiled Santa Fe™	1	630	35	8	1410	44	2	36
Chicken Sandwich, Spicy	1	420	27	5	930	33	2	12
Chicken Strips	5 pcs	610	43	9	1030	32	3	23
Chicken Strips	3 pcs	370	26	6	620	19	2	14
Chicken™ Sandwich, Crispy w/ Bacon & Swiss	1	750	40	9	1990	62	4	36
Chili Cheeseburger	1	780	41	19	1650	58	4	41
Famous Star™ w/ Cheese	1	660	39	13	1300	53	3	27
Fish Sandwich, Carl's Catch™	1	710	37	6	1280	74	4	20
Jalapeño Burger™	1	720	46	15	1340	50	3	27
Taco Salad, Green Burrito®	1	970	58	19	1850	76	17	42
SIDES AND SNACKS								
Chicken Stars™	4 pcs	210	16	4	310	10	1	8
Chicken Stars™	6 pcs	320	24	6	460	14	2	12
Chicken Stars™	9 pcs	480	36	9	690	21	2	18
Chili Cheese Fries	1 serv	990	56	19	2380	89	8	28
CrissCut® Fries	1 serv	450	29	5	900	42	4	5
Fish & Chips	1 serv	730	39	7	1630	72	6	22
French Fries	med	460	22	4.5	1180	60	5	5
Fried Zucchini	1 serv	330	18	3	610	36	2	6
Onion Rings	1 serv	530	28	4.5	590	61	3	8
Salad	side	50	2.5	1.5	55	4	2	3

For additional information visit www.carlsjr.com. The information contained in this guide is based on standard U.S. product formulations. Variations may occur due to a variety of factors and circumstances including, but not limited to, differences in suppliers, ingredient substitutions, recipe revisions, product assembly, and seasonal variances. Product participation may vary by location, and test products are not included. This information is current as of April 1, 2009. The information in this guide is reported for informational purposes only by Carl Karcher Enterprises, Inc. Neither CKE, its franchisees, its suppliers and/or vendors, or its employees assume any responsibility for sensitivity or allergy to any food product or ingredient provided by or in our restaurants. We do have an allergen-free cooking environment in our kitchen. All of our products are prepared in the same kitchen area. Anyone with any food sensitivity, allergies, special dietary needs, or specific dietary inquiries and/or concerns should consult a medical professional of their own selection regarding the suitability of our food products and/or ingredients, and should regularly review the information contained at www.carlsjr.com for content updates. The Dietary Guidelines for Americans recommend limiting saturated fat to 20 grams and sodium to 2,300 milligrams for a typical adult eating 2,000 calories daily. Recommended limits may be higher or lower depending on daily calorie consumption. © 2009 Carl Karcher Enterprises, Inc. All rights reserved.

CHILI'S

APPETIZERS

ITEM DESCRIPTION	Serving Size	Calories	Total Fat (g)	Saturated Fat (g)	Sodium (mg)	Carbohydrates (g)	Fiber (g)	Protein (g)
Fries, Texas Cheese	1 serv	1920	147	63	3570	67	7	84
Fries, Texas Cheese	half	1400	111	49	2500	41	4	64
Kickin' Jack Nachos	8	890	67	35	2070	46	6	40
Kickin' Jack Nachos	12	1290	97	50	3040	66	9	59
Kickin' Jack Nachos w/ Fajita Beef	8	1080	72	37	3000	47	6	67

ITEM DESCRIPTION	Serving Size	Calories	Total Fat (g)	Saturated Fat (g)	Sodium (mg)	Carbohydrates (g)	Fiber (g)	Protein (g)
Kickin' Jack Nachos w/ Fajita Beef	12	1480	102	52	3970	68	9	86
Kickin' Jack Nachos w/ Fajita Chicken	12	1440	100	50	3960	68	9	87
Kickin' Jack Nachos w/ Fajita Chicken	8	1040	70	35	2990	48	6	68
Onion String & Crispy Jalapeño Stack	1 serv	2130	213	31	1320	34	5	6
Skillet Queso w/ Chips	1 serv	940	77	32	3870	42	7	32
Southwestern Eggrolls w/ Avocado Ranch	1 serv	910	57	14	1960	72	7	27
Spinach & Artichoke Dip w/ Chips	1 serv	930	77	34	3130	39	3	24
Tostada Chips w/ Hot Sauce	1 serv	470	39	5	2790	26	5	4
Triple Dipper Big Mouth Bites	2 pcs	780	51	15	1440	46	2	30
Triple Dipper Buffalo Chicken Crisper Bites	2 pcs	620	34	8	2380	54	2	2
Triple Dipper Chicken Crisper Bites	2 pcs	690	40	9	1970	58	2	20
Triple Dipper™ Boneless Buffalo Wings w/ Bleu Cheese	5 pcs	730	57	9	2130	28	0	25
Triple Dipper™ Boneless Sweet Chile Glazed Wings w/ Ranch	5 pcs	750	48	8	1700	51	0	26
Triple Dipper™ Chicken Crispers® No Dressing	3 pcs	600	42	7	1300	20	2	34
Triple Dipper™ Hot Spinach & Artichoke Dip w/ Chips	1 serv	460	38	17	1560	20	2	12
Triple Dipper™ Southwestern Eggrolls w/ Avocado Ranch	2 pcs	640	42	10	1370	48	5	18
Triple Dipper™ Wings Over Buffalo® w/ Bleu Cheese	5 pcs	740	66	14	2090	2	0	33
DESSERTS								
Brownie, Sweet Shot Double Chocolate Fudge	1	420	24	14	25	51	1	1
Cake, Chocolate Chip Cookie Molten	1 pc	1240	64	33	680	152	4	14
Cake, Molten Chocolate	1 pc	1150	60	34	780	145	5	12
Cake, Sweet Shot Red Velvet	1 pc	250	9	4.5	200	39	1	3
Cake, White Molten Chocolate	1 pc	1290	68	25	470	152	0	15
Cheesecake	1 pc	700	42	26	460	67	0	12
Cinnamon Roll, Sweet Shot Warm	1	280	13	8	95	38	1	3
Pie, Chocolate Chip Paradise	1 pc	1590	76	37	910	220	5	19

ITEM DESCRIPTION	Serving Size	Calories	Total Fat (g)	Saturated Fat (g)	Sodium (mg)	Carbohydrates (g)	Fiber (g)	Protein (g)
Pie, Sweet Shot Key Lime	1 pc	240	12	8	75	30	0	4
Shake, Frosty Chocolate	1	740	35	21	210	100	0	8
DRESSINGS AND SPREADS								
Barbecue Sauce	1 serv	60	0	0	560	14	1	1
Dressing, Ancho Chile Ranch	1 serv	170	17	3.5	390	3	0	1
Dressing, Avocado Ranch	1 serv	110	11	2	210	2	1	1
Dressing, Bleu Cheese	1 serv	240	25	5	310	1	0	1
Dressing, Caesar	1 serv	260	27	4.5	390	2	0	2
Dressing, Citrus Balsamic Vinaigrette	1 serv	250	25	3.5	220	6	0	0
Dressing, Fire Roasted Tomato Vinaigrette	1 serv	90	9	1.5	320	2	0	0
Dressing, Honey Mustard	1 serv	180	21	3	380	1	0	0
Dressing, Honey Mustard, Fat Free	1 serv	70	0	0	510	11	0	0
Dressing, Jalapeño Ranch	1 serv	150	15	3	340	2	0	1
Dressing, Low Fat Ranch	1 serv	45	3	0	440	4	0	1
Dressing, Low Fat Vinaigrette	1 serv	60	2	0	230	8	0	0
Dressing, Ranch	1 serv	170	18	3.5	340	2	0	1
Guacamole	1 serv	35	3.5	0	65	2	1	1
Honey Barbecue Sauce	1 serv	80	0	0	600	20	1	0
Honey Chipotle Sauce	1 serv	150	0	0	720	37	0	0
KIDS MENU								
Apples w/ Cinnamon	side	190	7	2.5	65	34	4	0
Chicken Crispers, Fried	1 serv	560	37	5	1600	25	1	31
Chicken Platter, Grilled	1 serv	150	1	0	690	4	0	27
Chicken Sandwich, Grilled	1 serv	230	3.5	1	650	26	1	22
Corn	side	130	2	0	0	23	6	4
Corn Dog	1 serv	280	17	3.5	650	25	2	5
Corn on the Cob, no Butter	1 serv	150	1.5	0	5	32	3	5
French Fries	side	240	15	2.5	140	24	2	2
Grilled Cheese	1 serv	510	41	12	990	28	0	10
Kettle Black Beans	side	110	1	0	670	19	6	6
Little Chicken Crispers	1 serv	600	42	7	1300	20	2	34
Little Mouth Burger	1 serv	440	23	8	420	24	1	33
Little Mouth Cheeseburger	1 serv	510	29	12	740	25	1	36

ITEM DESCRIPTION	Serving Size	Calories	Total Fat (g)	Saturated Fat (g)	Sodium (mg)	Carbohydrates (g)	Fiber (g)	Protein (g)
Macaroni & Cheese	1 serv	500	18	6	930	69	3	16
Mandarin Oranges	side	70	0	0	10	17	0	0
Pizza, Cheese	1 serv	560	24	9	1130	67	3	23
Quesadilla, Cheese	1 serv	450	24	12	990	40	1	18
Rice	side	220	1	0	660	49	2	5
Shake, Chocolate	1 serv	550	26	16	150	75	0	6
Veggies, Seasonal	1 serv	35	0	0	30	6	3	3
MAIN MENU								
Big Mouth® Bites	1 serv	1579	97	28	2932	104	6	61
Buffalo Chicken Crisper Bites	1 serv	1622	100	21	5384	123	6	49
Buffalo Chicken Fajitas	1 skillet	1092	77	17	5236	50	5	48
Burger, Bacon	1 serv	1088	69	21	1801	57	3	56
Burger, Jalapeño Smokehouse Bacon Big Mouth Burger®	1 serv	1692	120	39	4052	68	4	84
Burger, Mushroom-Swiss	1 serv	1071	67	19	1667	65	4	52
Burger, Oldtimer®	1 serv	821	44	12	1310	59	3	45
Burger, Oldtimer® w/ Cheese	1 serv	901	51	16	1445	59	3	50
Burger, Smokehouse Bacon Triple Cheese Big Mouth Burger®	1 serv	1751	123	44	3861	66	3	94
Burger, Southern Smokehouse Bacon Big Mouth Burger®	1 serv	1650	108	36	4200	85	4	84
Cheesesteak	1 serv	860	40	16	2052	81	4	53
Chicken Crispers®	1 serv	1780	123	19	2910	107	10	65
Chicken Crispers®, Fried, no Sauce	1 serv	1490	90	13	3000	110	8	60
Chicken Crispers®, Crispy Honey-Chipotle	1 serv	1960	108	17	4780	187	8	61
Chicken Crisper™ Bites	1 serv	1412	79	18	3986	126	6	42
Chicken Pasta, Cajun	1 serv	1340	68	37	3650	106	6	67
Chicken Tacos	2 pcs	920	31	11	3440	121	13	42
Chicken, Margarita Grilled	1 serv	710	14	2	2530	88	9	54
Chicken, Margarita, Create Your Own	1 serv	310	9	1.5	1020	10	0	41
Chicken, Monterey ®	1 serv	860	43	15	3060	57	9	63
Chicken, Monterey, Create Your Own	1 serv	460	24	12	1700	14	1	45
Crispy Sweet Chile Glazed Chicken Crispers	1 serv	1860	108	17	4160	158	8	63

ITEM DESCRIPTION	Serving Size	Calories	Total Fat (g)	Saturated Fat (g)	Sodium (mg)	Carbohydrates (g)	Fiber (g)	Protein (g)
Fajita Condiments	1 serv	210	18	9	320	7	2	7
Fajita, Classic Chicken	1 serv	367	11	1.4	1995	25	4	39
Fajita, Classic Combo	1 serv	420	18	3.4	2256	25	4	42
Fajita, Classic Steak	1 serv	473	25	5	2517	25	4	45
Fajita, Mushroom Jack	1 skillet	724	41	13	3374	36	6	58
Fajita, Pita Beef	1 serv	489	21	4	1543	51	3	30
Fajita, Pita Chicken	1 serv	455	13	2	1401	52	3	31
Fajita, Quesadillas Beef w/ Rice & Beans	1 serv	1550	61	31	4780	167	12	78
Fajita, Quesadillas Chicken w/ Rice & Beans	1 serv	1510	59	29	4760	168	12	80
Fajita, Steak & Portobello	1 skillet	788	56	8.6	3430	33	6	46
Fajita, TRIO	1 serv	554	27	5	3056	28	4	54
Guiltless Black Bean Burger	1 serv	609	11	2	1791	91	18	37
Guiltless Buffalo Chicken Sandwich	1 serv	386	7	2	2301	46	9	36
Guiltless Carne Asada Steak	1 serv	371	10	7.5	1436	11	6	46
Guiltless Cedar Plank Tilapia	1 serv	199	4	2	689	8	5	34
Guiltless Chicken Platter	1 serv	371	2	1	1937	49	7	39
Guiltless Grilled Chicken Sandwich	1 serv	361	5	2	1385	44	9	36
Guiltless Grilled Salmon	1 serv	395	20	6	420	8	3	51
Guiltless Honey-Mustard Glazed Salmon	1 serv	416	20	6	605	13	2	50
Ribeye, Cajun	1 serv	1110	96	33	930	18	2	42
Ribeye, Flame-Grilled	1 serv	1090	95	32	1160	17	1	42
Ribs, Honey Barbecue	1/2 rack	600	34	13	2690	43	1	29
Ribs, Honey-Chipotle	1/2 rack	730	34	12	2930	78	0	28
Ribs, Memphis Dry Rub	1/2 rack	570	39	13	2480	23	2	29
Ribs, Original	1/2 rack	490	34	12	2050	17	1	28
Ribs, Original Baby Back, Create Your Own	1/2 rack	490	34	12	2050	17	1	28
Salmon w/ Garlic & Herbs, Grilled	1 serv	650	29	7	1130	56	5	48
Salmon, Grilled w/ Garlic & Herbs, Create Your Own	1 serv	380	25	7	300	1	0	40
Sandwich, Cajun Chicken	1 serv	927	49	12	2404	70	4	47
Sandwich, Chicken Caesar Pita	1 serv	701	41	8	1566	45	4	39

ITEM DESCRIPTION	Serving Size	Calories	Total Fat (g)	Saturated Fat (g)	Sodium (mg)	Carbohydrates (g)	Fiber (g)	Protein (g)
Sandwich, Chicken Ranch	1 serv	1174	71	11	2911	86	4	45
Sandwich, Grilled Chicken	1 serv	847	45	10	1925	62	2	47
Sandwich, Smoked Turkey	1 serv	877	48	12	2154	76	3	40
Sandwich, Smoked Turkey Combo	1 half	438	24	6	1077	38	1	20
Shrimp Alfredo, Grilled	1 serv	1320	76	38	3560	105	6	51
Shrimp, Spicy Garlic & Lime Grilled create your own	1 serv	170	11	2	1090	7	0	12
Sirloin, Chili's Classic	1 serv	680	50	18	990	16	1	38
Sirloin, Chili's Classic create your own	1 serv	540	43	15	700	1	0	36
Steak w/ Sides, Fried	1 serv	1430	82	15	2950	122	9	52
Tacos, Chicken Club	2 pcs	1180	57	15	3930	117	10	47
Tacos, Chicken Club	3 pcs	1520	76	21	5030	140	12	64
Tacos, Crispy Chicken Crisper™	2 pcs	1520	76	18	4600	157	10	50
Tacos, Crispy Chicken Crisper™	3 pcs	2020	104	25	6050	201	12	69
Tilapia, Southwest Cedar Plank	1 serv	600	27	4	1820	61	7	31
Tortillas, Flour	4 pcs	480	13	3.5	1290	79	2	9
Wings Over Buffalo® w/ Bleu Cheese	1 serv	1220	104	22	2580	3	0	65
Wings, Boneless Buffalo w/ Bleu Cheese	1 serv	1180	86	13	3870	52	1	46
Wings, Boneless Sweet Chile Glazed w/ Ranch	1 serv	1280	74	12	2990	98	1	48
SALADS								
Boneless Buffalo Chicken	1 serv	1070	77	15	4380	46	5	44
Caesar	side	350	31	6	550	13	2	6
Chicken Caesar	1 serv	900	71	13	1740	28	6	37
House, no Dressing	side	210	12	6	310	17	3	10
Mesquite Chicken	1 serv	960	62	18	2680	45	10	54
Quesadilla Explosion	1 serv	1260	76	23	2630	84	9	59
Southwestern Cobb	1 serv	1080	71	16	2650	57	9	55
Spicy Garlic & Lime Grilled Shrimp	1 serv	630	40	11	1850	43	9	29
SOUPS								
Broccoli Cheese	1 cup	120	8	3.5	650	9	1	5
Chicken Enchilada	1 cup	220	13	5	690	9	1	15
Chicken Noodle	1 cup	60	0.5	0	580	10	1	3
Chicken Tortilla	1 cup	130	7	2.5	1030	10	1	7

ITEM DESCRIPTION	Serving Size	Calories	Total Fat (g)	Saturated Fat (g)	Sodium (mg)	Carbohydrates (g)	Fiber (g)	Protein (g)
Chili's Terlingua Chili w/ Toppings	1 cup	210	14	5	620	9	1	12
New England Clam Chowder	1 cup	190	13	7	390	11	1	6
Potato, Baked	1 cup	250	18	10	890	13	1	9
Southwestern Vegetable	1 cup	100	4	1.5	630	13	2	4
TOPPINGS AND EXTRAS								
Bacon	2 pcs	50	4	1.5	220	0	0	3
Cheese, American	1 pc	70	6	3.5	320	1	0	3
Cheese, Cheddar	1 pc	80	7	4	135	0	0	5
Cheese, Provolone	1 pc	40	3	2	95	0	0	3
Cheese, Swiss	1 pc	50	4	2.5	35	0	0	4
Cinnamon Apples	1 serv	210	8	2.5	70	37	4	0
Corn on the Cob w/ Butter	1	190	7	1	120	32	3	5
French Fries	1 serv	410	25	4.5	240	41	4	4
Gravy	1 serv	35	1.5	0	350	4	0	1
Kettle Black Beans	1 serv	110	1	0	690	20	6	6
Mashed Potatoes w/ Black Pepper Gravy	1 serv	280	15	1.5	1050	33	5	5
Mashed Potatoes, Loaded	1 serv	390	25	8	940	29	5	13
Portobella Mushroom, Marinated	1 serv	90	8	1	75	3	0	1
Rice	1 serv	220	1	0	660	49	2	5
Rice & Kettle Black Beans, Added to Entrée	1 serv	330	2	0	1350	69	7	11
Shrimp, Spicy & Garlic Added to Entrée	3 pcs	70	4.5	1	400	1	0	6
Sour Cream	1 serv	80	8	5	75	3	0	1
Veggies, Seasonal	1 serv	60	4	1	170	7	3	3

The nutritional analysis is comprised of data from Analytical Food Laboratories (an independent testing facility commissioned by Chili's) combined with nutrient data from Chili's suppliers, the U.S. Agriculture and nutrient database analysis of Chili's recipes using Genesis SQL Nutritional Analysis Program from ESHA Research in Salem, Oregon. The rounding of figures is based on FDA guidelines. Chili's attempts to provide nutritional information regarding its products that is as complete as possible. Some menu items may not be at all restaurants; test products, test recipes, limited time offers, or regional items may not be included. While menu item ingredients information is based on standard product recipes, variations may occur due to ordinary differences inherent in the preparation of menu items, local suppliers, region of the country, and season of the year. Additionally, no products are certified as vegetarian. This listing is updated periodically in an attempt to reflect the current status of Chili's products. 040109

CHIPOTLE

Barbacoa	1 serv (4 oz)	170	7	2.5	510	2	0	24
Beans, Black	1 serv (4 oz)	120	1	0	250	23	11	7
Beans, Pinto	1 serv (4 oz)	120	1	0	330	22	10	7
Carnitas	1 serv (4 oz)	190	8	2.5	590	1	0	27
Cheese	1 serv (1 oz)	100	8.5	5	180	0	0	8

ITEM DESCRIPTION	Serving Size	Calories	Total Fat (g)	Saturated Fat (g)	Sodium (mg)	Carbohydrates (g)	Fiber (g)	Protein (g)
Chicken	1 serv (4 oz)	190	6.5	2	370	1	0	32
Chips	1 serv (4 oz)	570	27	3.5	420	73	8	8
Crispy Taco Shell	1	60	2	0.5	10	9	1	<1
Fajita Vegetables	1 serv (2.5 oz)	20	0.5	0	170	4	1	1
Guacamole	1 serv (3.5 oz)	150	13	2	190	8	6	2
Rice, Cilantro-Lime	1 serv (3 oz)	130	3	0.5	150	23	0	2
Romaine Lettuce (salad)	2.5 oz	10	0	0	5	2	1	1
Romaine Lettuce (tacos)	1 oz	5	0	0	0	1	1	0
Salsa, Corn	1 serv (3.5 oz)	80	1.5	0	410	15	3	3
Salsa, Green Tomatillo	1 serv (2 oz)	15	0	0	230	3	1	1
Salsa, Red Tomatillo	1 serv (2 oz)	40	1	0	510	8	4	2
Salsa, Tomato	1 serv (3.5 oz)	20	0	0	470	4	<1	1
Sour Cream	1 serv (2 oz)	120	10	7	30	2	0	2
Steak	1 serv (4 oz)	190	6.5	2	320	2	0	30
Tortilla (burrito)	1	290	9	3	670	44	2	7
Tortilla (taco)	1	90	2.5	1	200	13	<1	2
Vinaigrette	1 serv (2 oz)	260	24.5	4	700	12	1	0

We got these facts from analyzing our food. But nutritional content may vary because of changes in growing seasons, different suppliers, slight variations in our recipes, or the different places that we buy our ingredients. We may update this chart from time to time.

CHUCK E. CHEESE

DESSERTS

Cake, Chocolate	1 pc	290	13	4	220	41	2	3
Cake, Chocolate 1/4 Sheet	1 pc	310	14	5	200	41	2	3
Cake, Vanilla Buttercream	1 pc	310	18	6	230	35	0	2
Cinnamon Sticks w/ Cinnamon Topping & Sugar Icing	1 pc	70	2	1	87	11	0	1
Dessert Pizza w/ Cinnamon Apples, Shortbread & Sugar Icing	1 pc	192	5	2	164	33	1	2

MAIN MENU

Ciabatta w/ Chicken	1	715	28	7	1940	80	3	44
Pizza, Individual Cheese	1	540	19	8	1255	69	3	21
Pizza, Large All Meat Combo	1 pc	240	11	4	566	24	1	10
Pizza, Large Barbecue Chicken	1 pc	205	7	3	447	27	1	7
Pizza, Large Cheese	1 pc	170	6	3	404	23	1	7

ITEM DESCRIPTION	Serving Size	Calories	Total Fat (g)	Saturated Fat (g)	Sodium (mg)	Carbohydrates (g)	Fiber (g)	Protein (g)
Pizza, Large Super Combo	1 pc	205	9	3	508	24	1	8
Pizza, Large Veggie Combo	1 pc	175	6	2	402	24	1	10
Pizza, Medium All Meat Combo	1 pc	215	11	4	608	21	1	9
Pizza, Medium Barbecue Chicken	1 pc	185	6	2	460	24	1	8
Pizza, Medium Cheese	1 pc	155	5	2	360	21	1	6
Pizza, Medium Super Combo	1 pc	185	8	3	453	22	1	7
Pizza, Medium Veggie Combo	1 pc	160	6	2	366	22	2	6
Pizza, Small All Meat Combo	1 pc	180	9	3	508	19	1	9
Pizza, Small Barbecue Chicken	1 pc	150	5	2	394	21	1	7
Pizza, Small Cheese	1 pc	130	4	2	308	19	1	5
Pizza, Small Super Combo	1 pc	160	7	3	393	19	1	6
Pizza, Small Veggie Combo	1 pc	135	5	2	319	20	1	5
Sandwich Platter (Chicken, Ham & Cheese, or Italian)	1 pc	183	8	2	543	20	1	9
Sandwich w/ Ham & Cheese	1	685	27	8	2206	79	3	33
Sub, Italian	1	790	39	12	2374	78	3	34
Wings Platter	4 pcs	300	20	4	1308	16	4	16
SIDES AND SNACKS								
Breadsticks w/ Marinara & Light Ranch Dressing	1 pc	175	9	2	412	18	1	6
Buffalo Wings	1 pc	75	5	1	327	4	1	4
Carrot Sticks w/ Ranch	side	183	15	2	451	12	2	2
Celery & Bleu Cheese	4 pcs	269	26	5	606	6	2	3
French Fries w/ Ketchup & Light Ranch	1 serv	420	20	2	929	55	6	6
Fruit Garnish	1 serv	65	0	0	2	9	1	0
Hot Dogs w/ Mustard & Relish	1	310	19	7	1084	35	2	11
Mandarin Oranges	1 serv	56	0	0	6	15	1	0
Mozzarella Sticks w/ Marinara Sauce	1 pc	93	6	2	211	6	0	4
Pasta Salad	side	150	4	0.5	280	24	1	4
Sampler Platter	1 serv/ 7	329	19	5	840	25	2	13
Veggie Platter	1 serv/ 8	129	11	2	264	7	2	2

* All sandwiches served with Lettuce, Tomatoes, Onion, Balsamic Vinaigrette, Mayonnaise **

Chuck E. Cheese's attempts to provide nutrition and ingredient information regarding its products that is as complete as possible. While the nutrition and ingredient information is based on standard product formulations, variations may occur depending on the local supplier, the region of the country, and the season of the year. Further, product formulations change periodically. Serving sizes may vary from the quantity on which the analysis was completed. If you need further information or have food sensitivities and/or dietary concerns regarding specific ingredients in specific menu items, please visit our website (www.chuckecheese.com) or call us at 972-258-4255. This listing is effective as of January 2009.

DAIRY QUEEN

DESSERTS

ITEM DESCRIPTION	Serving Size	Calories	Total Fat (g)	Saturated Fat (g)	Sodium (mg)	Carbohydrates (g)	Fiber (g)	Protein (g)
Arctic Rush, All Flavors	sm	240	0	0	0	48	0	0
Banana Split	1 serv	520	13	10	160	94	3	9
Blizzard, Banana Cream Pie	sm	580	22	13	290	84	0	11
Blizzard, Banana Split	sm	440	13	9	190	71	0	11
Blizzard, Butterfinger®	sm	470	16	10	220	71	0	11
Blizzard, Cappuccino Heath®	sm	600	24	14	310	86	0	11
Blizzard, Cherry CheeseQuake®	sm	500	20	13	280	68	0	11
Blizzard, Choco Cherry Love	sm	500	21	10	190	68	0	11
Blizzard, Chocolate Chip	sm	590	29	12	190	70	1	11
Blizzard, Chocolate Xtreme	sm	660	29	15	340	88	1	13
Blizzard, Cookie Dough	sm	710	27	14	350	103	1	13
Blizzard, French Silk Pie	sm	680	31	18	260	88	1	12
Blizzard, Georgia Mud Fudge™	sm	690	35	12	400	82	2	13
Blizzard, Hawaiian	sm	440	15	10	180	67	1	10
Blizzard, Heath	sm	600	25	16	310	84	1	11
Blizzard, M&M's® Chocolate Candy	sm	660	22	14	230	101	1	13
Blizzard, Mint Oreo®	sm	580	20	10	410	89	1	12
Blizzard, Mocha Chip	sm	570	24	18	200	78	1	12
Blizzard, Oreo CheeseQuake	sm	590	25	14	410	78	1	12
Blizzard, Oreo Cookies	sm	550	20	10	410	81	1	12
Blizzard, Peanut Butter Butterfinger	sm	670	32	13	400	83	2	14
Blizzard, Reese's® Peanut Butter Cups®	sm	530	21	11	260	74	1	13
Blizzard, Snickers®	sm	670	25	13	310	99	1	14
Blizzard, Strawberry CheeseQuake	sm	510	21	13	280	69	0	12
Blizzard, Tropical	sm	500	24	10	220	62	3	11
Blizzard, Turtle Pecan Cluster	sm	680	32	11	320	86	2	13
Buster Bar® Treat	1	480	31	15	220	45	2	11
Cake, 10"	1 pc /10	500	19	13	260	72	1	11
Cake, 10" Chocolate Xtreme Blizzard	1 pc /10	820	33	20	360	97	2	12

ITEM DESCRIPTION	Serving Size	Calories	Total Fat (g)	Saturated Fat (g)	Sodium (mg)	Carbohydrates (g)	Fiber (g)	Protein (g)
Cake, 10" Cookie Dough Blizzard	1 pc /10	760	34	22	350	103	1	12
Cake, 10" Oreo Blizzard	1 pc /10	720	31	20	430	97	1	12
Cake, 10" Reese's® Peanut Butter Cups Blizzard	1 pc /10	730	34	22	340	93	2	13
Cake, 10" Strawberry CheeseQuake Blizzard	1 pc /10	630	27	18	320	84	1	12
Cake, 8"	1 pc /8	410	15	10	210	59	1	9
Cake, 8" Chocolate Xtreme Blizzard	1 pc /8	780	36	22	410	101	2	13
Cake, 8" Cookie Dough Blizzard	1 pc /8	740	32	20	340	100	1	12
Cake, 8" Oreo Blizzard	1 pc /8	760	33	20	460	104	2	13
Cake, 8" Reese's® Peanut Butter Cups Blizzard	1 pc /8	720	33	20	340	94	2	13
Cake, 8" Strawberry CheeseQuake Blizzard	1 pc /8	610	27	19	310	79	0	12
Cake, Heart	1 pc /10	290	11	7	150	42	1	6
Cake, Log	1 pc /8	310	12	8	160	44	1	6
Cake, Sheet	1 pc /24	320	12	9	170	47	1	6
Chocolate Dilly Bar	1	240	15	9	70	24	1	4
Cone, Chocolate	sm	240	7	5	115	32	0	6
Cone, Chocolate Coated Waffle w/ Soft Serve	1	540	21	13	170	77	1	10
Cone, Plain Waffle w/ Soft Serve	1	420	13	7	140	67	0	10
Cone, Vanilla	sm	230	7	4.5	100	31	0	6
Dilly Bar, Butterscotch	1	210	11	9	105	24	0	3
Dilly Bar, Cherry	1	210	12	8	80	24	0	3
Dilly Bar, Heath	1	220	13	10	95	25	0	3
Dilly Bar, no Sugar Added	1	190	13	10	60	24	5	3
Dilly Bar, Chocolate Mint	1	240	15	9	70	24	1	4
Dipped Cone, Butterscotch	sm	340	16	8	110	35	0	6
Dipped Cone, Cherry	sm	330	16	11	105	35	0	6
Dipped Cone, Chocolate	sm	330	15	6	105	36	0	6
DQ Fudge Bar, no Sugar Added	1	50	0	0	70	13	6	4
DQ Sandwich	1	190	5	3	135	31	1	4
DQ Vanilla Orange Bar, no Sugar Added	1	60	0	0	45	18	6	2
DQ Vanilla Take Home-Pak™	1/2 cup	140	4.5	3	65	21	0	4

ITEM DESCRIPTION	Serving Size	Calories	Total Fat (g)	Saturated Fat (g)	Sodium (mg)	Carbohydrates (g)	Fiber (g)	Protein (g)
Malt, Banana	sm	540	15	10	260	86	1	16
Malt, Caramel	sm	690	18	12	380	116	0	16
Malt, Cherry	sm	590	16	10	300	94	0	15
Malt, Chocolate	sm	650	16	10	310	110	0	15
Malt, Hot Fudge	sm	700	23	16	360	105	0	17
Malt, Marshmallow	sm	650	16	10	290	112	0	15
Malt, Pineapple	sm	550	15	10	280	89	0	15
Malt, Strawberry	sm	570	15	10	290	93	1	15
MooLatte, Cappuccino	16 oz	500	18	15	170	71	0	8
MooLatte, Caramel	16 oz	630	19	15	240	101	0	9
MooLatte, French Vanilla	16 oz	560	18	14	160	88	0	8
MooLatte, Mocha	16 oz	590	23	15	190	82	0	9
Oreo Brownie Earthquake®	1 serv	760	27	16	400	117	2	11
Parfait, Peanut Buster®	1 serv	700	30	16	360	94	2	16
Shake, Banana	sm	450	14	9	210	68	1	14
Shake, Caramel	sm	610	17	11	320	99	0	15
Shake, Cherry	sm	500	15	10	240	76	0	13
Shake, Chocolate	sm	570	15	10	250	92	0	13
Shake, Hot Fudge	sm	610	22	15	300	87	0	15
Shake, Marshmallow	sm	560	15	10	230	94	0	13
Shake, Pineapple	sm	480	15	10	220	71	0	13
Shake, Strawberry	sm	470	15	10	220	70	0	14
StarKiss® Bar, Cherry	1	80	0	0	10	21	0	0
StarKiss® Bar, Stars & Stripes™	1	80	0	0	10	21	0	0
Sundae, Banana	sm	230	7	4.5	90	37	1	6
Sundae, Caramel	sm	300	7	5	150	51	0	6
Sundae, Cherry	sm	250	7	4.5	110	40	0	5
Sundae, Chocolate	sm	280	7	4.5	115	48	0	5
Sundae, Hot Fudge	sm	300	10	7	140	46	0	6
Sundae, Marshmallow	sm	280	7	4.5	110	49	0	5
Sundae, Pineapple	sm	230	7	4.5	100	38	0	6
Sundae, Strawberry	sm	260	7	4.5	105	44	0	6
Waffle Bowl Sundae, Chocolate Covered Strawberry	1	790	40	27	180	99	2	10

ITEM DESCRIPTION	Serving Size	Calories	Total Fat (g)	Saturated Fat (g)	Sodium (mg)	Carbohydrates (g)	Fiber (g)	Protein (g)
Waffle Bowl Sundae, Fab Fudge	1	750	30	21	230	108	1	10
Waffle Bowl Sundae, Fudge Brownie Temptation	1	970	49	21	370	120	3	14
Waffle Bowl Sundae, Nut & Fudge	1	880	47	21	420	99	4	17
Waffle Bowl Sundae, Turtle	1	810	34	18	320	116	2	12
TOPPINGS AND EXTRAS								
Almond Pieces	1 serv	90	8	0.5	110	2	1	3
Banana Slices	1 serv	25	0	0	0	6	1	0
Blackberry Topping	1 serv	60	0	0	10	14	0	0
Blueberry Topping	1 serv	60	0	0	10	15	1	0
Butterfinger Pieces	1 serv	110	4.5	2	55	18	0	1
Butterscotch Topping	1 serv	90	0	0	85	20	0	1
Caramel Topping	1 serv	90	0.5	0.5	60	20	0	1
Cheesecake Pieces	1 serv	100	6	3.5	80	10	0	2
Cherry Topping	1 serv	40	0	0	20	9	0	0
Chewy Baked Brownie Pieces	1 serv	130	6	1.5	130	17	0	2
Choco Chunks	1 serv	150	10	8	0	17	1	1
Chocolate Topping	1 serv	70	0	0	25	17	0	0
Cocoa Fudge	1 serv	160	10	2	50	15	1	2
Coconut Flakes	1 serv	80	7	6	35	7	2	1
Cookie Dough Pieces	1 serv	130	6	1.5	70	18	0	1
Heath Pieces	1 serv	150	9	5	95	17	0	1
Hot Fudge Topping	1 serv	90	3	2.5	45	15	0	1
M&M's Chocolate Candies	1 serv	140	6	3.5	20	20	1	1
Maple Walnut Topping	1 serv	130	8	0.5	5	14	1	2
Marshmallow Topping	1 serv	70	0	0	15	18	0	0
Oreo Cookie Pieces	1 serv	140	6	1.5	190	20	1	1
Peanut Butter Topping	1 serv	180	15	2	170	8	1	3
Peanuts	1 serv	80	7	1	55	3	1	4
Pecan Pieces	1 serv	100	11	1	55	2	1	1
Pineapple Topping	1 serv	30	0	0	5	7	0	0
Rainbow Sprinkles	1 serv	70	2.5	1	0	10	0	0
Red Raspberry Topping	1 serv	50	0	0	5	14	2	0
Reese's® Peanut Butter Cups Pieces	1 serv	150	9	3	85	16	1	3

ITEM DESCRIPTION	Serving Size	Calories	Total Fat (g)	Saturated Fat (g)	Sodium (mg)	Carbohydrates (g)	Fiber (g)	Protein (g)
Snickers Pieces	1 serv	130	7	2.5	70	17	1	2
Strawberry Topping	1 serv	25	0	0	5	6	0	0
Whipped Topping	1 serv	90	7	7	0	7	0	0

DOMINO'S PIZZA

DRESSINGS AND SPREADS

ITEM DESCRIPTION	Serving Size	Calories	Total Fat (g)	Saturated Fat (g)	Sodium (mg)	Carbohydrates (g)	Fiber (g)	Protein (g)
Dipping Sauce, Blue Cheese	1 pkg	210	22	4	390	2	0	1
Dipping Sauce, Garlic	1 pkg	250	28	5	160	0	0	0
Dipping Sauce, Hot	1 pkg	50	4.5	0.5	1480	3	0	0
Dipping Sauce, Italian	1 pkg	25	0	0	270	5	1	1
Dipping Sauce, Marinara	1 pkg	25	0	0	270	5	1	1
Dipping Sauce, Parmesan Peppercorn	1 pkg	190	21	3	390	2	0	0
Dipping Sauce, Ranch	1 pkg	190	21	3	390	2	0	0
Dipping Sauce, Sweet Icing	1 pkg	250	2.5	0.5	0	57	0	0
Dressing, Blue Cheese	1 pkg	230	24	5	450	2	0	2
Dressing, Buttermilk Ranch	1 pkg	220	24	4	420	2	0	1
Dressing, Creamy Caesar	1 pkg	210	22	3.5	510	2	0	1
Dressing, Golden Italian	1 pkg	220	23	3.5	370	2	0	0
Dressing, Light Italian	1 pkg	20	1	0	780	2	0	0

PIZZAS

ITEM DESCRIPTION	Serving Size	Calories	Total Fat (g)	Saturated Fat (g)	Sodium (mg)	Carbohydrates (g)	Fiber (g)	Protein (g)
Hand Tossed Medium w/ Sauce & Cheese	1 pc/8	170	5	2.5	360	25	1	7
Thin Crust, Medium w/ Sauce & Cheese	1 pc/8	140	7	2.5	240	14	1	5
Deep Dish, Medium w/ Sauce & Cheese	1 pc /8	220	10	3.5	530	27	3	8
Brooklyn Style 14" w/ Sauce & Cheese	1 pc /6	240	10	5	560	27	2	12
Brooklyn Style 16" w/ Sauce & Cheese	1 pc /6	380	15	7	810	45	2	18

FEAST PIZZAS

ITEM DESCRIPTION	Serving Size	Calories	Total Fat (g)	Saturated Fat (g)	Sodium (mg)	Carbohydrates (g)	Fiber (g)	Protein (g)
America's Favorite Feast (Toppings Only): Pepperoni, Mushroom, Sausage	1 pc /8	120	10	4	470	4	1	6
Bacon Cheeseburger Feast (Toppings Only): Beef, Bacon, Cheddar Cheese	1 pc /8	140	11	5	450	3	1	8

ITEM DESCRIPTION	Serving Size	Calories	Total Fat (g)	Saturated Fat (g)	Sodium (mg)	Carbohydrates (g)	Fiber (g)	Protein (g)
Barbecue Feast (Toppings Only): Barbecue Sauce, Green Pepper, Onion, Bacon, Cheddar Cheese	1 pc /8	130	8	4	360	8	0	7
Deluxe Feast Pepperoni (Toppings Only): Green Pepper, Onion, Mushroom, Sausage	1 pc /8	100	8	3.5	380	4	1	5
ExtravaganZZa (Toppings Only): Pepperoni, Ham, Green Pepper, Onion, Black Olive, Mushroom, Sausage, Beef, Extra Cheese	1 pc /8	150	12	5	590	5	1	9
Feast Pizza Deep Dish (Shell Only)	1 pc /8	160	5	1	250	24	3	4
Feast Pizza Hand Tossed (Dough Only)	1 pc /8	120	1.5	0	125	22	1	4
Feast Pizza Thin Crust (Shell Only)	1 pc /8	80	3.5	0.5	15	12	1	2
Hawaiian Feast Ham (Toppings Only): Pineapple, Extra Cheese	1 pc /8	90	6	3	390	5	1	6
MeatZZa Feast (Toppings Only): Pepperoni, Ham, Sausage, Beef, Extra Cheese	1 pc /8	150	11	5	580	4	1	9
Pepperoni Feast (Toppings Only): Extra Pepperoni & Extra Cheese	1 pc /8	130	11	5	530	4	1	7
Philly Cheese Steak Feast (Toppings Only): Philly Meat, Mushroom, Green Pepper, Onion, Provolone Cheese, American Cheese	1 pc /8	100	7	4.5	360	1	0	7
Vegi Feast (Toppings Only): Green Pepper, Onion, Mushroom, Black Olive, Extra Cheese	1 pc /8	80	6	3	340	4	1	5
SANDWICHES								
Chicken Bacon Ranch	1	890	45	16	2210	72	2	49
Chicken Parm	1	770	30	16	2130	73	3	51
Italian	1	880	45	22	2560	71	3	47
Philly Cheese Steak	1	690	27	14	2080	72	3	41
SIDES AND SNACKS								
Breadsticks	1 pc	110	6	1.5	100	11	0	2
Buffalo Chicken Kickers	2 pcs	100	4.5	0.5	280	7	1	9
Buffalo Wings, Barbecue	2 pcs	230	14	3.5	410	6	0	17

ITEM DESCRIPTION	Serving Size	Calories	Total Fat (g)	Saturated Fat (g)	Sodium (mg)	Carbohydrates (g)	Fiber (g)	Protein (g)
Buffalo Wings, Hot	2 pcs	200	14	3.5	690	2	0	16
Cheesy Bread	1 pc	120	6	2	150	11	0	4
Chicken Caesar Salad, Grilled	half	100	4.5	2	310	6	2	10
Cinna Stix	1 pc	120	6	1	85	14	1	2
Croutons	1 pkg	45	2	0	70	6	0	1
Garden Fresh Salad	half	70	4	2.5	80	5	2	4
TOPPINGS AND EXTRAS (PER SLICE OR SANDWICH)								
Beef, Pizza Topping	1 serv	40	3	1.5	70	0	0	2
Black Olives, Pizza Topping	1 serv	10	1	0	65	1	0	0
Cheese, Pizza Topping	1 serv	25	2	1	85	1	0	2
Cheese, Sandwich Topping	1 serv	70	6	3.5	150	0	0	5
Chicken, Sandwich Topping	1 serv	70	3.5	1.5	310	1	0	10
Green Peppers, Pizza Topping	1 serv	0	0	0	0	0	0	0
Ham, Pizza Topping	1 serv	10	0	0	100	0	0	1
Italian Meat, Sandwich Topping	1 serv	120	10	3.5	560	0	0	7
Mushrooms, Pizza Topping	1 serv	0	0	0	0	0	0	0
Onions, Pizza Topping	1 serv	0	0	0	0	1	0	0
Pepperoni, Pizza Topping	1 serv	40	3.5	1	140	0	0	2
Philly Meat, Sandwich Topping	1 serv	45	1.5	0.5	250	1	0	6
Pineapple, Pizza Topping	1 serv	5	0	0	0	2	0	0
Sausage, Pizza Topping	1 serv	45	3.5	1.5	130	1	0	2
Veggies, Italian, Sandwich Topping	1 serv	5	0	0	30	1	0	0
Veggies, Philly, Sandwich Topping	1 serv	5	0	0	0	1	0	0

The pizza products listed in this publication, when made with approved Domino's Pizza ingredients, will provide the nutritional composition as indicated. Information may vary slightly depending on location and supplier. The availability of optional toppings may vary by size. Percent Daily Values (DV) are based on a 2,000 calorie diet. Your daily values may be higher or lower, depending on your calorie needs. The ingredient listings are provided by ingredient manufacturers. Domino's Pizza LLC, its franchisees and employees do not assume responsibility for a particular sensitivity or allergy to any food provided from our stores. This guide includes only standard menu items. For nutritional information on special menu product offers, visit www.dominos.com.

DUNKIN' DONUTS

BAKED ITEMS

ITEM DESCRIPTION	Serving Size	Calories	Total Fat (g)	Saturated Fat (g)	Sodium (mg)	Carbohydrates (g)	Fiber (g)	Protein (g)
Bagel, Blueberry	1	370	4	1	710	73	5	13
Bagel, Cinnamon Raisin	1	370	4	0.5	530	72	3	13
Bagel, Everything	1	360	5	0.5	780	74	3	15
Bagel, Garlic	1	350	3.5	0.5	780	76	4	15
Bagel, Multigrain	1	400	9	1	600	65	10	18
Bagel, Onion	1	340	3.5	0.5	660	65	3	12

ITEM DESCRIPTION	Serving Size	Calories	Total Fat (g)	Saturated Fat (g)	Sodium (mg)	Carbohydrates (g)	Fiber (g)	Protein (g)
Bagel, Plain	1	330	3	0.5	780	71	3	14
Bagel, Poppy Seed	1	370	6	0.5	780	73	3	15
Bagel, Salt	1	330	3	0.5	3540	71	3	14
Bagel, Sesame	1	370	7	0.5	780	72	3	16
Bagel, Wheat	1	350	4	0.5	650	66	5	13
Berries 'n Kreme	1	380	17	8	430	53	1	4
Biscuit	1	280	14	8	620	32	1	5
Bismark, Chocolate Iced	1	350	14	5	460	53	1	4
Bow Tie	1	310	15	7	400	39	1	4
Brownie	1	430	23	5	260	56	1	3
Cinnamon Twist	1	210	11	5	300	25	1	3
Coffee Roll	1	370	18	7	510	49	2	5
Coffee Roll w/ Chocolate Frosting	1	380	19	8	530	50	2	5
Coffee Roll w/ Maple Frosting	1	380	18	8	520	50	2	5
Coffee Roll w/ Vanilla Frosting	1	380	18	8	520	50	2	5
Cookie, Chocolate Chunk	1	540	23	13	550	80	3	7
Cookie, Oatmeal Raisin	1	480	14	7	310	83	5	8
Croissant	1	310	16	7	350	35	1	7
Danish, Apple	1	330	16	7	270	41	1	4
Danish, Cheese	1	330	17	8	270	39	1	5
Danish, Strawberry Cheese	1	320	16	7	260	40	1	4
Donut, Apple Crumb	1	460	14	8	330	80	2	4
Donut, Apple N' Spice	1	240	11	4.5	320	32	1	3
Donut, Bavarian Kreme	1	250	12	5	330	31	1	3
Donut, Blueberry Cake	1	330	18	8	460	38	1	3
Donut, Blueberry Crumb	1	470	14	8	330	84	2	4
Donut, Boston Kreme	1	280	12	5	350	38	1	3
Donut, Chocolate Coconut Cake	1	400	22	11	410	49	2	3
Donut, Chocolate Frosted	1	230	10	4	330	32	1	3
Donut, Chocolate Frosted Cake	1	340	19	8	330	38	1	3
Donut, Chocolate Glazed Cake	1	280	15	7	400	33	1	3
Donut, Chocolate Kreme Filled	1	310	16	7	340	37	1	4
Donut, Cinnamon Cake	1	290	18	8	310	30	1	3
Donut, Double Chocolate Cake	1	290	16	7	410	34	1	3

ITEM DESCRIPTION	Serving Size	Calories	Total Fat (g)	Saturated Fat (g)	Sodium (mg)	Carbohydrates (g)	Fiber (g)	Protein (g)
Donut, Glazed	1	220	9	4	320	31	1	3
Donut, Glazed Cake	1	320	18	8	310	37	1	3
Donut, Jelly Filled	1	260	11	5	330	36	1	3
Donut, Maple Frosted	1	230	10	4	330	33	1	3
Donut, Marble Frosted	1	230	10	4	330	32	1	3
Donut, Old Fashioned Cake	1	280	18	8	310	27	1	3
Donut, Powdered Cake	1	300	18	8	310	30	1	3
Donut, Pumpkin	1	320	18	8	270	36	1	3
Donut, Strawberry Frosted	1	230	10	4	330	33	1	3
Donut, Sugar Raised	1	190	9	4	320	22	1	3
Donut, Vanilla Kreme Filled	1	320	17	8	340	37	1	3
Eclair	1	350	14	5	460	53	1	4
English Muffin	1	160	1.5	0	340	31	2	6
French Cruller	1	250	20	9	105	18	0	2
Fritter, Apple	1	400	15	6	530	63	2	5
Fritter, Glazed	1	400	15	6	530	63	2	5
Muffin, Banana Walnut	1	530	23	2.5	500	72	3	8
Muffin, Blueberry	1	510	16	1.5	490	87	3	6
Muffin, Chocolate Chip	1	630	23	6	520	98	5	8
Muffin, Coffee Cake	1	620	25	7	530	93	2	7
Muffin, Corn	1	510	17	2	860	84	2	6
Muffin, Honey Bran Raisin	1	500	14	1.5	450	86	9	7
Muffin, Reduced Fat Blueberry	1	450	10	1.5	670	86	3	6
Munchkin, Cinnamon Cake	1	60	3	1.5	60	6	0	1
Munchkin, Glazed	1	50	2.5	1	65	7	0	1
Munchkin, Glazed Cake	1	60	3	1.5	65	8	0	1
Munchkin, Glazed Chocolate Cake	1	60	3	1.5	90	8	0	1
Munchkin, Jelly Filled	1	60	2.5	1	65	8	0	1
Munchkin, Plain Cake	1	50	3	1.5	60	5	0	1
Munchkin, Powdered Cake	1	60	3.5	1.5	60	6	0	1
Munchkin, Sugar Raised	1	40	2.5	1	65	5	0	1
Stick, Cinnamon Cake	1	310	20	9	300	30	1	3
Stick, Glazed Cake	1	340	20	9	300	38	1	3
Stick, Glazed Chocolate Cake	1	390	25	11	540	40	2	3

ITEM DESCRIPTION	Serving Size	Calories	Total Fat (g)	Saturated Fat (g)	Sodium (mg)	Carbohydrates (g)	Fiber (g)	Protein (g)
Stick, Jelly	1	400	20	9	320	54	1	3
Stick, Plain Cake	1	300	20	9	300	26	1	3
Stick, Powdered Cake	1	320	20	9	300	31	1	3
BEVERAGES								
Cappuccino	sm (10 oz)	80	4	2.5	70	7	0	4
Cappuccino w/ Sugar	sm (10 oz)	140	4	2.5	70	24	0	4
Chai, Vanilla	med (14 oz)	330	9	8	170	53	0	11
Coffee	sm (10 oz)	5	0	0	5	1	0	0
Coffee w/ Cream	sm (10 oz)	60	6	4	20	2	0	1
Coffee w/ Milk	sm (10 oz)	25	1	1	20	2	0	1
Coffee w/ Skim Milk	sm (10 oz)	15	0	0	25	3	0	2
Coffee w/ Splenda	sm (10 oz)	15	0	0	5	3	0	0
Coffee w/ Sugar	sm (10 oz)	60	0	0	5	18	0	0
Coffee, Blueberry	sm (10 oz)	15	0	0	5	2	0	0
Coffee, Caramel	sm (10 oz)	10	0	0	5	2	0	0
Coffee, Cinnamon	sm (10 oz)	15	0	0	5	2	0	0
Coffee, Coconut	sm (10 oz)	10	0	0	5	2	0	0
Coffee, French Vanilla	sm (10 oz)	10	0	0	10	2	0	0
Coffee, Hazelnut	sm (10 oz)	10	0	0	10	2	0	0
Coffee, Raspberry	sm (10 oz)	15	0	0	5	3	0	0
Coffee, Toasted Almond	sm (10 oz)	15	0	0	5	2	0	1
Coolatta®, Coffee w/ Cream	sm (16 oz)	330	23	14	60	28	0	3
Coolatta®, Coffee w/ Milk	sm (16 oz)	170	4	2.5	75	29	0	4
Coolatta®, Coffee w/ Skim Milk	sm (16 oz)	140	0	0	75	30	0	4
Coolatta®, Strawberry	sm (16 oz)	300	0	0	40	72	0	0
Coolatta®, Tropicana Orange	sm (16 oz)	220	0	0	35	52	0	1
Coolatta®, Vanilla Bean	sm (16 oz)	430	6	3.5	170	90	0	3
Dunkaccino®	sm (10 oz)	230	11	9	190	35	1	2
Espresso	1	0	0	0	0	0	0	0
Espresso w/ Sugar	1	30	0	0	5	7	0	0
Hot Chocolate	sm (10 oz)	210	7	7	270	39	2	2
Iced Caramel Swirl Latte	sm (16 oz)	220	6	3.5	150	35	0	8
Iced Caramel Swirl Latte w/ Skim Milk	sm (16 oz)	180	0	0	150	36	0	9

ITEM DESCRIPTION	Serving Size	Calories	Total Fat (g)	Saturated Fat (g)	Sodium (mg)	Carbohydrates (g)	Fiber (g)	Protein (g)
Iced Coffee	sm (16 oz)	10	0	0	5	2	0	1
Iced Coffee w/ Cream	sm (16 oz)	70	6	4	20	3	0	1
Iced Coffee w/ Milk	sm (16 oz)	30	1	1	20	3	0	2
Iced Coffee w/ Skim Milk	sm (16 oz)	20	0	0	25	3	0	2
Iced Coffee w/ Skim Milk & Splenda	sm (16 oz)	30	0	0	25	5	0	2
Iced Coffee w/ Sugar	sm (16 oz)	70	0	0	5	19	0	1
Iced Latte	sm (16 oz)	120	6	3.5	105	10	0	6
Iced Latte Lite	sm (16 oz)	80	0	0	110	13	0	7
Iced Latte w/ Skim Milk	sm (16 oz)	70	0	0	110	11	0	7
Iced Latte w/ Skim Milk & Sugar	sm (16 oz)	130	0	0	110	28	0	7
Iced Latte w/ Sugar	sm (16 oz)	170	6	3.5	100	27	0	6
Iced Latte, Mocha Raspberry	sm (16 oz)	230	6	4	110	36	1	7
Iced Latte, Mocha Spice	sm (16 oz)	220	6	4	95	35	1	7
Iced Mocha Swirl Latte	sm (16 oz)	220	6	4	115	35	1	7
Iced Mocha Swirl Latte w/ Skim Milk	sm (16 oz)	180	0	0	125	36	1	8
Iced Tea, Freshly Brewed Sweetened	16 fl oz	80	0	0	0	20	0	0
Iced Tea, Freshly Brewed Unsweetened	16 fl oz	5	0	0	0	1	0	0
Iced Tea, Peach Flavored	16 fl oz	15	0	0	0	3	0	0
Iced Tea, Peach Flavored Sweetened	16 fl oz	90	0	0	0	22	0	0
Iced Tea, Raspberry Flavored	16 fl oz	10	0	0	0	3	0	0
Iced Tea, Raspberry Flavored Sweetened	16 fl oz	90	0	0	0	22	0	0
Latte	sm (10 oz)	120	6	3.5	105	10	0	6
Latte Lite	sm (10 oz)	80	0	0	110	13	0	7
Latte w/ Sugar	sm (10 oz)	170	6	3.5	100	27	0	6
Latte, Caramel Swirl	sm (10 oz)	220	6	3.5	150	35	0	8
Latte, Mocha Raspberry	sm (10 oz)	230	6	4	110	36	1	7
Latte, Mocha Spice	sm (10 oz)	220	6	4	95	35	1	7
Latte, Mocha Swirl	sm (10 oz)	220	6	4	115	35	1	7
Latte, Vanilla Lite	sm (10 oz)	90	0	0	110	14	0	7
Tea, Decaffeinated	10 oz	0	0	0	5	0	0	0

ITEM DESCRIPTION	Serving Size	Calories	Total Fat (g)	Saturated Fat (g)	Sodium (mg)	Carbohydrates (g)	Fiber (g)	Protein (g)
Tea, Decaffeinated w/ Milk	10 oz	20	1	0.5	20	1	0	1
Tea, Decaffeinated w/ Skim Milk	10 oz	10	0	0	20	2	0	1
Tea, Decaffeinated w/ Sugar	10 oz	60	0	0	5	17	0	0
Tea, Earl Grey	10 oz	0	0	0	5	0	0	0
Tea, Earl Grey w/ Milk	10 oz	20	1	0.5	20	1	0	1
Tea, Earl Grey w/ Skim Milk	10 oz	10	0	0	20	2	0	1
Tea, Earl Grey w/ Sugar	10 oz	60	0	0	5	17	0	0
Tea, English Breakfast	10 oz	0	0	0	5	0	0	0
Tea, English Breakfast w/ Milk	10 oz	20	1	0.5	20	1	0	1
Tea, English Breakfast w/ Skim Milk	10 oz	10	0	0	20	2	0	1
Tea, English Breakfast w/ Sugar	10 oz	60	0	0	5	17	0	0
Tea, Freshly Brewed Unsweetened	10 oz	0	0	0	5	0	0	0
Tea, Freshly Brewed w/ Milk	10 oz	20	1	0.5	20	1	0	1
Tea, Freshly Brewed w/ Skim Milk	10 oz	10	0	0	20	2	0	1
Tea, Freshly Brewed w/ Sugar	10 oz	60	0	0	5	17	0	0
Tea, Green	10 oz	0	0	0	5	0	0	0
Tea, Green w/ Milk	10 oz	20	1	0.5	20	1	0	1
Tea, Green w/ Skim Milk	10 oz	10	0	0	20	2	0	1
Tea, Green w/ Sugar	10 oz	60	0	0	5	17	0	0
Tea, Sweet	16 oz	120	0	0	0	29	0	0
Turbo Shot™	1.75 oz	0	0	0	0	0	0	0
Turbo Shot™	3.5 oz	10	0	0	15	2	0	0
Turbo Shot™	2.5 oz	5	0	0	10	1	0	0
Turbo Shot™	4 oz	10	0	0	15	2	0	0
White Hot Chocolate	sm (10 oz)	230	9	7	310	38	0	2
BREAKFAST ITEMS								
Bagel w/ Bacon, Egg & Cheese	1	530	18	6	1370	76	3	26
Bagel w/ Bacon, Supreme Omelet & Cheese	1	560	20	8	1670	77	3	30
Bagel w/ Egg & Cheese	1	480	15	5	1180	75	3	22
Bagel w/ Ham, Egg & Cheese	1	520	17	6	1480	75	3	28
Bagel w/ Ham, Supreme Omelet & Cheese	1	560	18	8	1780	77	3	32
Bagel w/ Sausage, Egg & Cheese	1	660	29	11	1590	76	3	30
Bagel w/ Sausage, Supreme Omelet & Cheese	1	690	31	13	1890	78	3	34

ITEM DESCRIPTION	Serving Size	Calories	Total Fat (g)	Saturated Fat (g)	Sodium (mg)	Carbohydrates (g)	Fiber (g)	Protein (g)
Bagel w/ Supreme Omelet & Cheese	1	520	17	7	1480	77	3	26
Biscuit w/ Bacon, Egg & Cheese	1	470	29	14	1200	36	1	16
Biscuit w/ Bacon, Supreme Omelet & Cheese	1	510	31	16	1500	38	2	21
Biscuit w/ Egg & Cheese	1	430	26	13	1010	36	1	13
Biscuit w/ Ham, Egg & Cheese	1	470	28	14	1320	36	1	19
Biscuit w/ Ham, Supreme Omelet & Cheese	1	510	29	16	1620	38	2	23
Biscuit w/ Sausage, Egg & Cheese	1	600	40	18	1410	37	1	20
Biscuit w/ Sausage, Supreme Omelet & Cheese	1	640	42	20	1710	38	2	24
Biscuit w/ Supreme Omelet & Cheese	1	470	28	15	1310	37	2	17
Croissant w/ Bacon, Egg & Cheese	1	510	31	13	930	39	1	18
Croissant w/ Bacon, Supreme Omelet & Cheese	1	550	33	15	1230	41	2	22
Croissant w/ Egg & Cheese	1	470	28	12	750	39	1	15
Croissant w/ Ham, Egg & Cheese	1	510	30	12	1050	39	1	21
Croissant w/ Ham, Supreme Omelet & Cheese	1	540	31	14	1360	41	2	25
Croissant w/ Sausage, Egg & Cheese	1	640	42	17	1150	40	1	22
Croissant w/ Sausage, Supreme Omelet & Cheese	1	680	44	19	1450	41	2	26
Croissant w/ Supreme Omelet & Cheese	1	500	30	14	1050	41	2	19
English Muffin w/ Bacon, Egg & Cheese	1	360	16	6	920	35	2	18
English Muffin w/ Bacon, Supreme Omelet & Cheese	1	390	18	8	1220	36	3	22
English Muffin w/ Egg & Cheese	1	320	13	5	730	34	2	14
English Muffin w/ Ham, Egg & Cheese	1	350	15	6	1040	35	2	21
English Muffin w/ Ham, Supreme Omelet & Cheese	1	390	16	8	1340	36	3	25
English Muffin w/ Sausage, Egg & Cheese	1	490	28	10	1130	35	2	22
English Muffin w/ Sausage, Supreme Omelet & Cheese	1	520	29	12	1440	37	3	26
English Muffin w/ Supreme Omelet & Cheese	1	350	15	7	1040	36	3	19
Flatbread w/ Egg White Turkey Sausage	1	280	6	2.5	820	37	3	19

ITEM DESCRIPTION	Serving Size	Calories	Total Fat (g)	Saturated Fat (g)	Sodium (mg)	Carbohydrates (g)	Fiber (g)	Protein (g)
Flatbread w/ Egg White Veggie	1	290	9	4	680	39	3	11
Flatbread w/ Ham & Swiss	1	350	12	5	1040	41	2	20
Flatbread w/ Turkey Cheddar & Bacon	1	420	17	7	1270	41	2	24
Flatbread, Grilled Cheese	1	460	24	12	1000	42	2	20
Flatbread, Southwest Chicken	1	310	9	4	840	33	2	23
Hash Browns	9 pcs	200	11	1.5	730	22	3	2
Waffle Breakfast Sandwich	1	390	23	8	1000	28	1	16
Waffles	2 pcs	190	8	2	420	24	1	4
Wrap	1	170	10	4	450	14	1	7
Wrap w/ Bacon	1	190	12	4.5	540	14	1	9
DRESSINGS AND SPREADS								
Cream Cheese, Plain	1 serv	150	15	9	250	3	0	3
Cream Cheese, Reduced Fat	1 serv	100	8	5	250	5	0	4
Cream Cheese, Reduced Fat Blueberry	1 serv	150	9	6	210	15	0	2
Cream Cheese, Reduced Fat Onion & Chive	1 serv	130	11	7	250	6	0	3
Cream Cheese, Reduced Fat Smoked Salmon	1 serv	140	11	7	260	6	0	4
Cream Cheese, Reduced Fat Strawberry	1 serv	150	10	6	200	15	0	2
Cream Cheese, Reduced Fat Veggie	1 serv	120	10	6	240	6	0	2
SALADS								
Caesar	1	320	29	6	790	11	3	6
Chicken Caesar	1	440	33	7	1020	11	3	25
Garden	1	180	6	3	500	21	4	8
SANDWICHES								
Chicken Bruschetta	1	580	26	7	1200	49	2	37
Chipotle Chicken	1	600	25	8	1380	50	3	43
Pastrami Supreme	1	750	39	16	2060	51	3	48
Pressed Cuban	1	680	33	13	2000	50	2	46
Steak & Cheese	1	470	16	6	2040	50	2	31
Toasted Italian	1	560	25	9	2630	52	3	33
Tuna Melt	1	770	30	7	1560	57	3	36
Tuna, Albacore	1	660	19	2.5	1280	56	3	31

ITEM DESCRIPTION	Serving Size	Calories	Total Fat (g)	Saturated Fat (g)	Sodium (mg)	Carbohydrates (g)	Fiber (g)	Protein (g)
Turkey & Bacon Club	1	440	13	3	1800	51	3	35
Turkey & Cheese	1	450	13	4.5	1500	52	3	35
SOUPS								
Broccoli Cheddar	1	190	11	6	990	14	2	10
Chicken Noodle	1	130	3	1	970	19	1	7

Allergy sufferers should always read the product ingredient statement and allergen information available at www.DunkinDonuts.com/Nutrition. Please note that our restaurants prepare and serve products that contain allergens other than the products you select.

   Dunkin' Donuts has made a reasonable effort to provide nutritional and ingredient information based upon standard product formulations and following the FDA guidelines using formulation and nutrition labeling software. Variations may occur due to: seasonal conditions; regional differences; ingredient substitutions; and differences in product assembly or size at the restaurant. Test products, limited time offers, and regional menu variations may not be included and not all items listed may be available in all restaurants. The information on these printed materials may vary from that which may be available in our restaurants. We will update www.DunkinDonuts.com/Nutrition frequently, so please revisit this site for the most current information. Any customers with specific dietary concerns are advised to www.DunkinDonuts.com/Nutrition or call our customer care line at 800-859-5339.

HARDEE'S

BREAKFAST ITEMS

ITEM DESCRIPTION	Serving Size	Calories	Total Fat (g)	Saturated Fat (g)	Sodium (mg)	Carbohydrates (g)	Fiber (g)	Protein (g)
Big Country® Breakfast Platter w/ Bacon*	1	980	56	13	2080	90	3	28
Biscuit 'N' Gravy™	1	530	34	8	1550	47	0	8
Biscuit 'N' Gravy Breakfast Bowl™	1	770	54	14	1950	49	1	20
Biscuit w/ Bacon, Egg & Cheese	1	560	38	11	1360	37	0	16
Biscuit w/ Chicken Fillet	1	600	34	7	1680	50	1	24
Biscuit w/ Country Ham	1	440	26	6	1710	36	0	14
Biscuit w/ Country Steak	1	620	41	11	1360	44	0	16
Biscuit w/ Ham, Egg & Cheese	1	560	35	10	1800	37	0	23
Biscuit w/ Jelly	1	430	28	7	1110	35	0	8
Biscuit w/ Loaded Omelet	1	640	44	14	1510	37	0	21
Biscuit w/ Pork Chop	1	690	42	8	1330	48	1	29
Biscuit w/ Sausage	1	530	38	10	1240	36	0	11
Biscuit w/ Sausage & Egg	1	610	44	11	1290	36	0	17
Biscuit, Cinnamon 'N' Raisin™	1	280	12	3	650	40	0	3
Biscuit, Made from Scratch™	1	370	23	5	890	35	0	5
Biscuit, Monster Biscuit™	1	710	51	17	2250	37	0	24
Breakfast Burrito, Loaded	1	780	51	20	1620	38	2	40
Croissant, Sunrise Croissant™ w/ Ham	1	430	26	10	1050	28	0	23
Frisco Breakfast Sandwich®	1	420	20	7	1340	37	2	24
Grits	1 serv	110	5	1	480	16	0	2
Hash Rounds™	med	350	22	5	490	34	3	4
Low Carb Breakfast Bowl™	1	620	50	21	1380	6	2	36

ITEM DESCRIPTION	Serving Size	Calories	Total Fat (g)	Saturated Fat (g)	Sodium (mg)	Carbohydrates (g)	Fiber (g)	Protein (g)
Pancakes, no Syrup	3 pcs	300	5	1	830	55	2	8
DESSERTS								
Apple Turnover	1	290	15	5	350	36	1	2
Cookie, Chocolate Chip	1	290	11	5	270	44	0	4
Ice Cream Bowl†	1 scoop	235	13	8	85	27	0	5
Ice Cream Cone†	1 scoop	285	13	8	140	37	0	6
Malt †	1	780	35	24	325	98	0	17
Peach Cobbler	sm	285	7	1	235	56	1	1
Shake †	1	705	33	23	255	86	0	14
KIDS MENU								
Cheeseburger	kid	600	27	6	930	68	4	21
Chicken Strips, no Sauce	kid	500	25	5	1050	50	3	19
Hamburger	kid	560	24	6	710	67	4	18
SANDWICHES								
Big Hot Ham 'N' Cheese™	1	520	24	13	2190	40	2	40
Burger, Bacon Cheese Thickburger®**	1/3 lb	910	64	22	1550	50	3	33
Burger, Cheeseburger**	1/3 lb	680	39	19	1450	52	2	29
Burger, Double Bacon Cheese Thickburger®**	2/3 lb	1300	97	38	2200	50	3	54
Burger, Double Thickburger®**	2/3 lb	1250	90	35	2160	54	3	51
Burger, Grilled Sourdough Thickburger®**	1/2 lb	1030	77	28	1910	42	3	42
Burger, Low Carb Thickburger®**	1/3 lb	420	32	12	1010	5	2	30
Burger, Monster Thickburger®**	2/3 lb	1420	108	43	2770	46	2	60
Burger, Mushroom & Swiss Thickburger®**	1/3 lb	720	42	21	1570	48	2	35
Burger, Original Thickburger®**	1/3 lb	910	64	21	1560	53	3	30
Burger, Six Dollar Burger**	1/2 lb	1060	73	28	1950	58	3	40
Cheeseburger	sm	350	16	4	780	36	1	17
Chicken Club Sandwich, Charbroiled	1	550	30	8	1560	35	2	28
Chicken Club Sandwich, Low Carb Charbroiled	1	370	21	7	1170	10	2	35
Chicken Fillet Sandwich	1	800	37	6	1890	76	3	41
Chicken Sandwich, Barbecue	1	320	6	1	1200	43	3	33

ITEM DESCRIPTION	Serving Size	Calories	Total Fat (g)	Saturated Fat (g)	Sodium (mg)	Carbohydrates (g)	Fiber (g)	Protein (g)
Chicken Sandwich, Spicy	1	470	21	5	1220	46	3	11
Chicken Strips	3 pcs	380	21	4	1360	27	1	22
Chicken Strips	5 pcs	630	34	6	2260	45	2	37
Hamburger	sm	310	12	4	560	36	1	14
Hot Dog	1	420	30	12	1200	22	1	16
Hot Ham 'N' Cheese™	1	420	18	10	1600	39	2	30
Roast Beef	reg	330	16	7	860	29	2	19
Roast Beef	lg	470	23	10	1290	38	2	29
SIDES AND SNACKS								
Chicken Breast, Fried	1	370	15	4	1190	29	0	29
Chicken Leg, Fried	1	170	7	2	570	15	0	13
Chicken Thigh, Fried	1	330	15	4	1000	30	0	19
Chicken Wing, Fried	1	200	8	2	740	23	0	10
Cole Slaw	sm	170	10	2	140	20	2	1
Crispy Curls™	med	410	20	5	1020	52	4	5
French Fries	med	430	19	4	960	60	4	5
Mashed Potatoes	sm	90	2	0	410	17	0	1
Salad, no Dressing	sm	120	7	5	160	7	2	7

* Served w/ syrup, jam & butter (Not included in nutrition above)
  ** Weight before cooking
   † Nutrient amounts may vary slightly by flavor. Items may vary by restaurant.
   For additional information visit www.hardees.com.

The information contained in this guide is based on standard U.S. product formulations. Variations may occur due to differences in suppliers, ingredient substitutions, recipe revisions, product assembly, and seasonal variances. Test products are not included. This information is current as of January 25, 2008. The information in this guide is reported for informational purposes only by Carl Karcher Enterprises, Inc., Neither CKE, its franchisees, or its employees assume any responsibility for sensitivity or allergy to any food product provided in our restaurants. Anyone with food sensitivities, allergies, or special dietary needs should consult a medical professional regarding the suitability of our food products, and should regularly review the information contained at www.hardees.com for content updates. If you have specific questions about our menu, call 1-877-799-STAR.

© 2008 Hardee's Food Systems, Inc. All rights reserved.

JACK IN THE BOX

BEVERAGES

Coca Cola Classic®	20 oz	170	0	0	0	46	0	0
Coffee, Bold Roast, Regular or Decaf	1	5	0	0	5	1	0	0
Diet Coke®	20 oz	0	0	0	15	0	0	0
Dr Pepper®	20 oz	150	0	0	50	42	0	0
Fanta® Orange	20 oz	150	0	0	50	41	0	0
Fanta® Strawberry	20 oz	150	0	0	10	41	0	0
Iced Coffee, Caramel	16 oz	90	1.5	1	55	17	0	4

ITEM DESCRIPTION	Serving Size	Calories	Total Fat (g)	Saturated Fat (g)	Sodium (mg)	Carbohydrates (g)	Fiber (g)	Protein (g)
Iced Coffee, Original	16 oz	100	1.5	1	55	17	0	4
Iced Coffee, Vanilla	16 oz	100	2	1	55	18	0	4
Iced Tea, Fresh Brewed	20 oz	5	0	0	20	2	0	0
Lemonade, Minute Maid®	20 oz	160	0	0	65	42	0	0
Orange Juice	10 oz	140	0	0	25	32	2	2
Root Beer, Barq's®	20 oz	180	0	0	40	50	0	0
Smoothie, Mango	16 oz	290	0	0	75	72	0	2
Smoothie, Pomegranate-Berry	16 oz	280	0	0	70	69	0	2
Smoothie, Strawberry	16 oz	280	0	0	70	68	1	2
Smoothie, Strawberry Banana	16 oz	290	0	0	70	73	1	2
Sprite®	20 oz	160	0	0	40	42	0	0
BREAKFAST ITEMS								
Bacon Breakfast Jack®	1	300	14	5	730	29	1	16
Biscuit & Gravy	1	450	28	12	1320	39	2	9
Biscuit w/ Bacon, Egg & Cheese	1	440	26	11	1030	37	2	16
Biscuit w/ Homestyle Chicken	1	520	26	10	1230	52	2	20
Biscuit w/ Sausage, Egg & Cheese	1	590	40	16	1140	38	2	20
Breakfast Bowl	1	780	60	20	1350	34	4	26
Breakfast Burrito w/ Meat, no Salsa	1	610	36	14	1360	39	5	32
Breakfast Jack®	1	290	12	4.5	760	29	1	17
Croissant Supreme	1	450	25	9	860	36	1	20
Croissant w/ Sausage	1	580	39	13	770	37	2	21
Denver Breakfast Bowl	1	720	53	18	1310	37	5	25
Extreme Sausage® Sandwich	1	670	48	17	1300	31	2	29
Hash Brown Sticks	5 pcs	230	16	4	330	20	2	2
Original French Toast Sticks	4 pcs	470	23	5	450	58	4	7
Sausage Breakfast Jack®	1	450	28	10	840	29	1	20
Sourdough Breakfast Sandwich	1	420	24	8	980	31	2	20
Steak & Egg Burrito, no Salsa	1	790	48	15	1320	52	6	37
Ultimate Breakfast Sandwich	1	570	27	10	1700	49	2	34
DESSERTS								
Cake, Chocolate Overload™	1 pc	300	7	1.5	350	57	2	4
Cheesecake	1 pc	310	16	9	220	34	0	7
Churros, Mini	5 pcs	320	17	5	270	39	2	3

ITEM DESCRIPTION	Serving Size	Calories	Total Fat (g)	Saturated Fat (g)	Sodium (mg)	Carbohydrates (g)	Fiber (g)	Protein (g)
Shake, Chocolate Ice Cream	16 oz	750	36	24	280	95	1	12
Shake, Oreo® Cookie Ice Cream	16 oz	760	40	26	360	87	1	12
Shake, Strawberry Ice Cream	16 oz	730	35	24	240	90	0	11
Shake, Vanilla Ice Cream	16 oz	650	35	24	230	70	0	11
DRESSINGS AND SPREADS								
Chipotle Sauce	1 serv	110	12	2	230	1	0	0
Country Crock® Spread	1 pkg	25	2.5	0.5	45	0	0	0
Dipping Sauce, Barbecue	1 pkg	45	0	0	330	11	0	0
Dipping Sauce, Buttermilk House	1 pkg	130	13	2	210	3	0	0
Dipping Sauce, Franks® Red Hot® Buffalo	1 pkg	10	0	0	840	2	0	0
Dipping Sauce, Honey Mustard	1 pkg	60	2	0	220	11	0	0
Dipping Sauce, Sweet & Sour	1 pkg	45	0	0	160	11	0	0
Dipping Sauce, Teriyaki	1 pkg	60	1	0	530	11	0	1
Dressing, Asian Sesame	1 serv	190	14	2	630	16	0	1
Dressing, Bacon Ranch	1 serv	260	26	4	700	3	0	2
Dressing, Creamy Southwest	1 serv	220	22	3.5	850	3	0	1
Dressing, Lite Ranch	1 serv	150	15	2.5	560	3	0	1
Dressing, Low Fat Balsamic	1 serv	35	1.5	0	480	5	0	0
Dressing, Ranch	1 serv	310	33	5	470	3	0	1
Jelly, Grape	1 pkg	35	0	0	10	9	0	0
Jelly, Strawberry	1 pkg	35	0	0	5	9	0	0
Ketchup	1 pkg	10	0	0	105	2	0	0
Mayo, Peppercorn	1 serv	190	20	3.5	250	1	0	0
Mayo, Smoky Cheddar	1 serv	210	22	3.5	220	1	0	1
Mayonnaise	1 pkg	80	9	1.5	40	0	0	0
Mayo-Onion Sauce	1 serv	90	10	1.5	85	1	0	0
Mustard	1 pkg	5	0	0	50	1	0	0
Salsa, Fire Roasted	1 pkg	5	0	0	105	1	0	0
Sauce, Zesty Marinara	1 pkg	15	0	0	200	4	0	0
Sour Cream	1 pkg	60	5	3	25	2	<1	1
Soy Sauce	1 pkg	5	0	0	480	1	0	1
Syrup, Log Cabin®	1 pkg	190	0	0	35	49	0	0
Taco Sauce	1 pkg	0	0	0	80	0	0	0

ITEM DESCRIPTION	Serving Size	Calories	Total Fat (g)	Saturated Fat (g)	Sodium (mg)	Carbohydrates (g)	Fiber (g)	Protein (g)
Tartar Sauce	1 pkg	210	22	3.5	370	2	0	0
Vinegar	1 pkg	0	0	0	20	0	0	0
KIDS MENU								
Applesauce	1 pkg	100	0	0	0	25	1	0
Cheeseburger	1	280	12	4.5	540	29	1	14
Chicken Strips, Crispy	2 pcs	250	12	3	630	18	2	17
Chicken Strips, Grilled	2 pcs	250	12	3	630	18	2	17
French Fries	kid	210	11	2.5	380	25	3	3
Grilled Cheese Sandwich	1	330	18	6	730	31	2	11
Hamburger w/ Cheese	1	320	15	7	730	30	1	16
Milk, 1% Chocolate Low Fat	8 oz	200	2.5	1.5	230	34	1	11
Milk, 2% Reduced Fat Chug**	8 oz	130	5	3	130	13	0	10
MAIN MENU								
Chicken Breast Strips, Crispy	4 pcs	500	25	6	1260	36	3	35
Chicken Club w/ Homestyle Ranch	1	720	33	9	1860	74	3	33
Chicken Fajita Pita Made w/ Whole Grain, no Salsa	1	320	11	5	1110	33	4	24
Chicken Sandwich	1	400	21	4.5	740	38	2	15
Chicken Sandwich w/ Bacon	1	440	24	6	970	38	2	19
Chicken Strips, Grilled, no Sauce	4 pcs	180	2	0.5	700	3	0	37
Chicken Teriyaki Bowl	1	580	5	1	1460	106	4	26
Fish & Chips	sm	630	35	8	1290	61	5	19
Fruit Cup	1	50	0	0	10	14	1	1
Hamburger Deluxe	1	340	18	6	550	31	2	14
Jack's Spicy Chicken®	1	550	24	5	1050	59	4	24
Jack's Spicy Chicken® w/ Cheese	1	630	30	9	1360	61	4	29
Sourdough Grilled Chicken Club	1	530	28	7	1440	34	3	36
Sourdough Grilled Chicken Club, no Bun	1	230	10	4	1020	5	1	30
Steak Teriyaki Bowl	1	650	10	3	1740	106	4	30
SALADS								
Asian Chicken Salad, Crispy*	1	340	13	3	660	38	8	21
Asian Chicken Salad, Grilled*	1	180	1.5	0	380	22	6	22
Chicken Club Salad, Crispy*	1	480	27	10	1050	28	6	33
Chicken Club Salad, Grilled*	1	320	16	7	780	12	4	34

ITEM DESCRIPTION	Serving Size	Calories	Total Fat (g)	Saturated Fat (g)	Sodium (mg)	Carbohydrates (g)	Fiber (g)	Protein (g)
Side Salad*	1	50	3	1.5	60	5	2	3
Southwest Chicken Salad, Crispy*	1	470	23	8	1100	44	9	30
Southwest Chicken Salad, Grilled*	1	310	12	5	820	28	7	31
SANDWICHES								
Cheeseburger, Bacon Ultimate	1	980	67	27	1880	52	2	43
Cheeseburger, Big	1	650	40	15	1170	50	2	24
Cheeseburger, Ultimate	1	920	63	26	1530	52	2	38
Hamburger	1	280	12	4.5	540	29	1	14
Hamburger Deluxe w/ Cheese	1	430	25	10	920	33	2	19
Hamburger w/ Cheese	1	320	15	7	730	30	1	16
Jumbo Jack®	1	580	33	11	920	51	2	20
Jumbo Jack® w/ Cheese	1	670	40	15	1290	53	2	24
Jumbo Jack®, no Bun	1	230	19	9	270	2	1	12
Jumbo Jack®, no Sauce	1	470	23	10	790	47	2	20
Junior Bacon Cheeseburger	1	400	23	8	800	30	1	18
Sirloin Burger w/ Bacon, Swiss & Grilled Onions	1	990	64	20	2230	61	4	47
Sirloin Burger w/ Swiss & Grilled Onions	1	930	59	18	1880	60	4	42
Sirloin Cheeseburger	1	950	60	19	1920	61	4	41
Sirloin Cheeseburger w/ Bacon	1	1010	65	20	2270	62	4	46
Sourdough Jack®	1	680	46	17	1200	41	2	26
Sourdough Steak Melt	1	650	40	14	1500	34	3	37
SIDES AND SNACKS								
Egg Roll	1 pc	130	6	2	310	15	2	5
French Fries	med	460	24	6	850	55	6	6
Mozzarella Sticks	3 pcs	240	14	6	510	20	1	10
Onion Rings	8 pcs	500	30	6	420	51	3	6
Pita Snack, Crispy Chicken	1	390	19	4.5	780	39	3	17
Pita Snack, Fish	1	380	19	4.5	720	39	3	13
Pita Snack, Grilled Chicken	1	310	13	3	640	31	3	17
Pita Snack, Steak	1	350	16	4.5	640	31	3	19
Potato Wedges, Bacon Cheddar	1 serv	760	52	16	960	53	4	21
Sampler Trio	1	740	38	15	1720	72	7	26
Seasoned Curly Fries	med	420	24	5	920	46	5	6

ITEM DESCRIPTION	Serving Size	Calories	Total Fat (g)	Saturated Fat (g)	Sodium (mg)	Carbohydrates (g)	Fiber (g)	Protein (g)
Stuffed Jalapeños	3 pcs	230	13	6	690	22	2	7
Stuffed Jalapeños	7 pcs	530	30	13	1600	51	4	15
Taco, Beef	1	160	8	3	270	15	2	5
TOPPINGS AND EXTRAS								
Almonds, Roasted Slivered	1 serv	110	9	0.5	5	4	2	4
Cheese, American	1 pc	45	3.5	2	180	1	0	2
Cheese, Real Swiss	1 pc	70	6	3.5	80	0	n/a	5
Cheese, Swiss-Style	1 pc	40	3	2	150	1	0	2
Corn Sticks, Spicy	1 serv	130	5	1	150	20	<1	2
Croutons, Gourmet Seasoned	1 serv	100	5	1	230	11	0	2
Equal® Sweetener	1 pkg	5	0	0	0	1	0	0
Half & Half	1 pkg	10	1	0.5	0	0	0	0
Onion Rings, Red	1 serv	5	0	0	0	1	0	0
Onions, Short Sliced Grilled	1 serv	10	0	0	250	1	0	0
Splenda® No Calorie Sweetener	1 pkg	0	0	0	0	<1	0	0
Sugar	1 pkg	10	0	0	0	3	0	0
Sweet 'N Low® Sugar Substitute	1 pkg	5	0	0	0	1	0	0
Wonton Strips	1 serv	110	6	1.5	45	13	2	2

* Nutritional data does not include dressing or condiments.

  ** 37% fat reduction compared to whole milk.

  All data displayed follows the federal regulations regarding the rounding on nutritional data. Information may vary slightly from actual due to rounding of nutritional data.

  Variations within the nutritional values may occur due to the use of regional suppliers, seasonal influences, manufacturing tolerances, minor differences in product assembly at the restaurant level, recipe revisions, and other factors.

  Serving size designation for beverages refers to total cup capacity. The actual fill might be slightly different.

  Sodium and potassium values in drinks may vary due to local water supplies.

  To help our customers make better informed decisions about their menu choices at our restaurants, we have developed a Build Your Meal calculator on our website. You can combine menu items into a meal and view the complete nutritional information of each item. Once you have assembled your meal, you will be able to add or remove ingredients and choose from a list of common substitutes for each item. Jack in the Box invites you to go to www.jackinthebox.com/ourfood/ to build a meal of your favorite menu items.

KENTUCKY FRIED CHICKEN

BEVERAGES								
7UP®**	16 oz	200	0	0	50	52	0	0
Apple Juice	6.5 oz	100	0	0	10	24	0	0
Code Red Mountain Dew®*	16 oz	220	0	0	70	62	0	0
Diet Dr Pepper®**	16 oz	0	0	0	70	0	0	0
Diet Mountain Dew®*	16 oz	0	0	0	80	0	0	0
Diet Pepsi®*	16 oz	0	0	0	50	0	0	0
Diet Root Beer**, A&W®	16 oz	0	0	0	90	0	0	0

ITEM DESCRIPTION	Serving Size	Calories	Total Fat (g)	Saturated Fat (g)	Sodium (mg)	Carbohydrates (g)	Fiber (g)	Protein (g)
Dr Pepper®**	16 oz	200	0	0	70	54	0	0
Fruit Punch*, Tropicana®	16 oz	220	0	0	50	60	0	0
Lemonade*, Tropicana®	16 oz	200	0	0	210	54	0	0
Lemonade*, Tropicana® Pink	16 oz	200	0	0	210	54	0	0
Lemonade*, Tropicana® Sugar Free	16 oz	0	0	0	130	4	0	0
Lipton® Brisk® Green w/ Peach Tea*	16 oz	0	0	0	140	0	0	0
Lipton® Brisk® Lemon Tea*	16 oz	160	0	0	130	44	0	0
Lipton® Brisk® No Calorie Green Tea*	16 oz	0	0	0	140	0	0	0
Lipton® Brisk® Peach Tea*	16 oz	160	0	0	50	42	0	0
Lipton® Brisk® Raspberry Tea*	16 oz	160	0	0	50	42	0	0
Lipton® Brisk® Tea*	16 oz	0	0	0	60	0	0	0
Manzanita Sol®*	16 oz	220	0	0	50	58	0	0
Milk, 2%	16 oz	170	6	4	180	17	0	12
Miranda® Strawberry*	16 oz	220	0	0	100	58	0	0
Mountain Dew®*	16 oz	220	0	0	70	58	0	0
Orange Slice®*	16 oz	240	0	0	50	64	0	0
Pepsi®*	16 oz	200	0	0	50	56	0	0
Root Beer**, A&W®	16 oz	240	0	0	60	62	0	0
Root Beer®, Mug	16 oz	200	0	0	30	52	0	0
Sierra Mist® Free*	16 oz	0	0	0	50	0	0	0
Sierra Mist®*	16 oz	200	0	0	40	54	0	0
Twister® Orange* Tropicana®	16 oz	220	0	0	50	62	0	0
Wild Cherry Pepsi®*	16 oz	200	0	0	40	56	0	0
DESSERTS								
Apple Turnover	1	260	13	3	170	35	1	2
Cake, Café Valley Bakery® Chocolate Chip	1 pc	280	9	3.5	160	47	1	3
Cookie, Sweet Life® Chocolate Chip	1	170	8	4	90	23	1	2
Cookie, Sweet Life® Oatmeal Raisin	1	150	6	2.5	130	23	1	2
Cookie, Sweet Life® Sugar	1	160	7	3	125	22	0	2
Parfait Cup, Lil' Bucket™ Chocolate Crème	1	280	14	9	220	37	1	2
Parfait Cup, Lil' Bucket™ Lemon Crème	1	390	14	8	220	60	0	7
Parfait Cup, Lil' Bucket™ Strawberry Shortcake	1	230	8	4	220	39	1	2

ITEM DESCRIPTION	Serving Size	Calories	Total Fat (g)	Saturated Fat (g)	Sodium (mg)	Carbohydrates (g)	Fiber (g)	Protein (g)
Pie, Cookie Dough	1 pc	240	12	7	190	31	1	3
Pie, Dutch Apple	1 pc	320	14	6	300	47	1	2
Pie, Lemon Meringue	1 pc	250	7	3.5	210	42	0	4
Pie, Pecan	1 pc	410	21	6	220	52	1	4
Pie, Sara Lee® Apple	1 pc	310	13	5	290	48	1	2
Pie, Sara Lee® Pecan	1 pc	450	22	8	460	61	1	5
Pie, Sara Lee® Sweet Potato	1 pc	340	16	7	330	46	0	5
Pie, Strawberry Cream Cheese	1 pc	270	15	10	220	31	0	3
Teddy Grahams®, Graham Snacks, Cinnamon	1 pkg	90	3	0.5	95	15	1	1
DRESSINGS AND SPREADS								
Dipping Sauce, Creamy Ranch	1 serv	140	15	2.5	230	1	0	0
Dipping Sauce, Fiery Buffalo	1 serv	25	0	0	530	6	0	0
Dipping Sauce, Garlic Parmesan	1 serv	130	13	2.5	220	2	0	0
Dipping Sauce, Honey BBQ	1 serv	40	0	0	310	9	0	0
Dipping Sauce, Honey Mustard	1 serv	120	10	1.5	110	6	0	0
Dipping Sauce, Sweet & Sour	1 serv	45	0	0	95	12	0	0
Dressing, Heinz Buttermilk Ranch	1 serv	160	17	2	220	1	0	0
Dressing, Hidden Valley® The Original Ranch® Fat Free	1 serv	35	0	0	410	8	0	1
Dressing, KFC® Creamy Parmesan Caesar	1 serv	260	26	5	540	4	0	2
Dressing, Marzetti Light Italian	1 serv	10	0.5	0	510	2	0	0
MAIN MENU								
Chicken Little	1 pc	190	10	2	390	20	1	6
Chicken, Popcorn	reg	400	26	4.5	1160	22	3	21
Crispy Strips	3 pcs	380	22	6	720	12	1	33
Crispy Strips	2 pcs	250	15	4	480	8	1	22
EC Chicken, Breast	1	490	31	7	1080	17	0	38
EC Chicken, Drumstick	1	150	9	2	360	6	0	11
EC Chicken, Thigh	1	370	27	6	840	12	0	18
EC Chicken, Whole Wing	1	150	10	2	320	6	0	11
Gizzards	1 serv	200	11	2	800	15	1	11
Grilled Chicken, Breast	1	180	4	1	440	0	0	35

ITEM DESCRIPTION	Serving Size	Calories	Total Fat (g)	Saturated Fat (g)	Sodium (mg)	Carbohydrates (g)	Fiber (g)	Protein (g)
Grilled Chicken, Drumstick	1	70	4	1	200	0	0	10
Grilled Chicken, Thigh	1	140	9	2.5	320	0	0	15
Grilled Chicken, Whole Wing	1	80	4	1	160	0	0	10
Hot & Spicy, Breast	1	470	28	6	1310	15	4	38
Hot & Spicy, Drumstick	1	160	10	2	400	5	1	12
Hot & Spicy, Thigh	1	380	28	6	810	11	2	22
Hot & Spicy, Whole Wing	1	160	8	2.5	460	10	1	12
Kentucky Nuggets®	1 serv	45	3	0.5	135	2	0	3
Livers	1 serv	180	10	2	620	11	0	11
OR Chicken, Breast	1	370	21	5	1050	7	0	38
OR Chicken, Breast, no Skin or Breading	1	140	2	0	510	1	0	29
OR Chicken, Drumstick	1	110	7	1.5	290	2	0	10
OR Chicken, Thigh	1	260	19	5	670	6	0	16
OR Chicken, Whole Wing	1	110	7	1.5	310	3	0	9
OR Strips	3 pcs	310	15	5	990	11	2	32
OR Strips	2 pcs	200	10	3.5	660	7	1	21
Steak, Country Fried w/ Peppered White Gravy	1	390	26	8	1200	23	2	16
Steak, Country Fried, no Peppered White Gravy	1	360	24	8	1040	19	2	16
SALADS								
Caesar, no Dressing or Croutons	side	35	2	1	90	2	1	3
Chicken BLT Salad, Crispy, no Dressing	1	340	19	5	840	14	3	30
Chicken BLT Salad, OR, no Dressing	1	300	15	5	1020	13	4	29
Chicken BLT Salad, Roasted, no Dressing	1	200	7	2	720	7	3	30
Chicken Caesar Salad, Crispy, no Dressing & Croutons	1	320	19	6	660	12	3	28
Chicken Caesar Salad, OR, no Dressing & Croutons	1	280	14	6	840	11	4	28
Chicken Caesar Salad, Roasted, no Dressing & Croutons	1	190	6	3	530	5	2	29
House Side Salad, no Dressing	1	15	0	0	10	2	1	1
SANDWICHES								
Crispy Twister® w/ Crispy Strip	1	580	30	7	1250	49	3	28
Crispy Twister® w/ Crispy Strip, no Sauce	1	480	20	6	1100	48	2	28

ITEM DESCRIPTION	Serving Size	Calories	Total Fat (g)	Saturated Fat (g)	Sodium (mg)	Carbohydrates (g)	Fiber (g)	Protein (g)
Crispy Twister® w/ OR Strip	1	540	26	7	1430	48	4	28
Crispy Twister® w/ OR Strip, no Sauce	1	440	15	5	1280	47	3	28
Double Crunch Sandwich w/ Crispy Strip	1	510	27	6	840	36	1	27
Double Crunch Sandwich w/ Crispy Strip, no Sauce	1	410	16	4.5	690	34	1	27
Double Crunch Sandwich w/ OR Strip	1	470	23	6	1020	35	2	27
Double Crunch Sandwich w/ OR Strip, no Sauce	1	360	12	4	870	33	2	27
Honey Barbecue Sandwich	1	310	4	1	810	42	1	23
KFC Snacker® w/ Crispy Strip	1	300	14	3	470	28	2	15
KFC Snacker® w/ Crispy Strip, Buffalo	1	260	9	2.5	580	30	2	15
KFC Snacker® w/ Crispy Strip, no Sauce	1	250	9	2.5	410	27	2	15
KFC Snacker® w/ Crispy Strip, Ultimate Cheese	1	280	11	3	560	29	2	16
KFC Snacker® w/ OR Strip	1	270	12	3	560	28	2	15
KFC Snacker® w/ OR Strip, Buffalo	1	240	7	2	670	29	2	15
KFC Snacker® w/ OR Strip, no Sauce	1	230	7	2	500	27	2	15
KFC Snacker® w/ OR Strip, Ultimate Cheese	1	260	9	3	650	29	2	15
KFC Snacker®, Fish	1	320	14	3	640	31	2	16
KFC Snacker®, Fish, no Sauce	1	290	12	2.5	550	29	1	16
KFC Snacker®, Honey Barbecue	1	210	3	1	470	32	2	13
OR Filet Sandwich	1	480	23	4	1230	38	2	25
OR Filet Sandwich, no Sauce	1	370	12	2.5	1080	36	2	25
Tender Roast Twister®	1	440	18	4	1120	42	2	29
Tender Roast Twister®, no Sauce	1	340	7	2.5	980	41	2	29
Tender Roast® Sandwich	1	400	15	3	810	29	1	34
Tender Roast® Sandwich, no Sauce	1	300	4	1.5	660	28	0	34
Toasted Wrap w/ Crispy Strip	1	360	20	6	730	27	2	17
Toasted Wrap w/ Crispy Strip, no Sauce	1	300	14	5	640	27	1	17
Toasted Wrap w/ OR Strip	1	340	18	6	820	27	2	17
Toasted Wrap w/ OR Strip, no Sauce	1	270	11	5	730	26	2	17
Toasted Wrap w/ Tender Roast® Filet	1	310	14	5	740	24	2	22
Toasted Wrap w/ Tender Roast® Filet, no Sauce	1	250	8	3.5	650	24	1	22

SIDES AND SNACKS

ITEM DESCRIPTION	Serving Size	Calories	Total Fat (g)	Saturated Fat (g)	Sodium (mg)	Carbohydrates (g)	Fiber (g)	Protein (g)
Beans, Barbecue Baked	1 serv	200	1.5	0	680	39	9	8
Beans, Red w/ Sausage & Rice	1 serv	160	2.5	0.5	340	26	4	24
Biscuit	1	180	8	6	530	23	1	4
Chicken Pot Pie	1	690	40	31	1760	57	3	27
Cole Slaw	1 serv	180	10	1.5	270	22	3	1
Corn on the Cob	5.5 in	140	1	0	5	33	4	5
Corn, Sweet Kernel	1 serv	110	0.5	0	0	23	2	4
Cornbread Muffin	1	210	10	2	160	27	1	3
Croutons, Parmesan Garlic	1 pkg	70	3	0	140	8	1	2
Famous Bowls® w/ Mashed Potato w/ Gravy	1	700	32	8	2260	77	6	26
Famous Bowls® w/ Rice & Gravy	1	790	28	7	2690	106	5	29
Green Beans	1 serv	25	0	0	380	5	2	1
Jalapeño Peppers	1 serv	20	1.5	0	480	1	1	0
Macaroni & Cheese	1 serv	180	9	3	880	20	2	6
Macaroni Salad	1 serv	180	9	2	400	20	1	3
Mashed Potatoes w/ Gravy	1 serv	130	4.5	1	550	20	1	2
Mashed Potatoes, no Gravy	1 serv	100	3	0.5	350	16	1	2
Mean Greens®	1 serv	30	0	0	400	4	2	3
Popcorn Chicken Snack Box	1 serv	660	38	7	1900	55	5	25
Potato Salad	1 serv	200	10	2	540	24	3	2
Potato Wedges	1 serv	260	13	2.5	740	33	3	4
Rice, Seasoned	1 serv	140	0.5	0	560	31	1	3
Snack Bowl	1 serv	320	15	4.5	990	34	3	12
Three Bean Salad	1 serv	70	0	0	170	14	3	3
Wings, Boneless Fiery Buffalo	1	80	3.5	0.5	390	6	1	5
Wings, Boneless Honey BBQ	1	80	3.5	0.5	340	7	1	5
Wings, Fiery Buffalo	1	80	5	1	230	4	1	4
Wings, Fiery Buffalo Hot™	1	80	5	1	280	5	1	4
Wings, Fiery Buffalo Hot™ Snack Box	1	500	27	6	1580	46	4	16
Wings, Honey BBQ Hot™	1	90	5	1	260	7	0	4
Wings, Honey BBQ Hot™ Snack Box	1	520	27	6	1530	53	4	16
Wings, Honey BBQ Wings	1	80	5	1	170	5	1	4

ITEM DESCRIPTION	Serving Size	Calories	Total Fat (g)	Saturated Fat (g)	Sodium (mg)	Carbohydrates (g)	Fiber (g)	Protein (g)
Wings, Hot™	1	70	5	1	150	3	0	4
Wings, Hot™ Snack Box	1	470	27	6	1190	41	4	16

The Dietary Guidelines for Americans recommend limiting saturated fat to 20 grams and sodium to 2,300 milligrams for a typical adult eating 2,000 calories daily. Recommended limits may be higher or lower depending upon daily calorie consumption.

Substitution of ingredients may alter nutritional values. Menu items and hours of availability may vary at participating locations. Although this data is based on standard portion product guidelines, variation can be expected due to seasonal influences, minor differences in product assembly per restaurant, and other factors. Except for limited time offerings or test market items, menu products as of this printing are included in this brochure. Product data is based on current formulation as of date of publication. If you have any questions about KFC® and nutrition or are particularly sensitive to specific ingredients or foods, please contact us at 1-800-CALL-KFC. Nutrition values for fountain beverages do not account for ice. Depending on the sodium content of the water where the beverage is dispensed, the actual sodium content may be higher or lower than the listed values.

Please visit www.MyPyramid.gov for more information.
* Registered Trademark of PepsiCo, Inc.
** Registered Trademark of Dr Pepper/Seven Up, Inc

LONG JOHN SILVER'S

BEVERAGES

ITEM	Serving Size	Calories	Total Fat (g)	Saturated Fat (g)	Sodium (mg)	Carbohydrates (g)	Fiber (g)	Protein (g)
Diet Pepsi®	med (14 oz)	0	0	0	45	0	0	0
Mountain Dew®	med (14 oz)	190	0	0	60	51	0	0
Pepsi®	med (14 oz)	180	0	0	45	49	0	0
DESSERTS								
Pie, Chocolate Cream	1 pc	310	22	14	170	24	1	5
Pie, Pecan	1 pc	370	15	3	190	55	2	4
Pie, Pineapple Cream	1 pc	290	13	7	210	39	1	4
DRESSINGS AND SPREADS								
Cocktail Sauce	1 serv	25	0	0	250	6	0	0
Ginger Teriyaki Sauce	1 pkg	80	0	0	380	18	0	1
Ketchup	1 pkg	10	0	0	100	2	0	0
Louisiana Hot Sauce	1 pkg	0	0	0	140	0	0	0
Malt Vinegar	1 serv	0	0	0	35	0	0	0
Tartar Sauce	1 serv	100	9	1.5	250	4	0	0
MAIN MENU								
Alaskan Flounder	1 pc	250	11	2.5	910	26	2	12
Chicken Plank®	1 pc	140	8	2	480	9	0	8
Chicken Sandwich	1	360	15	3.5	900	40	3	14
Clam Strips, Breaded	1 serv	320	19	4.5	1190	29	2	9
Cod, Baked	1 pc	120	4.5	1	240	1	0	22
Crab Cake, Lobster Stuffed	1 pc	170	9	2	390	16	1	6
Fish Sandwich	1	470	23	5	1210	48	3	18
Fish Sandwich, Ultimate®	1	530	28	8	1400	49	3	21

ITEM DESCRIPTION	Serving Size	Calories	Total Fat (g)	Saturated Fat (g)	Sodium (mg)	Carbohydrates (g)	Fiber (g)	Protein (g)
Fish, Battered	1 pc	260	16	4	790	17	0	12
Lobster Bites, Buttered	1 serv	250	9	3	560	27	2	14
Pacific Salmon, Grilled	2 pcs	150	5	1	440	2	0	24
Salmon Bowl w/ Sauce	1	460	8	2.5	1660	65	4	30
Salmon Bowl, no Sauce	1	380	8	2	1270	47	4	29
Shrimp Bowl w/ Sauce	1	380	4.5	1.5	1580	64	4	21
Shrimp Bowl, no Sauce	1	300	4	1.5	1200	46	4	20
Shrimp Scampi	8 pcs	110	5	1	610	1	0	16
Shrimp, Battered	3 pcs	130	9	2.5	480	8	0	5
Shrimp, Popcorn	1 serv	270	16	4	570	23	1	9
Tilapia, Grilled	1 pc	110	2.5	1	250	1	0	22
SIDES AND SNACKS								
Breadstick	1	170	3.5	1	290	29	1	6
Broccoli Cheese Soup	1	220	18	8	650	8	1	5
Cole Slaw	1	200	15	2.5	340	15	3	1
Corn Cobbette w/ Butter Oil	1	150	10	2	30	14	3	3
Corn Cobbette, no Butter Oil	1	90	3	0.5	0	14	3	3
Crumblies®	1 serv	170	12	2.5	420	14	1	1
French Fries Basket	1	310	14	3.5	460	45	4	3
French Fries Platter	1	230	10	2.5	350	34	3	3
Hushpuppy	1 pc	60	2.5	0.5	200	9	1	1
Rice	1 serv	180	1	0.5	470	37	2	4
Vegetable Medley	1 serv	50	2	0.5	360	8	3	1

Recommended limits for a 2,000 calorie daily diet are 20 grams of saturated fat and 2,300 milligrams of sodium.
    Substitution of ingredients may alter nutritional values. Menu items and hours of availability may vary at participating locations. Although this data is based on standard portion product guidelines, variation can be expected due to seasonal influences, minor differences in product assembly per restaurant, and other factors. Except for limited time offerings, optional, or test market items, menu products as of this printing are included in this brochure.
    Please visit www.MyPyramid.gov for more information.
    Data Revised: January 2009

McDONALD'S

BEVERAGES

Apple Juice	1	100	0	0	15	23	0	0
Cappuccino w/ Sugar Free Vanilla Syrup§	med (16 oz)	120	6	3.5	130	18	0	6
Cappuccino§	med (16 oz)	140	8	4.5	105	11	0	8
Cappuccino§, Caramel	med (16 oz)	240	6	3.5	150	41	0	6

ITEM DESCRIPTION	Serving Size	Calories	Total Fat (g)	Saturated Fat (g)	Sodium (mg)	Carbohydrates (g)	Fiber (g)	Protein (g)
Cappuccino§, Hazelnut	med (16 oz)	240	6	3.5	85	42	0	6
Cappuccino§, Vanilla	med (16 oz)	240	6	3.5	85	42	0	6
Coca-Cola® Classic§	sm (16 oz)	150	0	0	10	40	0	0
Coffee Cream	1 pkg	20	2	1.5	15	0	0	0
Coffee§	sm (12 oz)	0	0	0	0	0	0	0
Diet Coke®§	sm (16 oz)	0	0	0	20	0	0	0
Equal® 0 Calorie Sweetener	1 pkg	0	0	0	0	1	0	0
Hi-C® Orange Lavaburst§	sm (16 oz)	160	0	0	5	44	0	0
Hot Chocolate w/ Nonfat Milk§	med (16 oz)	310	6	3.5	190	55	0	11
Hot Chocolate§	med (16 oz)	380	15	9	170	53	0	10
Iced Coffee w/ Sugar Free Vanilla Syrup§	med (11.5 oz)	90	8	5	100	11	0	2
Iced Coffee, Caramel§	med (11.5 oz)	190	8	5	115	27	0	2
Iced Coffee, Hazelnut§	sm (8 oz)	130	5	3.5	40	21	0	1
Iced Coffee, Hazelnut§	med (11.5 oz)	190	8	5	60	29	0	2
Iced Coffee, Vanilla§	med (11.5 oz)	190	8	5	60	29	0	2
Iced Coffee§	med (11.5 oz)	200	8	5	60	30	0	2
Iced Latte w/ Sugar Free Vanilla Syrup§	med (16 oz)	90	5	3	105	14	0	5
Iced Latte§	med (16 oz)	100	6	3.5	80	8	0	6
Iced Latte§, Caramel	med (16 oz)	180	4.5	2.5	120	31	0	4
Iced Latte§, Hazelnut	med (16 oz)	180	4.5	2.5	65	33	0	4
Iced Latte§, Vanilla	med (16 oz)	190	4.5	2.5	70	33	0	5
Iced Mocha w/ Nonfat Milk§	med (16 oz)	270	8	4.5	140	43	0	7
Iced Mocha§	med (16 oz)	310	13	8	140	42	0	7
Iced Nonfat Latte w/ Sugar Free Vanilla Syrup§	med (16 oz)	50	0	0	100	14	0	5
Iced Nonfat Latte§	med (16 oz)	60	0	0	90	9	0	6
Iced Nonfat Latte§, Caramel	med (16 oz)	150	0	0	120	32	0	5
Iced Nonfat Latte§, Hazelnut	med (16 oz)	150	0	0	70	33	0	5
Iced Nonfat Latte§, Vanilla	med (16 oz)	150	0	0	70	33	0	5
Iced Tea§	sm (16 oz)	0	0	0	10	0	0	0
Latte w/ Sugar Free Vanilla Syrup§	med (16 oz)	160	8	5	150	21	0	8

ITEM DESCRIPTION	Serving Size	Calories	Total Fat (g)	Saturated Fat (g)	Sodium (mg)	Carbohydrates (g)	Fiber (g)	Protein (g)
Latte§	med (16 oz)	180	10	6	130	13	0	10
Latte§, Caramel	med (16 oz)	280	8	4.5	170	43	0	8
Latte§, Hazelnut	med (16 oz)	280	8	4.5	110	45	0	8
Latte§, Vanilla	med (16 oz)	280	8	4.5	110	44	0	8
Milk, 1% Low Fat Chocolate	1	170	3	1.5	150	26	1	9
Milk, 1% Low Fat	1	100	2.5	1.5	125	12	0	8
Mocha w/ Nonfat Milk§	med (16 oz)	280	6	3.5	160	50	0	8
Mocha§	med (16 oz)	330	12	7	150	48	0	7
Nonfat Cappuccino w/ Sugar Free Vanilla Syrup§	med (16 oz)	70	0	0	130	19	0	7
Nonfat Cappuccino§	med (16 oz)	80	0	0	110	12	0	8
Nonfat Cappuccino§, Caramel	med (16 oz)	190	0	0	150	41	0	6
Nonfat Cappuccino§, Hazelnut	med (16 oz)	190	0	0	90	43	0	6
Nonfat Cappuccino§, Vanilla	med (16 oz)	190	0	0	90	42	0	6
Nonfat Latte w/ Sugar Free Vanilla Syrup§	med (16 oz)	90	0	0	160	22	0	9
Nonfat Latte§	med (16 oz)	110	0	0	140	15	0	10
Nonfat Latte§, Caramel	med (16 oz)	220	0	0	180	45	0	9
Nonfat Latte§, Hazelnut	med (16 oz)	220	0	0	115	46	0	9
Nonfat Latte§, Vanilla	med (16 oz)	220	0	0	115	46	0	9
Orange Juice§	med (16 oz)	180	0	0	5	42	0	3
Powerade® Mountain Blast§	sm (16 oz)	100	0	0	85	27	0	0
Splenda® No Calorie Sweetener	1 pkg	0	0	0	0	1	0	0
Sprite®§	sm (16 oz)	150	0	0	40	39	0	0
Sugar Packet	1 pkg	15	0	0	0	4	0	0
Sweet Tea†	sm (16 oz)	120	0	0	10	30	0	0
BREAKFAST ITEMS								
Big Breakfast®	1	740	48	17	1560	51	3	28
Biscuit	1	260	12	7	740	33	2	5
Biscuit w/ Bacon, Egg & Cheese	1	420	23	12	1160	37	2	15
Biscuit w/ Egg, Sausage	1	510	33	14	1170	36	2	18
Biscuit, Sausage	1	430	27	12	1080	34	2	11
Biscuit, Southern Style Chicken	1	410	20	8	1180	41	2	17
Burrito w/ Sausage	1	300	16	7	830	26	1	12

ITEM DESCRIPTION	Serving Size	Calories	Total Fat (g)	Saturated Fat (g)	Sodium (mg)	Carbohydrates (g)	Fiber (g)	Protein (g)
Deluxe Breakfast, no Syrup or Margarine	1	1090	56	19	2150	111	6	36
English Muffin	1	160	3	0.5	280	27	2	5
Hash Brown	1	150	9	1.5	310	15	2	1
Hotcakes & Sausage, no Syrup or Margarine	1 serv	520	24	7	930	61	3	15
Hotcakes, no Syrup or Margarine	1 serv	350	9	2	590	60	3	8
McGriddles® w/ Bacon, Egg & Cheese	1	420	18	8	1110	48	2	15
McGriddles® w/ Sausage, Egg & Cheese	1	560	32	12	1360	48	2	20
McGriddles®, Sausage	1	420	22	8	1030	44	2	11
McMuffin® w/ Egg	1	300	12	5	820	30	2	18
McMuffin® w/ Egg, Sausage	1	450	27	10	920	30	2	21
McMuffin® w/ Sausage	1	370	22	8	850	29	2	14
McSkillet™ Burrito w/ Sausage	1 serv	610	36	14	1390	44	3	27
McSkillet™ Burrito w/ Steak	1 serv	570	30	12	1470	44	3	32
Sausage Patty	1	170	15	5	340	1	0	7
Scrambled Eggs	2	170	11	4	180	1	0	15
DESSERTS								
Apple Dippers	1 pkg	35	0	0	0	8	0	0
Caramel Dip, Low Fat	1 serv	70	0.5	0	35	15	0	0
Cinnamon Melts	1 serv	460	19	9	370	66	3	6
Cookie, Chocolate Chip	1	160	8	3.5	90	21	1	2
Cookie, Oatmeal Raisin	1	150	6	2.5	135	22	1	2
Cookie, Sugar	1	160	7	3	120	21	0	2
Cookies, McDonaldland®	1 pkg	250	8	2	260	42	1	4
Fruit 'n Yogurt Parfait, no Granola»	1 serv	130	2	1	55	25	0	4
Fruit 'n Yogurt Parfait»	1 serv	160	2	1	85	31	0	4
Ice Cream Cone, Reduced Fat Vanilla	1	150	3.5	2	60	24	0	4
Kiddie Cone	1	45	1	0.5	20	8	0	1
McFlurry® w/ M&M'S® Candies	12 oz	620	20	12	190	96	1	14
McFlurry® w/ Oreo® Cookies	12 oz	550	17	9	250	88	1	13
Peanuts	1 serv	45	3.5	0.5	0	2	1	2
Pie, Baked Hot Apple	1	250	13	7	170	32	4	2
Shake, Chocolate Triple Thick®	16 oz	580	14	8	250	102	1	13
Shake, Strawberry Triple Thick®	16 oz	560	13	8	170	97	0	13

ITEM DESCRIPTION	Serving Size	Calories	Total Fat (g)	Saturated Fat (g)	Sodium (mg)	Carbohydrates (g)	Fiber (g)	Protein (g)
Shake, Vanilla Triple Thick®	16 oz	550	13	8	190	96	0	13
Sundae, Hot Caramel	1	340	8	5	160	60	1	7
Sundae, Hot Fudge	1	330	10	7	180	54	2	8
Sundae, Strawberry	1	280	6	4	95	49	1	6
DRESSINGS AND SPREADS								
Barbecue Sauce	1 pkg	50	0	0	260	12	0	0
Barbecue Sauce, Southwestern Chipotle	1 pkg	70	0	0	260	18	1	0
Buffalo Sauce, Spicy	1 pkg	70	7	1	960	1	2	0
Dressing, Newman's Own® Creamy Caesar	1 pkg	190	18	3.5	500	4	0	2
Dressing, Newman's Own® Creamy Southwest	1 pkg	100	6	1	340	11	0	1
Dressing, Newman's Own® Low Fat Balsamic Vinaigrette	1 pkg	40	3	0	730	4	0	0
Dressing, Newman's Own® Low Fat Family Recipe Italian	1 pkg	60	2.5	0	730	8	0	1
Dressing, Newman's Own® Ranch	1 pkg	170	15	2.5	530	9	0	1
Honey	1 pkg	50	0	0	0	12	0	0
Honey Mustard Sauce, Tangy	1 pkg	70	2.5	0	170	13	0	1
Jam, Grape	1 pkg	35	0	0	0	9	0	0
Margarine, Whipped	1 pkg	40	4.5	1.5	55	0	0	0
Mustard Sauce, Hot	1 pkg	60	2.5	0	250	9	2	1
Ranch Sauce, Creamy	1 pkg	200	22	3.5	320	2	0	0
Strawberry Preserves	1 pkg	35	0	0	0	9	0	0
Sweet 'N Sour Sauce	1 pkg	50	0	0	150	12	0	0
Syrup	1 pkg	180	0	0	20	45	0	0
MAIN MENU								
Big Mac®	1	540	29	10	1040	45	3	25
Big N' Tasty®	1	460	24	8	720	37	3	24
Big N' Tasty® w/ Cheese	1	510	28	11	960	38	3	27
Cheeseburger	1	300	12	6	750	33	2	15
Chicken Classic Sandwich, Premium Crispy	1	530	20	3.5	1150	59	3	28
Chicken Classic Sandwich, Premium Grilled	1	420	10	2	1190	51	3	32

ITEM DESCRIPTION	Serving Size	Calories	Total Fat (g)	Saturated Fat (g)	Sodium (mg)	Carbohydrates (g)	Fiber (g)	Protein (g)
Chicken Club Sandwich, Premium Crispy	1	630	28	7	1360	60	4	35
Chicken Club Sandwich, Premium Grilled	1	530	17	6	1410	52	4	39
Chicken McNuggets®	4 pcs	190	12	2	400	11	0	10
Chicken McNuggets®	6 pcs	280	17	3	600	16	0	14
Chicken McNuggets®	10 pcs	460	29	5	1000	27	0	24
Chicken Ranch BLT Sandwich, Premium Crispy	1	580	23	4.5	1400	62	3	31
Chicken Ranch BLT Sandwich, Premium Grilled	1	470	12	3	1440	54	3	36
Chicken Sandwich, Southern Style Crispy	1	400	17	3	1030	39	1	24
Chicken Selects® Premium Breast Strips	3 pcs	400	24	3.5	1010	23	0	23
Chicken Selects® Premium Breast Strips	5 pcs	660	40	6	1680	39	0	38
Double Cheeseburger	1	440	23	11	1150	34	2	25
Double Quarter Pounder® w/ Cheese++	1	740	42	19	1380	40	3	48
Filet-O-Fish®	1	380	18	3.5	640	38	2	15
Hamburger	1	250	9	3.5	520	31	2	12
McChicken®	1	360	16	3	830	40	2	14
McDouble	1	390	19	8	920	33	2	22
McRib®†	1	500	26	10	980	44	3	22
Quarter Pounder® w/ Cheese+	1	510	26	12	1190	40	3	29
Quarter Pounder®+	1	410	19	7	730	37	2	24
Snack Wrap® Chipotle Barbecue, Crispy	1	330	15	4.5	810	35	1	14
Snack Wrap® Chipotle Barbecue, Grilled	1	260	9	3.5	830	28	1	18
Snack Wrap® Honey Mustard, Crispy	1	330	16	4.5	780	34	1	14
Snack Wrap® Honey Mustard, Grilled	1	260	9	3.5	800	27	1	18
Snack Wrap® Ranch, Crispy	1	340	17	4.5	810	33	1	14
Snack Wrap® Ranch, Grilled	1	270	10	4	830	26	1	18
SALADS								
Bacon Ranch Salad w/ Crispy Chicken	1	370	20	6	970	20	3	29
Bacon Ranch Salad w/ Grilled Chicken	1	260	9	4	1010	12	3	33
Bacon Ranch Salad, no Chicken	1	140	7	3.5	300	10	3	9
Butter Garlic Croutons	1 serv	60	1.5	0	140	10	1	2

ITEM DESCRIPTION	Serving Size	Calories	Total Fat (g)	Saturated Fat (g)	Sodium (mg)	Carbohydrates (g)	Fiber (g)	Protein (g)
Caesar Salad w/ Crispy Chicken	1	330	17	4.5	840	20	3	26
Caesar Salad w/ Grilled Chicken	1	220	6	3	890	12	3	30
Caesar Salad, no Chicken	1	90	4	2.5	180	9	3	7
Side Salad	1	20	0	0	10	4	1	1
Snack Size Fruit & Walnut Salad	1	210	8	1.5	60	31	2	4
Southwest Salad w/ Crispy Chicken	1	430	20	4	920	38	6	26
Southwest Salad w/ Grilled Chicken	1	320	9	3	960	30	6	30
Southwest Salad, no Chicken	1	140	4.5	2	150	20	6	6
SIDES AND SNACKS								
French Fries	med	380	19	2.5	270	48	5	4
Ketchup	1 pkg	15	0	0	110	3	0	0
Salt	1 pkg	0	0	0	270	0	0	0

Note: Nutrient contributions from individual components may not equal the total due to federal rounding regulations. Percent Daily Values (DV) and RDIs are based on unrounded values.

    This list is effective 05-26-2009.

    * Contains less than 2% of the Daily Value of these nutrients

    † Available at participating McDonald's

    + Based on the weight before cooking 4 oz (113.4 g)

    ++ Based on the weight before cooking 8 oz (226.8 g)

    § The value represents the sodium derived from ingredients plus water. Sodium content of the water is based on the value listed for municipal water in the USDA National Nutrient Database. The actual amount of sodium may be higher or lower depending upon the sodium content of the water where the beverage is dispensed.

    • Made with low fat yogurt

    ** Percent Daily Values (DV) are based on a 2,000 calorie diet. Your daily values may be higher or lower depending on your calorie needs.

The nutrition information on this website is derived from testing conducted in accredited laboratories, published resources, or from information provided from McDonald's suppliers. The nutrition information is based on standard product formulations and serving sizes. All nutrition information is based on average values for ingredients from McDonald's suppliers throughout the U.S. and is rounded to meet current U.S. FDA NLEA guidelines. Variation in serving sizes, preparation techniques, product testing, and sources of supply, as well as regional and seasonal differences may affect the nutrition values for each product. In addition, product formulations change periodically. You should expect some variation in the nutrient content of the products purchased in our restaurants. None of our products is certified as vegetarian. This information is correct as of January 2007, unless stated otherwise.

    SPLENDA® No Calorie Sweetener is the registered trademark of McNeil Nutritionals, LLC

    EQUAL® 0 Calorie Sweetener is a registered trademark of Merisant Company

NATHAN'S FAMOUS

BEVERAGES								
Coca Cola	16 oz	130	0	0	10	36	0	0
Lemonade	16 oz	185	0	0	0	44	0	0
DRESSINGS AND SPREADS								
Barbecue Sauce	1 serv	45	0	0	281	11	1	0
Garlic Sauce	1 serv	60	5	1	420	4	1	0
Honey Mustard Dipping Sauce	1 serv	174	18	3	136	3	0	0
Mayonnaise	1 serv	110	12	2	70	0	0	0
Tartar Sauce	1 serv	100	8	1.5	240	5	0	0
Thousand Island Dressing	1 serv	220	21	3	350	6	0	0
Tzatziki Sauce	1 serv	50	5	3.5	125	2	0	1

ITEM DESCRIPTION	Serving Size	Calories	Total Fat (g)	Saturated Fat (g)	Sodium (mg)	Carbohydrates (g)	Fiber (g)	Protein (g)
Wing Sauce	1 serv	30	8	1	230	0	0	0
MAIN MENU								
Apple Pie	1 pc	310	19	4	310	33	0	3
Bacon Cheeseburger	1	783	50	20	1364	45	2	36
Burger w/ Cheese	1	705	43	16	1071	45	2	33
Burger, Double w/ Cheese	1	1178	84	32	1299	45	2	57
Cheese Dog, Nathan's Famous All Beef	1	390	25	8	1440	30	1	12
Cheeseburger, Super	1	987	72	23	1349	47	3	35
Chicken Tender Order	1	526	39	5.6	900	24	3	21
Chicken Tender Platter	1 serv	1245	90	14	1352	80	10	26
Chicken Tender Sandwich	1	706	43	6	1165	58	5	22
Chicken Wing Order w/ Bleu Cheese	1 serv	1478	137	26	2346	26	0	56
Chili Dog, Nathan's Famous All Beef	1	400	23	6	1000	33	2	16
Clams, Breaded	1 pc	470	27	4	470	40	6	18
Corn Dog on a Stick	1	380	21	5	730	39	1	7
Fish & Chips Platter	1 pc	1536	95	15.5	2743	163	11	35
Fish Sandwich	1	435	18	3	715	50	3	18
French Fries	med	492	34	5	66	42	4	4
French Fries w/ Cheese	med	562	39	6	486	46	4	5
Grilled Chicken Breast Platter	1	839	56	9	1134	58	7	24
Grilled Chicken Sandwich	1	554	32	5	1158	40	3	27
Hoagie Roll	1	290	3	0.5	560	58	2	11
Hot Dog Nuggets	6 pcs	350	28	6	400	20	0	5
Hot Dog Roll	1	120	2	0	240	23	0	4
Hot Dog, Nathan's Famous All Beef	1	297	18	7	692	24	1	11
Kaiser Roll	1	200	3	0.5	330	36	2	8
Mozzarella Sticks	1 serv	386	28	8	941	20	1	14
Onion Rings	reg	544	45	6	580	36	1	3
Pita Bread	1	240	5	1	510	41	2	7
Seafood Sampler	1 pc	1559	94	17	3325	166	13	44
Shrimp & Chips Platter	1 pc	1852	120	22	3406	185	12	32
SOUPS AND SIDES								
Chicken Noodle Soup	1	190	5	1.5	1560	27	3	10

ITEM DESCRIPTION	Serving Size	Calories	Total Fat (g)	Saturated Fat (g)	Sodium (mg)	Carbohydrates (g)	Fiber (g)	Protein (g)
Corn on the Cob	1	140	2	0	20	34	2	5
Hush Puppies	2 pcs	520	16	2	1960	84	4	10
Manhattan Clam Chowder	1	270	5	0	2730	48	6	9
New England Clam Chowder	1	250	5	3	1590	42	3	10
TOPPINGS AND EXTRAS								
Cheese Sauce, Cheddar	1 serv	100	8	2	720	6	0	1
Cheese, Swiss American	1 pc	110	9	6	300	1	0	5
Cheese, Yellow American	1 pc	110	9	6	300	1	0	5
Chili w/ Beans	1 serv	80	5	2	383	5	2	5
Cole Slaw	1	180	12	2.5	280	15	2	1
Ketchup	1 serv	15	0	0	190	4	0	0
Nathan's Mustard	1 serv	0	0	0	40	0	0	0
Relish	1 serv	10	0	0	65	3	0	0
Sauerkraut	1 serv	13	0	0	600	3	2	1

OLIVE GARDEN

BEVERAGES

ITEM DESCRIPTION	Serving Size	Calories	Total Fat (g)	Saturated Fat (g)	Sodium (mg)	Carbohydrates (g)	Fiber (g)	Protein (g)
Beer, Light	1	103	0	0	14	6	n/a	n/a
Beer, Non-Alcoholic	1	65	0	0	6	13	n/a	n/a
Beer, Reg	1	153	0	0	14	12	n/a	n/a
Bellini, Peach	1	170	0	0	0	33	n/a	n/a
Bellini, Peach-Raspberry Iced Tea	1	70	0	0	0	16	n/a	n/a
Bellini, Strawberry	1	220	0	0	0	46	n/a	n/a
Bellini, Wild Berry	1	160	0	0	10	31	n/a	n/a
Caffè La Toscana Coffee	1	0	0	0	5	0	n/a	n/a
Caffè Latte	1	130	4	2	85	15	n/a	n/a
Caffè Mocha	1	180	4	2.5	80	31	n/a	n/a
Cappuccino	1	150	8	4	65	14	n/a	n/a
Caramel Macchiato w/ Hazelnut	1	220	4.5	2.5	40	43	n/a	n/a
Chocolate Almond Amore	1	600	21	13	135	82	n/a	n/a
Coca-Cola Classic	1	99	0	0	6	27	n/a	n/a
Cream Soda	1	200	6	4	50	36	n/a	n/a
Daiquiri, Mango	1	240	0	0	10	43	n/a	n/a
Daiquiri, Peach	1	270	0	0	10	50	n/a	n/a

ITEM DESCRIPTION	Serving Size	Calories	Total Fat (g)	Saturated Fat (g)	Sodium (mg)	Carbohydrates (g)	Fiber (g)	Protein (g)
Daiquiri, Strawberry	1	250	0	0	15	47	n/a	n/a
Daiquiri, Wild Berry	1	270	0	0	5	50	n/a	n/a
Diet Coke	1	0	0	0	10	0	n/a	n/a
Dr Pepper	1	100	0	0	35	27	n/a	n/a
Espresso, Lavazza	1	0	0	0	25	0	n/a	n/a
Fresco, Lime-Mint	1	230	0	0	45	29	n/a	n/a
Fresco, Peach	1	200	1	0	10	22	n/a	n/a
Fresco, Sicilian Citrus	1	210	0	0	10	25	n/a	n/a
Fresco, Strawberry	1	230	0	0	5	31	n/a	n/a
Frozen Cappuccino	1	320	10	6	60	53	n/a	n/a
Frozen Margarita, Strawberry	1	340	0	0	25	66	n/a	n/a
Frozen Margarita, Strawberry-Mango	1	350	0	0	20	68	n/a	n/a
Frozen Margarita, Wild Berry	1	290	0	0	20	55	n/a	n/a
Frozen Tiramisu	1	410	14	8	54	95	n/a	n/a
Iced Tea, Fresh Brewed	1	0	0	0	1	0	n/a	n/a
Italian Sodas	1	120	0	0	5	30	n/a	n/a
Lemonade, Limoncello	1	260	0	0	5	42	n/a	n/a
Lemonade, Raspberry	1	110	0	0	15	29	n/a	n/a
Margarita, Italian	1	240	0	0	10	32	n/a	n/a
Martini, Chocolate	1	260	3.5	2	50	36	n/a	n/a
Martini, Mango	1	180	0	0	0	31	n/a	n/a
Martini, Pomegranate Margarita	1	290	0	0	5	44	n/a	n/a
Martini, Raspberry Sorbeto	1	350	6	3.5	40	42	n/a	n/a
Martini, Strawberry-Limoncello	1	300	0	0	15	42	n/a	n/a
Sangria, Berry	1	230	0	0	15	35	n/a	n/a
Sangria, Peach	1	250	0	0	50	40	n/a	n/a
Sangria, Tropical	1	220	0	0	10	32	n/a	n/a
Sicilian Splash	1	100	0	0	15	25	n/a	n/a
Sprite	1	97	0	0	22	26	n/a	n/a
Teas, Herbal & Flavored, Hot	1	0	0	0	1	0	n/a	n/a
Venetian Sunset	1	190	0	0	10	38	n/a	n/a
Wine, Bianco (White)	1	146	0	0	20	8	n/a	n/a
Wine, Rosato (Blush)	1	146	0	0	20	8	n/a	n/a
Wine, Rosso (Red)	1	146	0	0	20	8	n/a	n/a

ITEM DESCRIPTION	Serving Size	Calories	Total Fat (g)	Saturated Fat (g)	Sodium (mg)	Carbohydrates (g)	Fiber (g)	Protein (g)
Wine, Spumante Sparkling	1	126	0	0	20	8	n/a	n/a
DESSERTS								
Cake, Black Tie Mousse	1	760	48	27	270	73	8	n/a
Cake, Lemon Cream	1	620	35	16	430	69	2	n/a
Cheesecake, White Chocolate Raspberry	1	890	62	36	490	70	6	n/a
Chocolate Gelato	1	620	25	20	150	89	6	n/a
Tiramisu	1	510	32	19	75	48	2	n/a
Torta di Chocolate	1	800	51	29	125	75	4	n/a
DRESSINGS AND SPREADS								
Dipping Sauce, Alfredo	1 serv	380	35	22	510	9	1	n/a
Dipping Sauce, Marinara	1 serv	70	2.5	0	550	10	3	n/a
Parmesan-Peppercorn Sauce	1 serv	300	30	5	340	6	1	n/a
Sauce, Tomato	1 serv	45	1.5	0	270	6	1	n/a
KIDS MENU								
Broccoli	1	25	0	0	10	3	2	n/a
Chicken Fingers	1	330	16	1.5	940	23	0	n/a
Chicken, Grilled w/ Pasta & Broccoli	1	310	5	1	680	33	6	n/a
Fettuccine Alfredo	1	800	48	30	810	69	4	n/a
French Fries	1	400	21	2	880	47	4	n/a
Macaroni & Cheese	1	340	6	2.5	1000	58	3	n/a
Milkshake, Chocolate	1	520	22	14	230	72	7	n/a
Milkshake, Strawberry	1	500	24	15	160	62	10	n/a
Milkshake, Vanilla	1	530	23	14	170	73	16	n/a
Pizza, Cheese	1	470	14	6	1170	66	4	n/a
Spaghetti & Tomato Sauce	1	250	3	0.5	370	45	4	n/a
Sundae	1	180	9	6	21	45	0	n/a
LUNCH MENU								
Beef & Tortelloni, Braised	1	740	41	17	1280	60	5	n/a
Capellini Pomodoro	1	480	11	2	970	78	11	n/a
Chicken & Gnocchi Veronese	1	710	42	20	2040	50	3	n/a
Chicken Alfredo	1	910	52	31	1150	71	4	n/a
Chicken Parmigiana	1	570	18	5	1720	66	18	n/a
Chicken Scampi	1	720	34	14	1370	69	17	n/a
Chicken Spiedini, Grilled	1	460	13	2.5	1180	26	7	n/a

ITEM DESCRIPTION	Serving Size	Calories	Total Fat (g)	Saturated Fat (g)	Sodium (mg)	Carbohydrates (g)	Fiber (g)	Protein (g)
Chicken, Venetian Apricot	1	280	3	1	1180	32	8	n/a
Eggplant Parmigiana	1	620	26	8	1540	70	11	n/a
Fettuccine Alfredo	1	800	48	30	810	69	4	n/a
Five Cheese Ziti Al Forno	1	770	32	17	1450	89	5	n/a
Lasagna Classico	1	580	32	18	1930	35	7	n/a
Linguine Alla Marinara	1	310	4	1	670	55	5	n/a
Manicotti Formaggio	1	680	33	18	2100	58	7	n/a
Ravioli di Portobello	1	450	19	11	970	53	8	n/a
Ravioli w/ Marinara Sauce	1	530	18	9	1160	64	6	n/a
Ravioli w/ Meat Sauce	1	610	22	12	1210	65	8	n/a
Seafood Alfredo	1	670	36	21	1320	59	5	n/a
Shrimp Caprese, Grilled	1	820	39	17	2800	81	0	n/a
Shrimp Primavera	1	510	9	1.5	1130	79	12	n/a
Spaghetti & Italian Sausage	1	830	44	16	1920	61	9	n/a
Spaghetti & Meatballs	1	820	40	16	1600	65	6	n/a
Spaghetti w/ Meat Sauce	1	550	21	8	1040	59	6	n/a
Tour of Italy	1	1450	74	33	3830	97	10	n/a
MAIN MENU								
Beef & Tortelloni, Braised	1	1020	53	22	2060	82	10	n/a
Capellini Pomodoro	1	840	17	3	1250	141	19	n/a
Chicken & Gnocchi Veronese	1	1030	58	26	2580	72	8	n/a
Chicken & Shrimp Carbonara	1	1440	88	38	3000	80	9	n/a
Chicken Alfredo	1	1430	82	48	2030	103	5	n/a
Chicken con Broccoli, Garlic-Herb	1	960	41	18	2180	90	12	n/a
Chicken Marsala	1	770	37	5	1800	59	16	n/a
Chicken Marsala, Stuffed	1	800	36	16	2830	40	6	n/a
Chicken Parmigiana	1	1090	49	18	3380	79	27	n/a
Chicken Scampi	1	1020	53	22	1880	84	17	n/a
Chicken, Venetian Apricot	1	380	4	1.5	1420	32	8	n/a
Eggplant Parmigiana	1	850	35	10	1900	98	19	n/a
Fettuccine Alfredo	1	1220	75	47	1350	99	5	n/a
Five Cheese Ziti al Forno	1	1050	48	26	2370	112	9	n/a
Lasagna Classico	1	850	47	25	2830	39	19	n/a
Linguine Alla Marinara	1	430	6	1	900	76	9	n/a

ITEM DESCRIPTION	Serving Size	Calories	Total Fat (g)	Saturated Fat (g)	Sodium (mg)	Carbohydrates (g)	Fiber (g)	Protein (g)
Manicotti Formaggio	1	940	46	25	2530	81	8	n/a
Mixed Grill	1	770	24	5	1980	48	13	n/a
Pizza w/ Cheese & Sauce	1	910	28	12	2970	129	8	n/a
Pizza w/ Chicken Alfredo	1	1180	40	17	3330	144	11	n/a
Pork Filettino	1	640	19	3	840	44	14	n/a
Ravioli di Portobello	1	670	30	17	1400	74	15	n/a
Ravioli w/ Marinara Sauce	1	660	22	11	1440	84	7	n/a
Ravioli w/ Meat Sauce	1	790	28	14	1510	88	12	n/a
Salmon, Herb-Grilled	1	510	26	6	760	5	6	n/a
Seafood Alfredo	1	1020	52	31	2430	88	9	n/a
Seafood Portofino	1	800	33	14	1880	85	16	n/a
Short Ribs, Chianti Braised	1	1060	58	26	2970	71	17	n/a
Shrimp & Asparagus Risotto	1	620	30	17	2530	44	19	n/a
Shrimp Caprese, Grilled	1	900	41	17	3490	82	0	n/a
Shrimp Primavera	1	730	12	2	1620	110	14	n/a
Spaghetti & Italian Sausage	1	1270	68	24	3100	98	15	n/a
Spaghetti & Meatballs	1	1110	50	20	2180	103	9	n/a
Spaghetti w/ Meat Sauce	1	710	22	8	1340	94	9	n/a
Steak Gorgonzola-Alfredo	1	1310	73	41	2190	82	9	n/a
Steak Toscano	1	880	43	14	1700	45	12	n/a
Tilapia, Parmesan Crusted	1	590	25	10	910	42	6	n/a
Tour of Italy	1	1450	74	33	3830	97	10	n/a
SALADS								
Chicken Caesar, Grilled	1	850	64	13	1880	14	4	n/a
Garden-Fresh	1	120	3.5	0.5	550	17	3	n/a
Garden-Fresh w/ Dressing	1	350	27	4.5	1990	22	3	n/a
SIDES AND SNACKS								
Artichoke-Spinach Dip	1 serv	660	32	15	1450	68	6	n/a
Breadstick w/ Garlic-Butter Spread	1 pc	150	2.5	0.5	350	28	2	n/a
Bruschetta	1 serv	620	13	2.5	1760	100	10	n/a
Calamari	1 serv	890	54	5	2330	64	2	n/a
Calamari in Sampler Italiano	1 serv	440	27	2.5	1170	32	0	n/a
Caprese Flatbread	1 serv	600	33	10.5	1520	46	5	n/a
Chicken Fingers in Sampler Italiano	1 serv	330	16	1.5	940	23	0	n/a

ITEM DESCRIPTION	Serving Size	Calories	Total Fat (g)	Saturated Fat (g)	Sodium (mg)	Carbohydrates (g)	Fiber (g)	Protein (g)
Chicken Flatbread, Grilled	1 serv	760	44	14.5	1500	46	5	n/a
Fried Mozzarella in Sampler Italiano	1 serv	370	22	9	800	26	2	n/a
Fried Zucchini in Sampler Italiano	1 serv	370	20	1.5	630	42	4	n/a
Mozzarella Fonduta, Smoked	1 serv	940	48	28	1940	72	7	n/a
Mushrooms, Stuffed	1 serv	410	28	8	990	20	3	n/a
Mussels di Napoli	1 serv	180	8	4	1800	13	0	n/a
Ravioli, Toasted Beef & Pork in Sampler Italiano	1 serv	360	16	2.5	780	39	2	n/a
Sicilian Scampi	1 serv	500	22	10	1850	43	7	n/a
SOUPS								
Chicken & Gnocchi	1	250	8	3	1180	29	2	n/a
Minestrone	1	100	1.5	0	1090	19	3	n/a
Pasta E Fagioli	1	130	2.5	1	730	19	6	n/a
Zuppa Toscana	1	170	4	2	950	23	2	n/a
TOPPINGS AND EXTRAS								
Bell Peppers Pizza Topping	1	10	0	0	0	2	1	n/a
Black Olives Pizza Topping	1	45	4	0.5	350	3	1	n/a
Italian Sausage Pizza Topping	1	140	11	4	360	1	0	n/a
Mushrooms Pizza Topping	1	5	0	0	0	1	0	n/a
Onions Pizza Topping	1	15	0	0	0	4	1	n/a
Pepperoni Pizza Topping	1	120	11	4.5	460	1	0	n/a
Tomatoes Pizza Topping	1	10	0	0	0	2	1	n/a

Olive Garden has made an effort to provide complete and current nutrition information, but the handcrafted nature of our menu items and changes in recipes, ingredients, offerings, and kitchen procedures can cause variations from these values to occur. Therefore, the values shown here should be considered approximations. For more current information, please visit our website at www.olivegarden.com.

P.F. CHANG'S CHINA BISTRO

BEVERAGES

ITEM DESCRIPTION	Serving Size	Calories	Total Fat (g)	Saturated Fat (g)	Sodium (mg)	Carbohydrates (g)	Fiber (g)	Protein (g)
Beer, Light	12 oz	103	n/a	n/a	14	6	n/a	n/a
Beer, Regular	12 oz	153	n/a	n/a	14	13	n/a	n/a
Coke	16 oz	198	n/a	n/a	12	54	n/a	n/a
Diet Coke	16 oz	1	n/a	n/a	20	0.2	n/a	n/a
Distilled Spirits, 80 Proof	1.5 oz	96	n/a	n/a	n/a	n/a	n/a	n/a
Sprite	16 oz	194	n/a	n/a	44	52	n/a	n/a
Wine, Red or White	7 oz	171	n/a	n/a	10	6	n/a	n/a

ITEM DESCRIPTION	Serving Size	Calories	Total Fat (g)	Saturated Fat (g)	Sodium (mg)	Carbohydrates (g)	Fiber (g)	Protein (g)
DESSERTS								
Banana Spring Rolls	1	992	45	23	480	145	n/a	15
Cheesecake, New York-Style	1	870	56	35	620	70	n/a	16
Flourless Chocolate Dome	1	440	26	8	290	52	n/a	7
Mini Apple Pie	1	127	5	1	127	20	n/a	1
Mini Carrot Cake	1	170	7	3	110	25	n/a	1
Mini Great Wall	1	150	5	2	130	26	n/a	1
Mini Lemon Dream	1	164	6	2	60	25	n/a	3
Mini Red Velvet Cake	1	170	9	3	110	23	n/a	2
Mini S'Mores	1	268	10	3	184	44	n/a	2
Mini Strawberry Cheesecake	1	229	17	9	162	17	n/a	3
Mini Tiramisu	1	234	17	7	96	17	n/a	3
The Great Wall of Chocolate™	1	1440	61	20	1120	231	n/a	10
MAIN MENU								
Ahi Tuna*, Sesame Crusted	1	523	11	1	2130	63	n/a	42
Beef & Broccoli	1	345	14	3	2159	26	n/a	29
Beef & Broccoli w/ Brown Rice	1 bowl	766	24	5	4087	91	n/a	46
Beef & Broccoli w/ White Rice	1 bowl	790	23	5	4085	98	n/a	46
Beef A La Sichuan	1	518	22	5	2196	40	n/a	40
Beef Short Ribs w/ Pineapple Rice	1	427	22	9	892	31	n/a	24
Beef, Cantonese Chow Fun	1	338	12	2	1161	39	n/a	17
Beef, Mongolian	1	471	25	8	3094	27	n/a	33
Beef, Wok-Charred	1	170	6	3	2009	15	n/a	15
Buddha's Feast w/ Brown Rice	1 bowl	550	11	1	1833	95	n/a	22
Buddha's Feast w/ White Rice	1 bowl	574	10	1	1831	102	n/a	22
Buddha's Feast, Steamed	1	161	3	0	1073	24	n/a	12
Buddha's Feast, Stir-Fried	1	189	5	0	1064	28	n/a	12
Chicken w/ Black Bean Sauce	1	218	12	2	1295	12	n/a	17
Chicken, Almond & Cashew	1	280	12	2	2258	26	n/a	16
Chicken, Almond & Cashew w/ Brown Rice	1 bowl	965	38	6	4965	108	n/a	48
Chicken, Almond & Cashew w/ White Rice	1 bowl	991	37	6	4963	115	n/a	49
Chicken, Cantonese Chow Fun	1	352	13	2	995	39	n/a	17

ITEM DESCRIPTION	Serving Size	Calories	Total Fat (g)	Saturated Fat (g)	Sodium (mg)	Carbohydrates (g)	Fiber (g)	Protein (g)
Chicken, Chang's Spicy	1	300	12	2	800	29	n/a	18
Chicken, Crispy Honey	1	336	10	2	125	46	n/a	13
Chicken, Crispy Honey w/ Brown Rice	1 bowl	1210	51	9	610	135	n/a	55
Chicken, Crispy Honey w/ White Rice	1 bowl	1271	50	9	618	150	n/a	56
Chicken, Dali	1	276	13	2	300	24	n/a	20
Chicken, Ginger w/ Broccoli	1	283	13	2	1304	21	n/a	22
Chicken, Ground w/ Eggplant	1	188	6	1	1830	23	n/a	10
Chicken, Philip's Better Lemon	1	229	10	2	74	23	n/a	14
Chicken, Sesame	1	374	16	2	932	31	n/a	27
Chicken, Sesame w/ Brown Rice	1 bowl	979	27	4	2492	135	n/a	49
Chicken, Sesame w/ White Rice	1 bowl	1025	25	4	2489	148	n/a	49
Chicken, Sweet & Sour	1	276	13	2	280	29	n/a	11
Duck, VIP	1	495	18	5	1431	58	n/a	31
Eggplant, Stir-Fried	1	96	3	0	438	16	n/a	2
Fish, Hot	1	305	18	4	1395	18	n/a	20
Fried Rice Combo	1	401	18	4	1332	38	n/a	21
Fried Rice w/ Beef	1	384	16	3	1208	44	n/a	16
Fried Rice w/ Chicken	1	383	16	3	1137	41	n/a	18
Fried Rice w/ Pork	1	406	20	5	1603	41	n/a	14
Fried Rice w/ Shrimp	1	343	13	2	1251	41	n/a	13
Fried Rice, Vegetarian	1	214	2	1	421	43	n/a	6
Kung Pao Chicken	1	393	22	3	756	24	n/a	27
Kung Pao Scallops	1	269	12	2	878	16	n/a	26
Kung Pao Shrimp	1	258	12	2	844	16	n/a	24
Lamb, Chengdu Spiced	1	362	18	2	1173	16	n/a	33
Lamb, Wok-Seared	1	227	13	3	1102	7	n/a	20
Lo Mein Combo	1	492	24	3	1465	59	n/a	26
Lo Mein w/ Beef	1	483	21	2	1366	68	n/a	23
Lo Mein w/ Chicken	1	522	27	4	1581	59	n/a	26
Lo Mein w/ Pork	1	473	24	4	1723	56	n/a	24
Lo Mein w/ Shrimp	1	436	19	1	1415	65	n/a	20
Mahi-Mahi	1	325	16	4	749	22	n/a	23
Moo Goo Gai Pan	1	278	11	2	1880	26	n/a	19
Moo Goo Gai Pan w/ Brown Rice	1 bowl	809	25	4	4437	102	n/a	41

ITEM DESCRIPTION	Serving Size	Calories	Total Fat (g)	Saturated Fat (g)	Sodium (mg)	Carbohydrates (g)	Fiber (g)	Protein (g)
Moo Goo Gai Pan w/ White Rice	1 bowl	833	24	4	4435	109	n/a	41
Mu Shu Chicken	1	232	12	2	870	13	n/a	19
Mu Shu Pancake	1 pc	90	2	0	30	14	n/a	2
Mu Shu Pork	1	249	16	5	1541	10	n/a	17
Noodles, Dan Dan	1	472	24	1	1752	75	n/a	20
Noodles, Double Pan-Fried Combo	1	408	20	2	1918	39	n/a	18
Noodles, Double Pan-Fried w/ Beef	1	396	18	1	1911	43	n/a	15
Noodles, Double Pan-Fried w/ Chicken	1	403	19	1	1831	43	n/a	14
Noodles, Double Pan-Fried w/ Pork	1	395	18	1	1865	41	n/a	16
Noodles, Double Pan-Fried w/ Shrimp	1	364	17	1	1945	41	n/a	12
Noodles, Garlic	1	384	5	1	849	72	n/a	12
Noodles, Singapore Street	1	263	7	1	873	36	n/a	12
Orange Peel Beef	1	272	12	3	700	21	n/a	21
Orange Peel Chicken	1	295	15	2	454	21	n/a	21
Orange Peel Shrimp	1	182	7	1	794	15	n/a	14
Ponzu Sauce	1	38	0	0	881	6	n/a	2
Pork, Sweet & Sour	1	253	9	5	576	33	n/a	9
Prawns, Lemongrass w/ Garlic Noodles	1	608	44	10	1428	58	n/a	27
Prawns, Salt & Pepper	1	146	7	1	670	15	n/a	8
Salmon*, Wild Alaskan Citrus Soy	1	367	16	7	653	27	n/a	28
Salmon, Citrus Soy w/ Brown Rice*	1 bowl	761	36	16	1205	66	n/a	43
Salmon, Citrus Soy w/ White Rice*	1 bowl	785	35	16	1203	73	n/a	43
Salmon, Wild Alaskan Steamed w/ Ginger*	1	125	14	2	533	9	n/a	23
Scallops, Cantonese	1	297	14	2	1800	25	n/a	17
Scallops, Chang's Lemon	1	188	3	0	257	20	n/a	22
Sea Bass*, Oolong Marinated	1	291	15	4	1695	20	n/a	20
Shrimp w/ Candied Walnuts	1	412	26	1	754	30	n/a	18
Shrimp w/ Lobster Sauce	1	273	11	2	2712	27	n/a	18
Shrimp, Cantonese	1	262	10	2	1742	18	n/a	23
Shrimp, Crispy Honey	1	422	14	2	363	58	n/a	12
Shrimp, Lemon Pepper	1	227	10	2	1225	16	n/a	21
Shrimp, Lobster Sauce w/ Brown Rice	1 bowl	698	21	4	4747	95	n/a	31
Shrimp, Lobster Sauce w/ White Rice	1 bowl	722	20	4	4745	103	n/a	31
Sichuan from the Sea, Calamari	1	366	23	4	365	26	n/a	13

ITEM DESCRIPTION	Serving Size	Calories	Total Fat (g)	Saturated Fat (g)	Sodium (mg)	Carbohydrates (g)	Fiber (g)	Protein (g)
Sichuan from the Sea, Scallops	1	201	10	2	716	18	n/a	11
Sichuan from the Sea, Shrimp	1	177	7	1	676	13	n/a	16
Steak, Asian Marinated New York Strip	1	186	10	4	288	10	n/a	16
Steak, Pepper	1	314	13	3	1864	24	n/a	25
Steak, Pepper w/ Brown Rice	1 bowl	752	25	6	3491	89	n/a	42
Steak, Pepper w/ White Rice	1 bowl	776	23	5	3489	96	n/a	42
Tofu, Ma Po	1	260	15	5	1144	18	n/a	14
Vegetable Chow Fun	1	391	20	0	640	76	n/a	16
Vegetables, Coconut Curry	1	295	21	8	565	16	n/a	7
SALADS								
Chicken Chopped Salad w/ Ginger Dressing	1	940	68	10	2225	33	n/a	47
Shrimp Salad, Bikini	1	541	31	4	827	33	n/a	38
Wedge, Chang's	1	665	60	13	1080	17	n/a	12
Wedge, Chang's w/ Chicken	1	865	64	13	1900	19	n/a	52
Wedge, Chang's w/ Steak	1	984	74	13	2034	31	n/a	44
SIDES AND SNACKS								
Ahi Tuna*, Seared	1 serv	44	1	0	335	2	n/a	7
Asian Slaw	sm	302	29	4	646	8	n/a	3
Asparagus, Sichuan-Style	sm	107	5	1	131	11	n/a	3
Cabbage Slaw	1 serv	147	14	2	314	4	n/a	1
Calamari, Salt & Pepper	1 serv	362	10	2	1778	53	n/a	10
Crab Wontons	2 pcs	169	11	4	304	13	n/a	5
Cucumbers, Shanghai	sm	63	3	0	1109	5	n/a	3
Egg Rolls	1	174	8	1	673	22	n/a	5
Green Beans, Crispy	1 serv	167	14	13	27	8	n/a	2
Green Beans, Spicy	sm	96	5	1	13	10	n/a	3
Mushrooms, Wok-Seared	sm	251	19	8	949	12	n/a	6
Mustard Sauce, Spicy	1 serv	187	18	2	955	5	n/a	1
Noodles, Green Tea Soba	sm	407	18	2	1749	51	n/a	9
Peas, Garlic Snap	sm	100	3	0	162	12	n/a	3
Peking Dumplings, Pan-Fried	1	93	5	1	215	7	n/a	6
Peking Dumplings, Steamed	1	66	3	1	178	6	n/a	5
Plum Sauce	1 serv	247	0	0	1863	63	n/a	0
Rice, Brown Steamed	1/2 cup	109	1	0	1	23	n/a	2

ITEM DESCRIPTION	Serving Size	Calories	Total Fat (g)	Saturated Fat (g)	Sodium (mg)	Carbohydrates (g)	Fiber (g)	Protein (g)
Rice, White Steamed	1/2 cup	121	0	0	0	27	n/a	2
Shrimp Dumplings, Pan-Fried	1	68	2	1	347	8	n/a	6
Shrimp Dumplings, Steamed	1	58	1	0	347	8	n/a	6
Shrimp, Dynamite	1 serv	482	42	6	1133	10	n/a	19
Sichuan Flatbread, Chicken	1 serv	179	8	5	454	12	n/a	16
Sichuan Flatbread, Steak	1 serv	217	11	7	378	12	n/a	17
Sichuan Sauce	1 serv	335	36	5	556	4	n/a	0
Spare Ribs, Chang's Barbecue	1 serv	344	24	7	336	7	n/a	26
Spare Ribs, Northern Style	1 serv	342	19	2	985	11	n/a	31
Spinach, Stir-Fried w/ Garlic	sm	90	5	0	448	8	n/a	6
Spring Rolls	2	313	16	4	542	34	n/a	7
Vegetable Dumplings, Pan-Fried	1	66	2	0	172	11	n/a	2
Vegetable Dumplings, Steamed	1	56	0	0	172	11	n/a	2
Wraps, Chang's Chicken Lettuce	1 serv	322	6	1	347	52	n/a	12
Wraps, Chang's Vegetarian Lettuce	1 serv	269	6	1	511	49	n/a	5
SOUPS								
Chicken Noodle Soup, Chang's	1 bowl	759	24	4	4135	92	n/a	38
Egg Drop Soup	1 bowl	366	12	2	6731	58	n/a	4
Hot & Sour Soup	1 bowl	534	20	4	6878	52	n/a	31
Wonton Soup	1 bowl	693	24	4	5328	49	n/a	68

The Dietary Guidelines for Americans recommend limiting saturated fat to 20 grams and sodium to 2,300 milligrams for a typical adult eating 2,000 calories daily. Recommended limits may be higher or lower depending upon daily calorie consumption.

All entrées served with a choice of steamed brown or white rice.

* These items are cooked to order and may be served raw or undercooked. Consuming raw or undercooked meats, poultry, seafood, shellfish, or eggs may increase your risk of foodborne illness.

Signature drinks or liqueurs with added ingredients may increase caloric content.

PANDA EXPRESS

ITEM DESCRIPTION	Serving Size	Calories	Total Fat (g)	Saturated Fat (g)	Sodium (mg)	Carbohydrates (g)	Fiber (g)	Protein (g)
DESSERTS								
Fortune Cookie	1	32	0	0	8	7	0	1
DRESSINGS AND SPREADS								
Mandarin Sauce	1 serv	70	0	0	740	17	0	1
Potsticker Sauce	1 serv	35	0	0	970	8	0	1
Sweet & Sour Sauce	1 serv	80	0	0	135	19	0	0
MAIN MENU								
Beef, Beijing	1 serv	400	25	5	700	35	1	13
Beef & Broccoli	1 serv	170	8	2	570	12	4	12

ITEM DESCRIPTION	Serving Size	Calories	Total Fat (g)	Saturated Fat (g)	Sodium (mg)	Carbohydrates (g)	Fiber (g)	Protein (g)
Beef, Mongolian	1 serv	180	11	2	800	15	2	11
Chicken Breast, String Bean	1 serv	190	9.5	2	650	12	5	14
Chicken Potsticker	3 pcs	220	12	1.5	360	25	4	6
Chicken, Black Pepper	1 serv	215	13	3	880	12	2	14
Chicken, Kung Pao	1 serv	260	16	3	580	13	5	17
Chicken, Mandarin	1 serv	260	11	3	1215	8	0	33
Chicken, Mushroom	1 serv	150	7	2	600	9	3	13
Chicken, Orange	1 serv	545	29	6	880	46	3	25
Chicken, Potato	1 serv	220	11	2	1080	23	2	12
Chicken, Sweet & Sour	1 serv	340	13	2	320	41	1	13
Chow Mein	1 serv	440	14	2	1150	66	8	12
Cream Cheese Rangoon	3 pcs	190	8	5	180	24	2	5
Egg Roll, Chicken	1	170	8	1.5	410	17	2	8
Eggplant & Tofu	1 serv	220	12	2	830	24	5	6
Fried Rice	1 serv	480	15	3	760	72	6	14
Pork, Barbecue	1 serv	420	22	8.5	1485	14	1	39
Pork, Sweet & Sour	1 serv	400	23	4.5	360	35	2	13
Rice, Steamed	1 serv	430	3	1	35	92	5	10
Shrimp, Crispy	6 pcs	260	13	2.5	810	26	1	9
Shrimp, Kung Pao	1 serv	210	13	2	870	10	5	18
Shrimp, Tangy	1 serv	160	5	1	600	17	2	10
Soup, Egg Flower	1 serv	88	2.2	0	895	16	0	2
Soup, Hot & Sour	1 serv	100	3.5	0.5	940	12	1	6
Veggie Spring Roll	2	160	7	2	540	22	4	4
Veggies, Mixed	reg	90	7	1	110	8	3	2
Veggies, Mixed	side	140	11	1.5	165	12	4.5	3

Entrées may vary by location.

The Dietary Guidelines for Americans recommend limiting saturated fat to 20 grams and sodium to 2,300 milligrams for a typical adult eating 2,000 calories daily. Recommended limits may be higher or lower depending upon daily calorie consumption. These values are based on standard product formulation. Minor acceptable variations can be expected due to sampling differences, product assembly, seasonal influences, and regional suppliers. Promotional entrées have not been included.

* Not applicable in Hawaii where Trans Fat (g) equals 1. Please contact Panda Guest Relations at (800) 877-8988 for more information.

PANERA BREAD

BAKED ITEMS

Bagel, Asiago Cheese	1	330	6	3.5	570	55	2	13
Bagel, Blueberry	1	330	1.5	0	490	67	2	10

ITEM DESCRIPTION	Serving Size	Calories	Total Fat (g)	Saturated Fat (g)	Sodium (mg)	Carbohydrates (g)	Fiber (g)	Protein (g)
Bagel, Chocolate Chip	1	370	6	4	480	69	2	10
Bagel, Cinnamon Crunch	1	430	8	5	430	81	3	9
Bagel, Dutch Apple & Raisin	1	360	3	1	620	77	2	8
Bagel, Everything	1	300	2.5	0	630	59	2	10
Bagel, French Toast	1	350	5	2	610	67	2	9
Bagel, Plain	1	290	1.5	0	450	59	2	10
Bagel, Salt	1	290	1.5	0	2790	59	2	10
Bagel, Sesame	1	310	3	0	450	59	2	10
Bagel, Whole Grain	1	370	3.5	0	420	70	6	13
Baguette, French	2 oz	160	2	0	330	31	1	6
Baguette, French Artisan	2 oz	150	0.5	0	370	29	1	5
Baguette, Sourdough	2 oz	160	0.5	0	320	31	1	6
Baguette, Whole Grain	2 oz	140	1	0	320	28	3	6
Challah Bread	2 oz	180	2.5	1	290	34	1	6
Ciabatta	1	460	5	1	760	84	3	16
Demi, Asiago Cheese	2 oz	160	4	2.5	320	22	1	7
Demi, Three Cheese	2 oz	140	2	1	300	26	1	6
Demi, Three Seed	2 oz	160	3.5	0	300	27	2	6
Focaccia	2 oz	180	4.5	0.5	320	28	1	5
Focaccia w/ Asiago Cheese	2 oz	160	5	1.5	230	23	1	5
Loaf, Asiago Cheese	2 oz	160	4	2.5	320	22	1	7
Loaf, Cinnamon Raisin	2 oz	180	3	1.5	140	34	1	5
Loaf, Country	2 oz	140	0.5	0	310	27	1	5
Loaf, French	2 oz	150	2	0	310	29	1	5
Loaf, French XL	2 oz	150	2	0	300	29	1	5
Loaf, Honey Wheat	2 oz	160	3	1.5	240	30	2	5
Loaf, Sesame Semolina	2 oz	140	0.5	0	350	29	1	4
Loaf, Sourdough	2 oz	140	0.5	0	290	28	1	5
Loaf, Stone-Milled Rye	2 oz	140	0.5	0	380	28	2	5
Loaf, Three Cheese	2 oz	140	2	1	300	26	1	6
Loaf, Tomato Basil	2 oz	140	0.5	0	330	27	1	5
Loaf, White Whole Grain	2 oz	140	2.5	1	310	27	2	5
Loaf, Whole Grain	2 oz	130	1	0	240	26	3	6
Miche, Country	2 oz	140	0.5	0	330	28	1	5

ITEM DESCRIPTION	Serving Size	Calories	Total Fat (g)	Saturated Fat (g)	Sodium (mg)	Carbohydrates (g)	Fiber (g)	Protein (g)
Miche, French	2 oz	140	0.5	0	360	28	1	5
Miche, Sesame Semolina	2 oz	140	1	0	360	30	1	5
Miche, Stone-Milled Rye	2 oz	140	0.5	0	410	27	2	5
Miche, Three Cheese	2 oz	150	2	1	320	27	1	6
Miche, Whole Grain	2 oz	130	1	0	240	25	3	5
Roll, French	1	180	2	0	370	35	1	6
Roll, Sourdough	1	200	1	0	400	39	1	7
Soup Bowl, Sourdough	1	590	2.5	0	1210	117	4	22
BEVERAGES								
Apple Juice	1	120	0	0	25	29	0	0
Caffe Latte	1	110	4.5	3	95	11	0	7
Caffe Mocha	1	380	17	11	160	48	2	11
Cappuccino	1	110	4.5	3	95	11	0	7
Frozen Drink, Caramel	16 oz	580	25	17	170	83	1	6
Frozen Drink, Mango Smoothie	18 oz	330	10	7	30	61	3	2
Frozen Drink, Mocha	16 oz	550	25	16	140	78	2	7
Frozen Drink, Strawberry Smoothie	18 oz	240	1.5	0.5	190	51	3	5
Hot Chocolate	1	390	17	12	170	49	2	11
Iced Green Tea	16 oz	110	0	0	10	23	0	0
Iced Latte, Chai Tea	1	150	3.5	2	75	25	0	6
Latte, Caramel	1	410	18	12	190	54	0	9
Latte, Chai Tea	1	190	4	2.5	85	31	0	7
Lemonade	16 oz	90	0	0	10	22	0	0
Milk, Organic	1	120	4.5	3	120	12	0	8
Milk, Organic Chocolate	1	180	5	3	160	27	0	8
Orange Juice	sm	110	0	0	0	25	0	2
BREAKFAST ITEMS								
Egg Soufflé, Four Cheese	1	480	31	16	700	34	2	16
Egg Soufflé, Spinach & Artichoke	1	500	32	18	830	35	2	19
Egg Soufflé, Spinach & Bacon	1	570	37	20	990	36	2	21
Egg Soufflé, Turkey Sausage & Potato	1	460	28	15	600	35	2	15
Granola Parfait, Strawberry	1	310	12	3.5	100	41	4	3
Sandwich w/ Bacon, Egg & Cheese	1	510	24	10	1060	44	2	28
Sandwich w/ Egg & Cheese	1	380	14	6	620	43	2	18

ITEM DESCRIPTION	Serving Size	Calories	Total Fat (g)	Saturated Fat (g)	Sodium (mg)	Carbohydrates (g)	Fiber (g)	Protein (g)
Sandwich w/ Sausage, Egg & Cheese	1	540	27	11	980	44	2	26
DESSERTS								
Bear Claw	1	460	24	13	400	54	2	9
Brownie, Caramel Pecan	1	490	25	6	170	64	2	5
Brownie, Very Chocolate	1	460	22	5	180	61	2	5
Bundt Cake Mini, Lemon Poppyseed	1	460	20	4	440	63	0	6
Bundt Cake Mini, Pineapple Upside-Down	1	520	25	10	570	74	2	6
Cinnamon Roll	1	620	24	14	480	89	3	13
Cobblestone	1	650	13	5	410	123	3	12
Cookie, Chocolate Chipper	1	440	23	14	320	59	2	5
Cookie, Chocolate Duet w/ Walnuts	1	450	24	13	330	55	3	6
Cookie, Nutty Chocolate Chipper	1	460	27	13	300	54	3	5
Cookie, Nutty Oatmeal Raisin	1	390	16	8	300	58	2	6
Cookie, Petite Chocolate Chipper	1	110	6	3.5	80	15	1	1
Cookie, Petite Chocolate Duet w/ Walnuts	1	110	6	3	80	14	1	2
Cookie, Petite Nutty Oatmeal Raisin	1	100	4	2	75	14	1	1
Cookie, Petite Shortbread	1	90	5	3	40	9	0	1
Cookie, Shortbread	1	350	21	12	160	36	1	3
Croissant, French	1	290	17	11	220	31	1	6
Muffie, Chocolate Chip	1	270	12	3	140	40	1	4
Muffie, Pumpkin	1	250	10	2	200	39	1	3
Muffin, Carrot Walnut	1	430	19	4	380	61	2	8
Muffin, Pumpkin	1	530	20	4	430	82	2	6
Muffin, Reduced Fat Wild Blueberry	1	360	10	2	220	61	1	6
Muffin, Wild Blueberry	1	390	15	2.5	290	58	1	5
Pastry Ring, Cherry Cheese	1	210	11	6	120	26	1	3
Pastry, Cheese	1	380	22	13	330	39	1	7
Pastry, Cherry	1	450	22	13	340	55	2	8
Pastry, Chocolate	1	340	20	12	230	37	2	6
Pastry, Fresh Apple	1	440	23	14	340	51	3	9
Pastry, Gooey Butter	1	350	19	12	250	39	1	7
Pastry, Pecan Braid	1	440	25	11	270	46	2	8
Pecan Roll	1	720	38	11	310	88	2	11
Scone, Cinnamon Chip	1	530	27	16	310	67	2	8

ITEM DESCRIPTION	Serving Size	Calories	Total Fat (g)	Saturated Fat (g)	Sodium (mg)	Carbohydrates (g)	Fiber (g)	Protein (g)
Scone, Orange	1	460	20	11	290	65	1	8
Wild Blueberry	1	410	15	10	360	63	2	6
DRESSINGS AND SPREADS								
Asian Sesame Vinaigrette, Reduced-Sugar	.75 oz	45	4	0.5	190	3	0	0
Balsamic Vinaigrette, Cherry	.75 oz	70	6	1	135	3	0	0
Balsamic Vinaigrette, Reduced Fat	.75 oz	60	5	1	120	4	0	0
Caesar Dressing	.75 oz	80	8	1.5	95	1	0	0
Cream Cheese, Plain	2 oz	180	18	11	210	2	0	3
Cream Cheese, Reduced Fat Hazelnut	2 oz	140	11	6	210	6	1	5
Cream Cheese, Reduced Fat Honey Walnut	2 oz	150	11	6	200	8	1	5
Cream Cheese, Reduced Fat Plain	2 oz	130	12	7	230	2	1	5
Cream Cheese, Reduced Fat Raspberry	2 oz	130	10	6	190	7	1	4
Cream Cheese, Reduced Fat Sun-Dried Tomato	2 oz	130	11	7	220	4	1	5
Cream Cheese, Reduced Fat Veggie	2 oz	120	10	6	200	3	1	4
Greek Dressing	.75 oz	110	12	2	190	1	0	0
Light Buttermilk Ranch	.75 oz	40	2	0	170	4	0	0
Poppyseed Dressing, Reduced-Sugar	.75 oz	5	0	0	80	2	1	0
Raspberry Dressing, Fat-Free	.75 oz	15	0	0	45	4	0	0
White Balsamic Apple Vinaigrette	.75 oz	80	6	1	160	6	0	0
KIDS MENU								
Sandwich, Grilled Cheese	1	310	12	7	900	35	3	15
Sandwich, Peanut Butter & Jelly	1	410	17	3	410	56	5	14
Sandwich, Roast Beef	1	320	10	5	790	35	3	23
Sandwich, Smoked Ham	1	310	10	5	1250	34	3	21
Sandwich, Smoked Turkey	1	310	9	4.5	1160	35	3	21
Yogurt, Organic (Blueberry, Strawberry, or Orange)	1	70	1	0.5	40	12	0	2
SALADS								
Caesar	half	200	14	4	310	13	2	6
Chicken Caesar, Grilled	half	250	14	4	500	13	1	18
Chicken, Asian Sesame	half	210	10	1.5	450	16	2	16
Classic Cafe	half	90	5	1	135	9	2	1

ITEM DESCRIPTION	Serving Size	Calories	Total Fat (g)	Saturated Fat (g)	Sodium (mg)	Carbohydrates (g)	Fiber (g)	Protein (g)
Fruit Cup	sm	70	0	0	15	19	1	1
Fuji Apple	half	200	14	3	310	16	3	4
Fuji Apple w/ Chicken	half	260	15	3	450	17	3	16
Greek	half	220	20	4	690	7	3	5
Orchard Harvest	half	210	16	3.5	360	15	3	5
Orchard Harvest w/ Chicken	half	270	16	4	570	16	3	17
SANDWICHES								
Bacon Turkey Bravo® on Tomato Basil	half	420	16	5	1460	43	2	25
Chicken Caesar on Focaccia	half	430	19	4	820	41	2	22
Chicken Caesar on Three Cheese	half	400	16	5	820	42	2	23
Chicken Salad on Sesame Semolina	half	360	13	2.5	970	50	7	15
Chicken Salad on Whole Grain	half	320	13	2.5	770	40	9	16
Chicken, Chipotle on Artisan French	half	530	28	7	1280	43	2	27
Chicken, Chipotle on French	half	450	28	7	1050	26	2	25
Ham & Swiss, Smoked on Rye	half	350	18	7	940	28	2	20
Ham & Swiss, Smoked on Stone-Milled Rye	half	390	14	5	1290	41	3	24
Italian Combo on Ciabatta	half	520	23	9	1530	47	2	30
Panini, Chicken Bacon Dijon on Country	half	470	18	7	1010	48	2	29
Panini, Chicken Bacon Dijon on French	half	390	18	7	770	32	1	27
Panini, Frontega Chicken® on Focaccia	half	430	20	4.5	1080	40	2	23
Panini, Smokehouse Turkey® on Focaccia	half	430	18	6	1310	41	2	26
Panini, Smokehouse Turkey® on Three Cheese	half	390	14	5	1320	40	2	27
Panini, Tomato & Mozzarella on Ciabatta	half	390	15	5	650	50	4	15
Panini, Turkey Artichoke on Focaccia	half	370	13	3.5	1170	44	3	20
Roast Beef, Asiago on Asiago Cheese	half	360	16	6	640	29	1	24
Tuna Salad on Honey Wheat	half	380	23	4.5	570	32	3	10
Turkey Breast, Smoked on Country	half	310	9	1.5	1040	40	2	17
Turkey Breast, Smoked on Sourdough	half	240	9	1.5	840	25	1	15
Turkey, Sierra on Focaccia w/ Asiago Cheese	half	480	27	6	990	40	2	19

ITEM DESCRIPTION	Serving Size	Calories	Total Fat (g)	Saturated Fat (g)	Sodium (mg)	Carbohydrates (g)	Fiber (g)	Protein (g)
Veggie, Mediterranean on Tomato Basil	half	310	7	1.5	730	51	5	11
SOUPS								
Baked Potato, You Pick Two®	sm	230	14	9	720	21	2	5
Broccoli Cheddar, You Pick Two®	sm	230	16	9	970	14	1	8
Chicken Noodle, Low-Fat, You Pick Two®	sm	100	2	0	1110	16	1	6
Cream of Chicken & Wild Rice, You Pick Two®	sm	200	12	6	970	19	1	5
Creamy Tomato Soup w/ Croutons, You Pick Two®	sm	300	18	9	580	31	4	4
Creamy Tomato Soup, You Pick Two®	sm	210	15	8	770	20	3	3
Forest Mushroom, You Pick Two®	sm	170	12	6	770	14	1	3
French Onion w/ Cheese & Croutons, You Pick Two®	sm	210	9	4.5	1670	23	2	8
French Onion, no Cheese or Croutons, You Pick Two®	sm	90	3	1.5	1560	13	1	2
New England Clam Chowder, You Pick Two®	sm	320	28	18	740	11	1	6
Vegetarian Black Bean, Low-Fat, You Pick Two®	sm	150	1	0	920	28	6	8
Vegetarian Garden Vegetable, Low-Fat, You Pick Two®	sm	70	0.5	0	1200	15	4	3

Based on federal rounding and other applicable regulations. Nutritional information is calculated based on Panera's standardized recipes. Because our menu items are handcrafted and may be customized, variations in serving sizes, preparation techniques, ingredient substitutions, product testing, and sources of supply, as well as regional and seasonal differences may affect the nutrition values for each product. In addition, testing of new recipes of existing products may be conducted from time to time in certain markets. These new recipes may contain different/additional ingredients, including allergens, as compared to the original version. Some bakery-cafes may serve menu items which are not listed on this Site. Panera cannot guarantee that the nutritional information provided on this Site or available in any bakery-cafe is completely accurate as it relates to the prepared menu items in every bakery-cafe. For the most up-to-date information, please call or visit your nearest bakery-cafe to speak with a manager.

PIZZA HUT

BEVERAGES								
Diet Pepsi®	16 oz	0	0	0	50	0	0	0
Mountain Dew®	16 oz	220	0	0	70	58	0	0
Pepsi®	16 oz	200	0	0	50	56	0	0
Sierra Mist®	16 oz	200	0	0	40	54	0	0
DESSERTS								
Cinnamon Sticks	2 pcs	170	6	1.5	200	26	1	4
Hershey's® Chocolate Dunkers™	2 pcs	200	9	4	210	26	1	5
Hershey's® Chocolate Sauce	1 pkg	120	2.5	1	75	24	1	1

ITEM DESCRIPTION	Serving Size	Calories	Total Fat (g)	Saturated Fat (g)	Sodium (mg)	Carbohydrates (g)	Fiber (g)	Protein (g)
White Icing	1 pkg	190	0	0	0	47	0	0
MAIN MENU								
Fit 'n Delicious Pizza w/ Chicken, Mushrooms & Jalapeño	1 pc /8	170	4.5	2	760	23	2	10
Fit 'n Delicious Pizza w/ Chicken, Red Onion & Green Pepper	1 pc /8	180	4.5	2	550	24	2	10
Fit 'n Delicious Pizza w/ Diced Red Tomato, Mushroom & Jalapeño	1 pc /8	150	4	1.5	610	23	2	6
Fit 'n Delicious Pizza w/ Green Pepper, Red Onion & Diced Red Tomato	1 pc /8	150	4	1.5	400	24	2	6
Fit 'n Delicious Pizza w/ Ham, Pineapple & Diced Red Tomato	1 pc /8	160	4.5	1.5	560	24	1	7
Fit 'n Delicious Pizza w/ Ham, Red Onion & Mushroom	1 pc /8	160	4.5	1.5	550	23	1	8
Hand-Tossed Pizza w/ Cheese, Medium	1 pc /8	220	8	4.5	550	26	1	10
Hand-Tossed Pizza w/ Ham & Pineapple, Medium	1 pc /8	200	6	3	550	27	1	9
Hand-Tossed Pizza w/ Italian Sausage & Red Onion, Medium	1 pc /8	240	10	4.5	590	27	2	10
Hand-Tossed Pizza w/ Pepperoni & Mushroom, Medium	1 pc /8	210	8	3.5	550	26	2	9
Hand-Tossed Pizza w/ Pepperoni, Medium	1 pc /8	230	10	4.5	620	25	1	10
Hand-Tossed Pizza, Meat Lover's®, Medium	1 pc /8	310	17	7	860	26	2	14
Hand-Tossed Pizza, Supreme, Medium	1 pc /8	260	12	5	660	26	2	11
Hand-Tossed Pizza, Veggie Lover's®, Medium	1 pc /8	200	7	3	530	27	2	8
Pan Pizza w/ Cheese, Medium	1 pc /8	230	9	4	520	27	1	10
Pan Pizza w/ Ham & Pineapple, Medium	1 pc /8	220	8	3	520	28	1	9
Pan Pizza w/ Italian Sausage & Red Onion, Medium	1 pc /8	260	11	4.5	550	28	2	11
Pan Pizza w/ Pepperoni & Mushroom, Medium	1 pc /8	230	9	3.5	510	27	1	10

ITEM DESCRIPTION	Serving Size	Calories	Total Fat (g)	Saturated Fat (g)	Sodium (mg)	Carbohydrates (g)	Fiber (g)	Protein (g)
Pan Pizza w/ Pepperoni, Medium	1 pc /8	250	11	4.5	590	26	1	10
Pan Pizza, Meat Lover's®, Medium	1 pc /8	330	18	7	820	27	1	15
Pan Pizza, Supreme, Medium	1 pc /8	280	13	5	630	27	2	12
Pan Pizza, Veggie Lover's®, Medium	1 pc /8	220	8	3	490	28	2	9
Pasta, Bacon Mac N Cheese	1	520	22	12	1170	54	4	24
Pasta, Chicken Alfredo	1	630	33	11	1250	56	4	26
Pasta, Lasagna	1	570	30	13	1670	45	5	29
Pasta, Meaty Marinara	1	510	24	10	1310	48	5	25
Personal Pizza w/ Cheese	1	640	27	12	1420	70	3	29
Personal Pizza w/ Ham & Pineapple	1	590	22	9	1380	71	3	26
Personal Pizza w/ Italian Sausage & Red Onion	1	710	34	13	1540	71	4	30
Personal Pizza w/ Pepperoni	1	660	31	12	1580	68	3	28
Personal Pizza w/ Pepperoni & Mushroom	1	610	26	10	1380	69	4	27
Personal Pizza, Meat Lover's®	1	900	50	19	2250	70	4	41
Personal Pizza, Supreme	1	760	38	15	1740	71	4	33
Personal Pizza, Veggie Lover's®	1	580	22	9	1280	71	4	24
Pizza Mia Pizza w/ Cheese	1 pc /8	200	7	4	480	24	1	9
Pizza Mia Pizza w/ Pepperoni	1 pc /8	200	8	3.5	510	24	1	8
P'Zone®, Classic	1	630	23	11	1480	77	3	28
P'Zone®, Meaty	1	740	33	15	1840	76	3	34
P'Zone®, Pepperoni	1	630	24	11	1580	76	2	28
Stuffed Crust Pizza w/ Cheese, Large	1 pc /8	340	14	8	910	39	2	15
Stuffed Crust Pizza w/ Ham & Pineapple, Large	1 pc /8	330	13	7	940	41	2	15
Stuffed Crust Pizza w/ Italian Sausage & Red Onion, Large	1 pc /8	390	18	8	980	40	2	17
Stuffed Crust Pizza w/ Pepperoni & Mushroom, Large	1 pc /8	350	15	7	940	39	2	15
Stuffed Crust Pizza w/ Pepperoni, Large	1 pc /8	380	18	8	1060	39	2	16
Stuffed Crust Pizza, Meat Lover's®, Large	1 pc /8	480	26	12	1370	39	2	22
Stuffed Crust Pizza, Supreme, Large	1 pc /8	410	20	9	1090	40	3	18
Stuffed Crust Pizza, Veggie Lover's®, Large	1 pc /8	330	13	6	890	40	3	14

ITEM DESCRIPTION	Serving Size	Calories	Total Fat (g)	Saturated Fat (g)	Sodium (mg)	Carbohydrates (g)	Fiber (g)	Protein (g)
The Natural Pizza w/ Cheese	1 pc /8	220	8	4	460	26	2	10
The Natural Pizza w/ Pepperoni	1 pc /8	230	9	4	530	26	2	10
The Natural Pizza, Classicana	1 pc /8	260	11	5	570	27	2	11
The Natural Pizza, Veggie Lover's®, no Olives	1 pc /8	190	6	3	380	27	2	9
Thin 'N Crispy® Pizza w/ Cheese, Medium	1 pc /8	190	8	4	540	22	1	9
Thin 'N Crispy® Pizza w/ Ham & Pineapple, Medium	1 pc /8	180	6	2.5	530	23	1	8
Thin 'N Crispy® Pizza w/ Italian Sausage & Red Onion, Medium	1 pc /8	220	10	4	570	23	1	9
Thin 'N Crispy® Pizza w/ Pepperoni & Mushroom, Medium	1 pc /8	190	7	3	530	22	1	8
Thin 'N Crispy® Pizza w/ Pepperoni, Medium	1 pc /8	200	9	4	610	21	1	9
Thin 'N Crispy® Pizza, Meat Lover's®, Medium	1 pc /8	290	16	7	850	22	1	13
Thin 'N Crispy® Pizza, Supreme, Medium	1 pc /8	230	11	4.5	650	23	1	10
Thin 'N Crispy® Pizza, Veggie Lover's® Medium	1 pc /8	180	6	2.5	520	23	1	7
SIDES AND SNACKS								
Breadsticks	1 pc	140	6	1.5	240	18	1	4
Breadsticks w/ Cheese	1 pc	180	7	3.5	370	20	1	7
Dipping Sauce, Breadstick	1 pkg	60	0	0	440	12	2	2
Dipping Sauce, Wing Blue Cheese	1 pkg	230	24	4.5	430	2	0	1
Dipping Sauce, Wing Ranch	1 pkg	220	23	4	400	3	0	1
Wings, Hot	2 pcs	120	7	2	500	1	0	11
Wings, Mild	2 pcs	110	7	2	440	1	0	11

This data reflects U.S. products and builds only.

Substitution of ingredients/standard toppings combinations may alter nutritional values. Menu items and hours of availability may vary at participating locations. Although this data is based on standard portion product guidelines, variation can be expected due to seasonal influences, minor differences in products assembly per restaurant, and other factors. Except for limited time offerings or test market items, menu products as of this printing are included in this brochure. Product data is based on current formulation as of date of publication. Nutritional data is based on standard portion product guidelines and formulations as of date of printing. If you have any questions about Pizza Hut and nutrition or are particularly sensitive to specific ingredients or goods, please contact Pizza Hut at 1.800.948.8488 or visit us on the web at www.pizzahut.com.

The Dietary Guidelines for Americans recommend limiting saturated fat to 20 grams and sodium to 2,300 milligrams for a typical adult eating 2000 calories daily. Recommended limits may be higher or lower depending on daily calorie consumption.

For more information, go to www.MyPyramid.gov.

The HERSHEY'S® trademark and trade dress are used under license.

Pepsi, Diet Pepsi, Mountain Dew, and Sierra Mist are registered trademarks of PepsiCo, Inc.

© March 2009 Pizza Hut, Inc. The Pizza Hut name, logos, and related marks are trademarks of Pizza Hut, Inc.

POPEYES

ITEM DESCRIPTION	Serving Size	Calories	Total Fat (g)	Saturated Fat (g)	Sodium (mg)	Carbohydrates (g)	Fiber (g)	Protein (g)
MAIN MENU								
Breast, Mild	1	350	20	7	1130	8	0	33
Breast, Mild Skinless	2 pcs	120	2	1	540	0	0	24
Breast, Spicy	1	360	22	8	760	8	1	31
Breast, Spicy Skinless	1	120	2	1	380	<1	<1	25
Chicken Bowl	1	570	29	10	1600	44	8	35
Chicken Etouffee	1	160	10	3	870	6	2	12
Chicken Strips, Naked	3 pcs	220	10	4	720	2	0	30
Chicken Biscuit	1	350	20	9	930	30	<1	13
Chicken Sausage Jambalaya	1	220	11	3	760	20	1	10
Chicken, Smothered	1	210	8	2	743	24	1	10
Crawfish Etouffee	1	180	5	1	640	25	2	7
Delta Mini	1	300	13	4	780	30	1	15
Leg, Mild	1	110	7	2.5	280	3	0	11
Leg, Mild Skinless	1	50	2	0.5	190	0	0	9
Leg, Spicy	1	100	5	2	230	3	0	9
Leg, Spicy Skinless	1	50	1.5	0.5	135	0	0	9
Nuggets	6 pcs	220	12	5	500	13	<1	15
Sandwich, Crispy Chicken	1	560	23	8	1690	56	3	33
Sandwich, Deluxe Mild or Spicy w/ Mayo	1	630	31	8	1480	53	3	35
Sandwich, Deluxe Mild, no Mayo	1	480	15	6	1290	54	3	33
Sandwich, Po Boy	1	330	17	3	560	36	0	8
Shrimp, Butterfly	1	310	19	8	800	22	2	13
Shrimp, Popcorn	1	280	16	6	1110	22	<1	12
Strips, Mild Skinless	2 pcs	130	2.5	1	620	3	0	25
Strips, Spicy Skinless	2 pcs	150	4	1.5	820	5	0	23
Tenders, Mild	3 pcs	375	17	7	1620	24	0	33
Tenders, Spicy	3 pcs	405	17	7	2160	30	0	33
Thigh, Mild	1	280	20	7	710	7	0	16
Thigh, Mild Skinless	1	80	4	1	230	0	0	11
Thigh, Spicy	1	300	24	8	490	7	0	15
Thigh, Spicy Skinless	1	80	3	1	170	2	0	12

ITEM DESCRIPTION	Serving Size	Calories	Total Fat (g)	Saturated Fat (g)	Sodium (mg)	Carbohydrates (g)	Fiber (g)	Protein (g)
Wing, Mild	1	150	10	3.5	690	5	0	9
Wing, Mild Skinless	1	40	1.5	0.5	400	0	<1	7
Wing, Spicy	1	140	9	3.5	290	5	0	8
Wing, Spicy Skinless	1	40	2	0.5	125	0	<1	6
Wings, Cajun	6 pcs	595	43	15	1274	19	0	34
Wrap, Loaded Chicken	1	400	17	6	1100	44	4	19
SIDES AND SNACKS								
Apple Turnover, Cinnamon	1	250	12	4	320	34	2	3
Beans, Red & Rice	reg	320	19	6	710	31	17	10
Biscuits	1	240	13	7	490	26	1	4
Coleslaw	reg	260	23	3.5	260	14	9	<1
Corn on the Cob	1	190	2	0.5	0	37	4	6
French Fries	1	310	17	7	660	35	3	4
Green Beans	reg	70	1	0	400	14	2	2
Mashed Potatoes w/ Gravy	reg	120	4	2	570	18	2	3
Mashed Potatoes, no Gravy	reg	100	3	1	380	17	<1	1
Rice, Cajun	reg	170	6	2	530	22	2	8

The nutritional information provided in the "Nutrition Guide" and otherwise on the Popeyes® website or in its restaurants is comprised from data provided by an independent testing company commissioned by Popeyes (Silliker, Inc.) and our suppliers, and is current as of January of 2009. The data is based on standard product formulations and portion sizes, which can vary due to sampling differences, seasonal differences, ingredient substitutions, supplier variations, slight differences in product assembly on a restaurant by restaurant basis, and other factors.

All standard domestic Popeyes menu items are listed in the "Nutrition Guide." Some products may not be available at all restaurants. Products currently being tested & other limited time offerings and other regional menu alternatives may not be listed. Servings sizes may also vary slightly.

We encourage anyone with food sensitivities, allergies, or other special dietary needs or concerns to consult with your local physician or dietitian prior to eating at any Popeyes restaurant. Please periodically review the "Nutrition Guide" and our Popeyes website as information may be updated.

Updated January 16, 2009

RED LOBSTER

APPETIZERS

ITEM DESCRIPTION	Serving Size	Calories	Total Fat (g)	Saturated Fat (g)	Sodium (mg)	Carbohydrates (g)	Fiber (g)	Protein (g)
Calamari, Crispy w/ Vegetables	1 serv	1520	98	12	3060	116	n/a	n/a
Calamari, Crispy w/ Vegetables, in Combo platter	1 serv	775	49	6	1530	58	n/a	n/a
Chicken Breast Strips	1 serv	690	40	3.5	2200	46	n/a	n/a
Chicken Breast Strips, in Combo platter	1 serv	414	24	2	1320	28	n/a	n/a
Chicken Wings, Buffalo*	1 serv	680	39	9	1750	0	n/a	n/a
Clam Strips, in Combo platter	1 serv	370	22	2	820	31	n/a	n/a
Clams, Steamed*	1 serv	430	15	3.5	1120	10	n/a	n/a
Crab Cakes, Pan-Seared	1 serv	360	22	3.5	1200	15	n/a	n/a
Crawfish, Fried*	1 serv	1180	75	8	2050	88	n/a	n/a

ITEM DESCRIPTION	Serving Size	Calories	Total Fat (g)	Saturated Fat (g)	Sodium (mg)	Carbohydrates (g)	Fiber (g)	Protein (g)
Fondue, Ultimate	1 serv	1490	80	40	3580	124	n/a	n/a
Lobster Pizza	1 serv	720	30	13	1390	69	n/a	n/a
Lobster Rolls, Southwestern	1 serv	870	51	13	1430	74	n/a	n/a
Lobster, Artichoke & Seafood Dip	1 serv	1200	74	20	1950	101	n/a	n/a
Mozzarella Cheese Sticks	1 serv	680	39	14	1910	49	n/a	n/a
Mozzarella Cheese Sticks, in Combo platter	1 serv	340	20	7	955	25	n/a	n/a
Mushrooms Stuffed w/ Lobster, Crab & Seafood	1 serv	380	21	11	1050	20	n/a	n/a
Mushrooms, Stuffed, in Combo platter	1 serv	220	12	6	740	12	n/a	n/a
Oysters, Fried*	1 serv	590	32	3.5	1100	58	n/a	n/a
Oysters, Hand-Shucked*	12 pcs	100	2	0	340	8	n/a	n/a
Scallops, Peach-Bourbon Barbecue	1 serv	580	35	5	1880	40	n/a	n/a
Seafood Sampler, New England	1 serv	760	42	11	2270	46	n/a	n/a
Shrimp Cocktail, Chilled Jumbo	1 serv	120	1	0	590	9	n/a	n/a
Shrimp, Parrot Bay Jumbo Coconut	1 serv	588	33	7	1170	54	n/a	n/a
BEVERAGES								
Amaretto Sour	1	170	0	0	0	30	n/a	n/a
Appletini, Caramel	1	160	0	0	10	18	n/a	n/a
Bahama Mama	1	350	0	0	20	51	n/a	n/a
Bahama Mama, Non-alcoholic	1	230	0	0	25	57	n/a	n/a
Baileys® & Coffee	1	180	8	5	50	15	n/a	n/a
Baileys® Irish Cream	1	270	4.5	0	0	5.7	n/a	n/a
Biscayne Bay Breeze	1	240	0	0	10	47	n/a	n/a
Bloody Mary	1	140	0	0	1170	16	n/a	n/a
Bud Light®	18 oz	158	0	0	20	19	n/a	n/a
Coffee Nudge	1	130	2	1.5	15	14	n/a	n/a
Coffee, Harbor Café™	1	3	0	0	5	0	n/a	n/a
Cognac	1	73	0	0	0	0	n/a	n/a
Coke®	1	105	0	0	35	27	n/a	n/a
Colada, Alotta	1	700	16	14	55	95	n/a	n/a
Colada, Piña	1	320	6	5	35	55	n/a	n/a
Colada, Piña, Non-alcoholic	1	280	8	7	20	53	n/a	n/a
Colada, Red Passion	1	310	4.5	4	35	56	n/a	n/a

ITEM DESCRIPTION	Serving Size	Calories	Total Fat (g)	Saturated Fat (g)	Sodium (mg)	Carbohydrates (g)	Fiber (g)	Protein (g)
Colada, Sunset Passion	1	360	8	7	15	62	n/a	n/a
Colada, Sunset Passion, Non-alcoholic	1	330	8	7	25	62	n/a	n/a
Cosmopolitan	1	220	0	0	0	15	n/a	n/a
Daiquiri, Berry Mango, Non-alcoholic	1	210	0	0	20	52	n/a	n/a
Daiquiri, Big Berry	1	350	0.45	0.36	30	62	n/a	n/a
Daiquiri, Strawberry	1	250	0	0	15	47	n/a	n/a
Daiquiri, Strawberry, Non-alcoholic	1	230	0	0	5	56	n/a	n/a
Diet Coke®	1	0	0	0	28	<1	n/a	n/a
Disaronno Amaretto®	1	80	0	0	0	12	n/a	n/a
Distilled Spirits, 80 Proof	1	96	0	0	0	0	n/a	n/a
Dr Pepper®	1	150	0	0	35	27	n/a	n/a
Frangelico®	1	70	0	0	0	12.3	n/a	n/a
Grand Marnier®	1	76	0	0	0	6.5	n/a	n/a
Iced Tea, Boston	1	50	0	0	10	13	n/a	n/a
Irish Coffee	1	90	2	1	25	4	n/a	n/a
Kahlua®	1	90	0	0	3	14.7	n/a	n/a
Lemonade, Minute Maid® Light	1	3	0	0	54	<1	n/a	n/a
Lemonade, Minute Maid® Raspberry	1	178	0	0	20	30	n/a	n/a
Liqueurs	1	86	0	0	6	6 to 15	n/a	n/a
Lobsterita®, Raspberry	1	690	0.47	0.31	50	131	n/a	n/a
Lobsterita®, Strawberry	1	700	0	0	55	135	n/a	n/a
Lobsterita®, Traditional	1	890	0	0	890	183	n/a	n/a
Long Island Iced Tea, Top-Shelf	1	190	0	0	0	22	n/a	n/a
Malibu Hurricane	1	200	0	0	15	36	n/a	n/a
Manhattan w/ Bourbon	1	150	0	0	0	5	n/a	n/a
Manhattan w/ Whiskey	1	150	0	0	0	5	n/a	n/a
Margarita, Classic Frozen	1	470	0	0	590	96	n/a	n/a
Margarita, Classic Frozen, Non-alcoholic	1	278	0	0	560	75	n/a	n/a
Margarita, Classic On the Rocks	1	246	0	0	770	22	n/a	n/a
Margarita, Classic On the Rocks, Non-alcoholic	1	150	0	0	750	22	n/a	n/a
Margarita, Frozen Raspberry	1	320	0	0	0	61	n/a	n/a
Margarita, Frozen Strawberry	1	350	0	0	20	68	n/a	n/a
Margarita, Raspberry, Non-alcoholic	1	330	0	0	0	81	n/a	n/a

ITEM DESCRIPTION	Serving Size	Calories	Total Fat (g)	Saturated Fat (g)	Sodium (mg)	Carbohydrates (g)	Fiber (g)	Protein (g)
Margarita, Strawberry, Non-alcoholic	1	330	0	0	20	70	n/a	n/a
Margarita, Top-Shelf Frozen	1	520	0	0	640	97	n/a	n/a
Margarita, Top-Shelf On the Rocks	1	296	0	0	810	25	n/a	n/a
Martini, Classic w/ Gin	1	140	1.5	0.33	330	<1	n/a	n/a
Martini, Classic w/ Vodka	1	130	2	0	400	1	n/a	n/a
Mudslide	1	520	21	13	160	52	n/a	n/a
Rob Roy	1	160	0	0	10	3	n/a	n/a
Scotches, Single Malt	1	69	0	0	0	0	n/a	n/a
Screwdriver	1	100	0	0	0	8	n/a	n/a
Smoothie, Banana Bay Chocolate	1	460	14	9	10	78	n/a	n/a
Smoothie, Berry Strawberry Banana	1	340	9	6	85	63	n/a	n/a
Smoothie, Sunset Strawberry	1	250	6	4	45	47	n/a	n/a
Sparkling Wine	1	105	0	0	0 to 20	1 to 8	n/a	n/a
Sprite®	1	98	0	0	47	26	n/a	n/a
Tea, Iced or Hot, Unsweetened	1	3	0	0	0	<1	n/a	n/a
Tequila Sunrise	1	170	0	0	10	24	n/a	n/a
Tropical Freeze, Orange	1	250	6	5	20	49	n/a	n/a
Tropical Freeze, Pineapple	1	250	5	4.5	180	50	n/a	n/a
Wine, White, Blush or Red	1	122	0	0	0 to 20	1 to 8	n/a	n/a
DESSERTS								
Apple Crumble, Warm a La Mode	1	770	31	13	200	117	n/a	n/a
Cheesecake, New York-Style w/ Strawberries	1	520	36	21	270	39	n/a	n/a
Chocolate Wave	1	1490	81	25	950	172	n/a	n/a
Cookie, Warm Chocolate Chip Lava	1	1070	51	23	470	142	n/a	n/a
Pie, Key Lime	1	580	22	12	450	88	n/a	n/a
DRESSINGS AND SPREADS								
Dipping Sauce, Butter, Melted	1 serv	230	25	15	20	1	n/a	n/a
Dipping Sauce, Cocktail	1 serv	25	0	0	320	6	n/a	n/a
Dipping Sauce, Honey Mustard	1 serv	240	22	4	320	10	n/a	n/a
Dipping Sauce, Ketchup	1 serv	30	0	0	310	8	n/a	n/a
Dipping Sauce, Marinara	1 serv	30	1	0	220	6	n/a	n/a
Dipping Sauce, Pico de Gallo	1 serv	10	0	0	170	2	n/a	n/a
Dipping Sauce, Piña Colada Sauce	1 serv	120	5	4	20	16	n/a	n/a

ITEM DESCRIPTION	Serving Size	Calories	Total Fat (g)	Saturated Fat (g)	Sodium (mg)	Carbohydrates (g)	Fiber (g)	Protein (g)
Dipping Sauce, Remoulade	1 serv	150	15	2.5	150	4	n/a	n/a
Dipping Sauce, Sweet & Spicy Glaze	1 serv	90	0	0	220	21	n/a	n/a
Dipping Sauce, Tartar	1 serv	130	13	2	110	4	n/a	n/a
Dressing, Balsamic Vinaigrette	1 serv	60	5	0.5	190	4	n/a	n/a
Dressing, Blue Cheese	1 serv	170	18	3.5	190	1	n/a	n/a
Dressing, Caesar	1 serv	200	21	3.5	370	<1	n/a	n/a
Dressing, French	1 serv	120	11	1.5	300	7	n/a	n/a
Dressing, Honey Mustard	1 serv	100	11	2	160	5	n/a	n/a
Dressing, Ranch	1 serv	110	11	2	210	1	n/a	n/a
Dressing, Ranch, Fat-Free	1 serv	40	0	0	340	10	n/a	n/a
Dressing, Thousand Island	1 serv	130	13	2	180	5	n/a	n/a
FRESH FISH—WOOD-FIRE GRILLED OR BROILED								
Arctic Char	half	335	19.5	4	255	10	n/a	n/a
Barramundi	half	235	5.5	1.5	275	9	n/a	n/a
Cobia	half	405	27.5	9	255	6	n/a	n/a
Cod	half	175	2	0.26	270	8	n/a	n/a
Corvina	half	185	1.5	0.33	305	8	n/a	n/a
Flounder	half	195	1.5	0.16	350	9	n/a	n/a
Grouper	half	205	1.5	0.29	285	6	n/a	n/a
Haddock	half	175	1.5	0.21	270	6	n/a	n/a
Mahi-Mahi	half	205	1	0.16	305	6	n/a	n/a
Monchong	half	195	1.5	21	290	8	n/a	n/a
Opah	half	275	12.5	3	290	6	n/a	n/a
Perch	half	175	2	0.32	290	6	n/a	n/a
Pompano	half	235	6.5	2.5	295	7	n/a	n/a
Rainbow Trout	half	225	9.5	2.5	390	6	n/a	n/a
Red Rockfish	half	175	2.5	0.43	290	8	n/a	n/a
Salmon	half	265	8.5	2	320	8	n/a	n/a
Seabass	half	225	6.5	1.5	280	6	n/a	n/a
Snapper	half	205	1.5	0.28	335	8	n/a	n/a
Sole	half	145	2	0.37	260	6	n/a	n/a
Tilapia	half	205	3	1	235	9	n/a	n/a
Tuna	half	205	1	0.14	420	7	n/a	n/a
Wahoo	half	225	2	0.5	390	8	n/a	n/a

ITEM DESCRIPTION	Serving Size	Calories	Total Fat (g)	Saturated Fat (g)	Sodium (mg)	Carbohydrates (g)	Fiber (g)	Protein (g)
Walleye	half	175	2	0.35	410	8	n/a	n/a
CHEF'S CREATIONS, ADD:								
Chef's Creations, Cajun Spices	1	40	0.5	0	140	1	n/a	n/a
Chef's Creations, Honey Barbecue Shrimp	1	180	11	4.5	890	11	n/a	n/a
Chef's Creations, In a Bag	1	110	5	1	790	6	n/a	n/a
Chef's Creations, Lobster Butter Sauce	1	260	12.5	7	660	21.5	n/a	n/a
Chef's Creations, Maple-Glaze & Shrimp	1	200	10	2	685	17	n/a	n/a
Chef's Creations, New Orleans	1	250	19	8	770	0	n/a	n/a
KIDS MENU								
Biscuit, Cheddar Bay ™	1	150	8	2.5	350	16	n/a	n/a
Broccoli	1 serv	45	0.5	0	200	6	n/a	n/a
Butter for Baked Potato	1	90	10	6	80	1	n/a	n/a
Caesar Salad	1	270	21	4.5	560	13	n/a	n/a
Chicken Fingers	1 serv	414	24	2.1	1320	28	n/a	n/a
Chicken, Grilled	1 serv	215	4	1.25	705	14	n/a	n/a
Crab Legs, Snow	1 serv	80	0.5	0	950	0	n/a	n/a
Fish, Broiled	1 serv	150	1	0.16	150	3	n/a	n/a
French Fries	1 serv	330	17	1.5	740	40	n/a	n/a
Garden Salad	1	90	3	0.46	105	13	n/a	n/a
Macaroni & Cheese	1	280	7	2	590	42	n/a	n/a
Potato, Baked	1	190	1	0	900	40	n/a	n/a
Potatoes, Mashed	1	180	9	4	610	22	n/a	n/a
Rice Pilaf, Wild	1 serv	180	3	0.5	650	34	n/a	n/a
Shrimp, Popcorn	1 serv	140	7	1	620	12	n/a	n/a
Sour Cream for Baked Potato	1 serv	30	2.5	1.5	10	1	n/a	n/a
Sundae, Surf's Up	1	170	9	6	45	20	n/a	n/a
MAIN MENU								
Admiral's Feast	1 serv	1506	93.4	8.63	4662	101	n/a	n/a
Cajun Chicken Linguini Alfredo	half	630	27	10	1550	45	n/a	n/a
Catfish, Blackened Farm-Raised	1 serv	380	18	3	300	0	n/a	n/a
Catfish, Fried Farm-Raised	1 serv	440	24	3	560	5	n/a	n/a
Chicken & Shrimp, Honey Barbecue Grilled	1 serv	710	30	12	2630	26	n/a	n/a
Chicken, Maple-Glazed	1 serv	570	10	2.5	1950	62	n/a	n/a

ITEM DESCRIPTION	Serving Size	Calories	Total Fat (g)	Saturated Fat (g)	Sodium (mg)	Carbohydrates (g)	Fiber (g)	Protein (g)
Crab Crackin' Monday	1 lb	160	1	0	1900	0	n/a	n/a
Crab Legs, North Pacific King	1 serv	390	3	0	3570	3	n/a	n/a
Crab Legs, Snow	1 serv	160	1	0	1900	0	n/a	n/a
Crab Legs, Steamed Snow, Create Your Own Feast	1 serv	80	0.5	0	950	0	n/a	n/a
Crab Linguini Alfredo	half	560	25	12	1310	47	n/a	n/a
Crawfish, Fried*, Create Your Own Feast	1 serv	755	46	5	1395	64	n/a	n/a
Flounder, Broiled	1 serv	280	3	0.64	560	0	n/a	n/a
Flounder, Fried	1 serv	440	16	1	520	4	n/a	n/a
Flounder, Seafood-Stuffed	1 serv	320	11	3.5	1550	13	n/a	n/a
Flounder, Seafood-Stuffed, Create Your Own Feast	1 serv	160	6	1.5	780	6	n/a	n/a
Lobster & Shrimp Pasta, Chef's Signature	half	510	25	11	1090	43	n/a	n/a
Lobster, Live Maine	1 serv	45	0.48	0.12	350	0	n/a	n/a
Lobster, Shrimp & Scallops, Wood-Grilled	1 serv	720	33	17	2630	59	n/a	n/a
Oysters, Fried, Create Your Own Feast	1 serv	590	32	3.5	1100	58	n/a	n/a
Rainbow Trout, Wood-Grilled or Broiled	1 serv	225	9.5	2.5	390	6	n/a	n/a
Rock Lobster Tail	1 serv	90	1	0.2	300	2	n/a	n/a
Rockzilla*	1 serv	125	1	0	475	2.5	n/a	n/a
Salmon, Wood-Grilled Fresh, Create Your Own Feast	1 serv	210	9	2	235	<1	n/a	n/a
Scallops, Shrimp & Chicken, Wood-Grilled	1 serv	580	10	2.5	2580	58	n/a	n/a
Seafood Platter, Broiled	1 serv	280	8	2.02	1660	10	n/a	n/a
Seafood Platter, Classic Fried	1 serv	1090	62	6.5	2830	90	n/a	n/a
Shrimp & Salmon, Maui Luau	1 serv	790	16	3.5	2150	101	n/a	n/a
Shrimp & Scallops, Peach-Bourbon Barbecue	1 serv	490	12	3.5	1880	55	n/a	n/a
Shrimp Linguini Alfredo	half	550	29	10	1580	41	n/a	n/a
Shrimp Lover's Tuesday Coconut Shrimp Bites	1 serv	290	18	3	830	19	n/a	n/a
Shrimp Lover's Tuesday Fried Shrimp	1 serv	190	11	1	560	9	n/a	n/a

ITEM DESCRIPTION	Serving Size	Calories	Total Fat (g)	Saturated Fat (g)	Sodium (mg)	Carbohydrates (g)	Fiber (g)	Protein (g)
Shrimp Lover's Tuesday Popcorn Shrimp	1 serv	180	9	1	670	16	n/a	n/a
Shrimp Lover's Tuesday Scampi	1 serv	130	9	1.5	690	1	n/a	n/a
Shrimp Scampi, Garlic, Create Your Own Feast	1 serv	195	13.5	2.5	1035	1.5	n/a	n/a
Shrimp, Coconut Bites	1 serv	290	18	3	830	19	n/a	n/a
Shrimp, Crunchy Popcorn	1 serv	560	29	3	2144	52	n/a	n/a
Shrimp, Fried	1 serv	190	11	1	1010	9	n/a	n/a
Shrimp, Garlic-Grilled Jumbo	1 serv	365	6	1.5	1850	42	n/a	n/a
Shrimp, Garlic-Grilled Jumbo, Create Your Own Feast	1 serv	105	1	0.12	900	6.6	n/a	n/a
Shrimp, Jumbo w/ Lobster Butter	1 serv	590	23	12	2260	61	n/a	n/a
Shrimp, Maple-Glazed	1 serv	60	0.5	0	370	0	n/a	n/a
Shrimp, Parrot Bay Jumbo Coconut	1 serv	980	36	8	1038	50	n/a	n/a
Shrimp, Parrot Bay Jumbo Coconut, Create Your Own Feast	1 serv	784	44	9	1560	72	n/a	n/a
Shrimp, Popcorn	1 serv	180	9	1	670	16	n/a	n/a
Shrimp, Scampi	1 serv	130	9	1.5	690	1	n/a	n/a
Shrimp, Seaside Trio	1 serv	1030	58	13	3490	68	n/a	n/a
Shrimp, Walt's Favorite	1 serv	700	40	3	2440	52	n/a	n/a
Shrimp, Walt's Favorite, Create Your Own Feast	1 serv	466	26.4	2	1628	35	n/a	n/a
Sirloin & Shrimp, Wood-Grilled	1 serv	500	12	4	1750	35	n/a	n/a
Sirloin, Wood-Grilled, Create Your Own Feast	1 serv	250	7	3	640	0	n/a	n/a
Steak, Center-Cut New York Strip	1 serv	480	26	11	820	0	n/a	n/a
Steak, Lobster & Shrimp Oscar	1 serv	990	60	26	2410	20	n/a	n/a
Steak, New York Strip & Rock Lobster Tail	1 serv	570	27	11	1330	0	n/a	n/a
Tilapia, Wood-Grilled or Broiled	1 serv	205	3	1	235	9	n/a	n/a
Ultimate Feast®	1 serv	638	40.18	16.4	2524	20	n/a	n/a
Walleye, Frozen Beer Battered*	1 serv	700	42	4	1200	24	n/a	n/a
Walleye, Frozen Blackened*	1 serv	300	8	1	420	10	n/a	n/a
Walleye, Frozen Broiled*	1 serv	260	4	1	560	0	n/a	n/a
Walleye, Frozen Fried*	1 serv	600	30	3	1000	36	n/a	n/a

SIDES AND SNACKS

ITEM DESCRIPTION	Serving Size	Calories	Total Fat (g)	Saturated Fat (g)	Sodium (mg)	Carbohydrates (g)	Fiber (g)	Protein (g)
Asparagus	1 serv	60	3	1.5	270	5	n/a	n/a
Broccoli	1 serv	45	0.5	0	200	6	n/a	n/a
Butter for Potato	n/a	90	10	6	80	1	n/a	n/a
Cheddar Bay Biscuit™	1	150	8	2.5	350	16	n/a	n/a
Clam Chowder, Manhattan*	1 cup	80	1	0	690	12	n/a	n/a
Clam Chowder, New England	1 cup	240	16	10	680	13	n/a	n/a
Coleslaw	1 serv	200	15	2.5	250	13	n/a	n/a
Crab Legs, North Pacific King	1/2 lb	130	1	0	1190	1	n/a	n/a
Crab Legs, Snow	1/2 lb	80	0.5	0	950	0	n/a	n/a
French Fries	1 serv	330	17	1.5	740	40	n/a	n/a
Lobster Tail, Maine	1 serv	60	0.5	0	610	0	n/a	n/a
Potato, Baked	1 serv	190	1	0	900	40	n/a	n/a
Potato, Baked w/ Creamy Lobster	1 serv	370	12	7	1110	48	n/a	n/a
Potato, Mashed w/ Creamy Lobster	1 serv	360	22	12	1110	23	n/a	n/a
Potatoes, Mashed Home-Style	1 serv	180	9	4	610	22	n/a	n/a
Rice Pilaf, Wild	1 serv	180	3	0.5	650	34	n/a	n/a
Salad, Caesar	1 serv	270	21	4.5	560	13	n/a	n/a
Salad, Garden	1 serv	90	3	0.46	105	13	n/a	n/a
Salad, Hand-Tossed Caesar w/ Wood-Grilled Chicken	1	670	51	10	1710	14	n/a	n/a
Salad, Hand-Tossed Caesar w/ Wood-Grilled Shrimp	1	620	51	10	1370	14	n/a	n/a
Saltines	1 serv	25	0.5	0	80	4	n/a	n/a
Seafood Gumbo*	1 cup	230	8	2.5	1180	26	n/a	n/a
Seafood Gumbo, Bayou	1 cup	190	6	2	1130	15	n/a	n/a
Shrimp, Parrot Bay Jumbo Coconut	4 pcs	392	48	11	1384	67	n/a	n/a
Shrimp, Petite for Salad	1 serv	15	0	0	130	0	n/a	n/a
Shrimp, Walt's Favorite	6 pcs	349	20	1.5	1220	26	n/a	n/a
Soup, Creamy Potato Bacon	1 cup	220	15	9	790	19	n/a	n/a
Soup, Spicy Shrimp*	1 cup	160	6	2.5	1010	15	n/a	n/a
Sour Cream for Potato	1 serv	30	2.5	1.5	10	1	n/a	n/a

* = Regional Items availability varies by restaurant. Due to the handcrafted nature of our menu items and the inherent size variations of seafood, nutritional content may vary. Guests who have special food sensitivities or dietary needs should not rely solely on this information. Nutritional information valid only for U.S. restaurants. Nutritional content does not include condiments, dipping sauces, or optional accompaniments.

RUBY TUESDAY

ITEM DESCRIPTION	Serving Size	Calories	Total Fat (g)	Saturated Fat (g)	Sodium (mg)	Carbohydrates (g)	Fiber (g)	Protein (g)
APPETIZERS								
Asian Dumplings	1/4 dish	110	5	n/a	n/a	11	1	n/a
Chicken Strips, Barbecue	1/4 dish	203	9	n/a	n/a	17	1	n/a
Chicken Strips, Buffalo	1/4 dish	236	14	n/a	n/a	13	2	n/a
Chicken Strips, Thai Phoon	1/4 dish	262	18	n/a	n/a	12	1	n/a
Chicken Strips, Traditional	1/4 dish	177	9	n/a	n/a	11	1	n/a
Crab Cake, Jumbo Lump	1/4 dish	68	4	n/a	n/a	3	1	n/a
Dip, Fresh Guacamole	1/4 dish	347	23	n/a	n/a	22	9	n/a
Dip, Spinach Artichoke	1/4 dish	300	19	n/a	n/a	23	2	n/a
French Fries w/ Cheddar	1/4 dish	314	18	n/a	n/a	24	2	n/a
Mozzarella, Fried	1/4 dish	182	11	n/a	n/a	11	2	n/a
Quesadilla, Chicken	1/4 dish	139	7	n/a	n/a	10	0	n/a
Quesadilla, Fresh Avocado	1/4 dish	215	14	n/a	n/a	11	2	n/a
Queso Dip	1/4 dish	306	19	n/a	n/a	25	3	n/a
Sampler, Four Way	1/4 dish	354	20	n/a	n/a	20	2	n/a
Shrimp, Buffalo	1/4 dish	126	6	n/a	n/a	11	1	n/a
Shrimp, Thai Phoon	1/4 dish	191	13	n/a	n/a	11	1	n/a
Spring Rolls, Southwestern	1/4 dish	173	10	n/a	n/a	14	1	n/a
Wings, Fire	1/4 dish	159	9	n/a	n/a	1	1	n/a
BEVERAGES								
Cream Soda, Orange Creamsicle	1	202	7	n/a	n/a	33	0	n/a
Cream Soda, Peaches 'n Cream	1	244	7	n/a	n/a	44	0	n/a
Cream Soda, Strawberry	1	245	7	n/a	n/a	44	1	n/a
Float, Classic Coke	1	384	14	n/a	n/a	64	0	n/a
Float, Root Beer	1	399	14	n/a	n/a	68	0	n/a
Fruit Tea, Blackberry	1	162	0	n/a	n/a	39	2	n/a
Fruit Tea, Mango	1	104	0	n/a	n/a	26	1	n/a
Fruit Tea, Mixed Berry	1	162	0	n/a	n/a	39	1	n/a
Fruit Tea, Peach	1	162	0	n/a	n/a	41	0	n/a
Fruit Tea, Raspberry	1	162	0	n/a	n/a	39	2	n/a
Lemonade, Blackberry	1	190	0	n/a	n/a	46	2	n/a
Lemonade, Mixed Berry	1	190	0	n/a	n/a	46	1	n/a

ITEM DESCRIPTION	Serving Size	Calories	Total Fat (g)	Saturated Fat (g)	Sodium (mg)	Carbohydrates (g)	Fiber (g)	Protein (g)
Lemonade, Pomegranate	1	235	0	n/a	n/a	59	0	n/a
Lemonade, Raspberry	1	185	0	n/a	n/a	46	0	n/a
Lemonade, Strawberry	1	192	0	n/a	n/a	48	1	n/a
RT Palmer	1	125	0	n/a	n/a	31	1	n/a
Ruby T	1	114	0	n/a	n/a	29	0	n/a
DESSERTS								
Blondie	1	626	27	n/a	n/a	86	2	n/a
Cake, Double Chocolate	1 pc	988	50	n/a	n/a	118	6	n/a
Cheesecake, New York	1 pc	736	60	n/a	n/a	82	2	n/a
Cookie, Chocolate Chip	1	320	15	n/a	n/a	40	2	n/a
Cookie, Chocolate Chip Mini	1	80	4	n/a	n/a	10	1	n/a
Cookie, White Chocolate Macadamia Nut	1	340	20	n/a	n/a	38	1	n/a
Cookie, White Chocolate Macadamia Nut Mini	1	85	5	n/a	n/a	10	0	n/a
Strawberries & Ice Cream	1 serv	900	50	n/a	n/a	98	4	n/a
Tallcake, Chocolate	1 pc	1,276	60	n/a	n/a	173	2	n/a
DRESSING AND SPREADS								
Dressing, Balsamic Vinaigrette	1 serv	35	3	n/a	n/a	4	0	n/a
Dressing, Blue Cheese	1 serv	170	18	n/a	n/a	1	0	n/a
Dressing, French	1 serv	113	10	n/a	n/a	6	0	n/a
Dressing, Honey Mustard	1 serv	85	8	n/a	n/a	5	0	n/a
Dressing, Italian	1 serv	60	6	n/a	n/a	2	0	n/a
Dressing, Ranch	1 serv	94	10	n/a	n/a	1	0	n/a
Dressing, Ranch Lite	1 serv	47	5	n/a	n/a	1	0	n/a
Dressing, Signature Parmesan	1 serv	150	16	n/a	n/a	1	0	n/a
Dressing, Thousand Island	1 serv	70	7	n/a	n/a	3	0	n/a
Salsa	1 serv	9	0	n/a	n/a	1	0	n/a
Sauce, Asian Barbecue	1 serv	60	3	n/a	n/a	7	0	n/a
Sauce, Barbecue	1 serv	47	0	n/a	n/a	12	0	n/a
Sauce, Lemon Butter	1 serv	88	9	n/a	n/a	1	0	n/a
Sauce, Marinara	1 serv	17	1	n/a	n/a	1	1	n/a
Sauce, Orange Peanut	1 serv	62	3	n/a	n/a	8	0	n/a
Sauce, Parmesan Cream	1 serv	60	5	n/a	n/a	1	0	n/a
Sauce, Sam Adams Steak	1 serv	51	0	n/a	n/a	12	0	n/a

ITEM DESCRIPTION	Serving Size	Calories	Total Fat (g)	Saturated Fat (g)	Sodium (mg)	Carbohydrates (g)	Fiber (g)	Protein (g)
Sauce, Sweet Chile	1 serv	170	17	n/a	n/a	2	0	n/a
Sour Cream	1 serv	22	1	n/a	n/a	2	0	n/a
KIDS MENU								
Cheese Sticks	1 serv	704	34	n/a	n/a	73	9	n/a
Chicken Breast	1 serv	217	9	n/a	n/a	5	3	n/a
Chicken Tenders	1 serv	714	31	n/a	n/a	74	7	n/a
Grilled Cheese	1 serv	749	32	n/a	n/a	90	7	n/a
Macaroni & Cheese	1 serv	680	37	n/a	n/a	58	3	n/a
Minis	1 serv	917	46	n/a	n/a	88	7	n/a
Minis, Turkey	1 serv	873	41	n/a	n/a	88	8	n/a
Pasta Marinara	1 serv	490	6	n/a	n/a	79	10	n/a
Pasta w/ Butter	1 serv	622	25	n/a	n/a	74	8	n/a
Shrimp, Fried	1 serv	571	21	n/a	n/a	71	6	n/a
Steak Chop	1 serv	403	30	n/a	n/a	15	2	n/a
Sundae	1 serv	574	29	n/a	n/a	70	1	n/a
MAIN MENU								
Burger, Alpine Swiss	1	1,207	83	n/a	n/a	64	3	n/a
Burger, Avocado Turkey	1	1,130	68	n/a	n/a	62	5	n/a
Burger, Bella Turkey	1	1,008	56	n/a	n/a	65	3	n/a
Burger, Blackened Fish	1	861	53	n/a	n/a	44	2	n/a
Burger, Boston Blue	1	1,424	96	n/a	n/a	84	6	n/a
Burger, Brewmaster	1	1,221	82	n/a	n/a	74	3	n/a
Burger, Buffalo Chicken	1	994	62	n/a	n/a	72	3	n/a
Burger, Chicken BLT	1	1,012	61	n/a	n/a	72	3	n/a
Burger, Jumbo Lump Crab	1	820	54	n/a	n/a	54	5	n/a
Burger, Ruby's Classic	1	1,090	75	n/a	n/a	61	3	n/a
Burger, Smokehouse	1	1,434	97	n/a	n/a	84	5	n/a
Burger, Three Cheese	1	1,320	94	n/a	n/a	62	3	n/a
Burger, Triple Prime	1	998	69	n/a	n/a	48	2	n/a
Burger, Triple Prime Bacon Cheddar	1	1,226	88	n/a	n/a	48	2	n/a
Burger, Triple Prime Cheddar	1	1,158	83	n/a	n/a	48	2	n/a
Burger, Triple Prime Havarti	1	1,306	94	n/a	n/a	48	2	n/a
Burger, Turkey	1	890	48	n/a	n/a	62	3	n/a
Burger, Ultimate Chicken	1	1,161	66	n/a	n/a	59	3	n/a

ITEM DESCRIPTION	Serving Size	Calories	Total Fat (g)	Saturated Fat (g)	Sodium (mg)	Carbohydrates (g)	Fiber (g)	Protein (g)
Burger, Veggie	1	952	53	n/a	n/a	95	3	n/a
Cheeseburger	1	1,160	81	n/a	n/a	62	3	n/a
Cheeseburger, Bacon	1	1,227	86	n/a	n/a	62	3	n/a
Cheeseburger, Bison Bacon	1	1,107	71	n/a	n/a	62	3	n/a
Chesapeake Catch	1 serv	536	32	n/a	n/a	7	1	n/a
Chicken & Broccoli Pasta	1 serv	1,167	55	n/a	n/a	90	11	n/a
Chicken Bella	1 serv	387	17	n/a	n/a	6	0	n/a
Chicken Fresco	1 serv	426	22	n/a	n/a	8	1	n/a
Chicken Pasta w/ Parmesan	1 serv	1,318	70	n/a	n/a	101	10	n/a
Chicken Piccata	1 serv	1,272	70	n/a	n/a	101	12	n/a
Chicken Salad, Grilled	1 serv	489	28	n/a	n/a	4	3	n/a
Chicken Tender Dinner	1 serv	n/a	n/a	n/a	n/a	n/a	n/a	n/a
Chicken, Grilled	1 serv	257	7	n/a	n/a	0	0	n/a
Chili, White Bean Chicken	1 serv	318	11	n/a	n/a	29	11	n/a
Clam Chowder	1 serv	437	28	n/a	n/a	23	2	n/a
Crab Cake Dinner	1 serv	271	17	n/a	n/a	10	3	n/a
Creole Catch	1 serv	320	16	n/a	n/a	1	1	n/a
Lobster Ravioli	1 serv	853	53	n/a	n/a	56	5	n/a
New Orleans Seafood	1 serv	443	25	n/a	n/a	2	0	n/a
Rib Eye	1 serv	683	45	n/a	n/a	5	1	n/a
Rib Eye, Cowboy	1 serv	932	56	n/a	n/a	28	4	n/a
Ribs & Louisiana Fried Shrimp	1 serv	916	49	n/a	n/a	53	2	n/a
Ribs, Classic Barbecue	half	493	32	n/a	n/a	14	0	n/a
Ribs, Memphis Dry Rub	half	538	40	n/a	n/a	3	0	n/a
Ribs, Triple Play	1 serv	n/a	n/a	n/a	n/a	n/a	n/a	n/a
Salmon & Shrimp, Asian	1 serv	466	28	n/a	n/a	7	0	n/a
Salmon, Asian Glazed	1 serv	433	27	n/a	n/a	8	1	n/a
Salmon, Grilled	1 serv	365	23	n/a	n/a	0	0	n/a
Shrimp Pasta, Parmesan	1 serv	1,030	48	n/a	n/a	85	9	n/a
Shrimp Scampi & Steak	1 serv	1,049	54	n/a	n/a	73	6	n/a
Shrimp, Louisiana Fried	1 serv	423	17	n/a	n/a	38	2	n/a
Sirloin, Bayou	1 serv	387	16	n/a	n/a	5	0	n/a
Sirloin, House	1 serv	298	15	n/a	n/a	2	0	n/a
Sirloin, Peppercorn Mushroom	1 serv	414	18	n/a	n/a	10	0	n/a

ITEM DESCRIPTION	Serving Size	Calories	Total Fat (g)	Saturated Fat (g)	Sodium (mg)	Carbohydrates (g)	Fiber (g)	Protein (g)
Sirloin, Petite	1 serv	298	15	n/a	n/a	2	0	n/a
Sirloin, Plain Grilled Petite	1 serv	206	5	n/a	n/a	2	0	n/a
Sirloin, Plain Grilled Top	1 serv	256	6	n/a	n/a	2	0	n/a
Sirloin, Top	1 serv	349	16	n/a	n/a	2	0	n/a
Tilapia, Herb Crusted	1 serv	402	24	n/a	n/a	9	2	n/a
Wrap, Grilled Chicken	1	436	17	n/a	n/a	40	2	n/a
Wrap, Turkey Burger	1	551	19	n/a	n/a	44	2	n/a
SIDES AND SNACKS								
Bread, Entrée	1 serv	140	7	n/a	n/a	14	1	n/a
Broccoli, Fresh Steamed	1 serv	89	6	n/a	n/a	5	3	n/a
Cauliflower, Creamy Mashed	1 serv	136	8	n/a	n/a	9	5	n/a
Chicken Salad, Carolina	1 serv	n/a	n/a	n/a	n/a	n/a	n/a	n/a
Chili, White Bean Chicken	1 serv	318	11	n/a	n/a	29	11	n/a
Cole Slaw	1 serv	159	13	n/a	n/a	8	1	n/a
French Fries	1 serv	359	13	n/a	n/a	52	5	n/a
Green Beans, Premium Baby	1 serv	85	5	n/a	n/a	5	3	n/a
Mini Trio	1 serv	856	47	n/a	n/a	64	5	n/a
Minis Combo	2 pcs	589	36	n/a	n/a	37	2	n/a
Minis Combo, Buffalo Chicken	1 serv	n/a	n/a	n/a	n/a	n/a	n/a	n/a
Minis Combo, Turkey	2 pcs	529	29	n/a	n/a	40	3	n/a
Minis, Bacon Cheese	4 pcs	1,268	79	n/a	n/a	75	4	n/a
Minis, Buffalo Chicken	4 pcs	n/a	n/a	n/a	n/a	n/a	n/a	n/a
Minis, Double Bacon Cheese	1 serv	987	69	n/a	n/a	38	2	n/a
Minis, Double Ruby	1 serv	897	62	n/a	n/a	38	2	n/a
Minis, Double Smokehouse	1 serv	1,045	70	n/a	n/a	49	2	n/a
Minis, Double Turkey	1 serv	853	54	n/a	n/a	40	4	n/a
Minis, Ruby	4 pcs	1,178	72	n/a	n/a	75	4	n/a
Minis, Turkey	4 pcs	1,058	58	n/a	n/a	79	6	n/a
Onion Straws	1 serv	298	21	n/a	n/a	20	4	n/a
Portabella Mushrooms, Sautéed Baby	1 serv	75	4	n/a	n/a	6	0	n/a
Potato, Baked w/ Butter & Sour Cream	1 serv	488	17	n/a	n/a	56	12	n/a
Potato, Loaded Baked	1 serv	668	31	n/a	n/a	56	12	n/a
Potato, Plain Baked	1 serv	329	2	n/a	n/a	54	12	n/a
Potatoes, White Cheddar Mashed	1 serv	130	7	n/a	n/a	15	2	n/a

ITEM DESCRIPTION	Serving Size	Calories	Total Fat (g)	Saturated Fat (g)	Sodium (mg)	Carbohydrates (g)	Fiber (g)	Protein (g)
Quiche, Chicken & Broccoli	1 serv	721	48	n/a	n/a	33	2	n/a
Quiche, Spinach & Mushroom	1 serv	673	44	n/a	n/a	39	15	n/a
Quiche, Tomato Basil	1 serv	734	44	n/a	n/a	52	11	n/a
Rice Pilaf, Brown	1 serv	226	7	n/a	n/a	33	2	n/a
Salad, Club House	1 serv	840	53	n/a	n/a	2	7	n/a
Salad, Signature House	1 serv	391	30	n/a	n/a	19	3	n/a
Soup, Broccoli & Cheese	1 serv	403	29	n/a	n/a	21	1	n/a

SONIC DRIVE-IN

BEVERAGES

ITEM DESCRIPTION	Serving Size	Calories	Total Fat (g)	Saturated Fat (g)	Sodium (mg)	Carbohydrates (g)	Fiber (g)	Protein (g)
Apple Juice, Minute Maid®	reg (14 oz)	160	0	0	20	40	0	0
Coca-Cola®	sm (14 oz)	140	0	0	10	39	0	0
Coffee	reg (14 oz)	10	0	0	35	2	1	1
Cranberry Juice, Minute Maid®	reg (14 oz)	170	0	0	20	46	0	0
Diet Coke®	sm (14 oz)	0	0	0	15	0	0	0
Diet Dr Pepper®	sm (14 oz)	0	0	0	70	0	0	0
Dr Pepper®	sm (14 oz)	130	0	0	45	37	0	0
Fruit Punch, Hi-C®	sm (14 oz)	150	0	0	15	40	0	0
Hot Chocolate	reg (14 oz)	120	2.5	2	170	23	1	1
Ice Tea	sm (14 oz)	5	0	0	10	1	0	0
Ice Tea, Peach	sm (14 oz)	5	0	0	15	1	0	0
Ice Tea, Raspberry	sm (14 oz)	5	0	0	15	1	0	0
Ice Tea, Sweet	sm (14 oz)	150	0	0	10	39	0	0
Iced Latté, Caramel	14 oz	260	8	6	190	44	0	3
Iced Latté, Caramel/Hazelnut	14 oz	260	8	5	140	44	0	3
Iced Latté, Chocolate	14 oz	260	7	5	150	45	0	3
Iced Latté, Chocolate/Caramel	14 oz	260	8	5	170	45	0	3
Iced Latté, Chocolate/Hazelnut	14 oz	250	7	5	120	45	0	3
Iced Latté, Hazelnut	14 oz	260	7	5	90	44	0	3
Java Chiller, Caramel	14 oz	540	18	12	300	86	0	7
Java Chiller, Caramel/Hazelnut	14 oz	530	18	11	230	85	0	7
Java Chiller, Chocolate	14 oz	540	18	11	260	87	0	7
Java Chiller, Chocolate/Caramel	14 oz	540	18	11	280	85	0	7
Java Chiller, Chocolate/Hazelnut	14 oz	540	18	11	250	86	0	7

ITEM DESCRIPTION	Serving Size	Calories	Total Fat (g)	Saturated Fat (g)	Sodium (mg)	Carbohydrates (g)	Fiber (g)	Protein (g)
Java Chiller, Hazelnut	14 oz	530	18	11	200	86	0	7
Latté, Caramel	14 oz	210	5	4.5	190	36	1	3
Latté, Caramel/Chocolate	14 oz	210	5	4.5	170	38	1	3
Latté, Caramel/Hazelnut	14 oz	210	5	4.5	160	38	1	3
Latté, Chocolate	14 oz	210	4.5	4	160	38	1	3
Latté, Hazelnut	14 oz	200	4.5	4	125	38	1	3
Latté, Hazelnut/Chocolate	14 oz	210	5	4.5	170	38	1	3
Lemonade, Minute Maid® Light	sm (14 oz)	5	0	0	5	1	0	0
Limeade	sm (14 oz)	140	0	0	30	38	0	0
Limeade, Apple Juice Minute Maid®	sm (14 oz)	160	0	0	35	42	0	0
Limeade, Cherry	sm (14 oz)	170	0	0	35	45	0	0
Limeade, Cranberry, Minute Maid®	sm (14 oz)	150	0	0	35	41	0	0
Limeade, Lo-Cal Diet	sm (14 oz)	5	0	0	10	1	0	0
Limeade, Lo-Cal Diet Cherry	sm (14 oz)	10	0	0	10	2	0	0
Limeade, Strawberry	sm (14 oz)	170	0	0	35	45	0	0
Mello Yello®	sm (14 oz)	150	0	0	10	42	0	0
Milk, 1%	1	110	2.5	1.5	130	13	0	8
Milk, 1% Chocolate	1	160	2.5	1.5	210	27	0	8
Ocean Water®	sm (14 oz)	150	0	0	35	41	0	0
Orange Juice, Minute Maid®	reg (14 oz)	150	0	0	20	36	0	2
Orange Soda, Minute Maid®	sm (14 oz)	150	0	0	0	42	0	0
Powerade® Mountain Blast®	sm (14 oz)	90	0	0	75	24	0	0
Powerade® Mountain Blast® Slush	sm (14 oz)	200	0	0	50	53	0	0
Root Beer, Barq's®	sm (14 oz)	160	0	0	35	43	0	0
Slush, Apple Juice, Minute Maid®	sm (14 oz)	190	0	0	30	51	0	0
Slush, Blue Coconut	sm (14 oz)	190	0	0	30	52	0	0
Slush, Bubble Gum	sm (14 oz)	190	0	0	35	52	0	0
Slush, Cherry	sm (14 oz)	200	0	0	30	53	0	0
Slush, Cranberry Juice, Minute Maid®	sm (14 oz)	190	0	0	30	52	0	0
Slush, Grape	sm (14 oz)	190	0	0	35	52	0	0

ITEM DESCRIPTION	Serving Size	Calories	Total Fat (g)	Saturated Fat (g)	Sodium (mg)	Carbohydrates (g)	Fiber (g)	Protein (g)
Slush, Green Apple	sm (14 oz)	200	0	0	30	54	0	0
Slush, Lemon	sm (14 oz)	200	0	0	30	53	0	0
Slush, Lemon-Berry	sm (14 oz)	210	0	0	30	55	0	0
Slush, Lime	sm (14 oz)	200	0	0	30	52	0	0
Slush, Orange	sm (14 oz)	200	0	0	30	52	0	0
Slush, Strawberry	sm (14 oz)	210	0	0	30	55	0	0
Slush, Watermelon	sm (14 oz)	200	0	0	30	53	0	0
Smoothie, Strawberry	reg (14 oz)	500	0	0	170	124	4	1
Smoothie, Strawberry-Banana	reg (14 oz)	460	0	0	180	113	8	1
Smoothie, Tropical	reg (14 oz)	440	0	0	160	108	3	1
Sonic Sunrise®	reg (14 oz)	180	0	0	30	46	0	1
Sprite®	sm (14 oz)	140	0	0	30	37	0	0
Sprite® Zero	sm (14 oz)	5	0	0	10	0	0	0
Strawberry Soda, Minute Maid®	sm (14 oz)	160	0	0	0	45	0	0
BREAKFAST ITEMS								
Breakfast Bistro w/ Bacon, Egg & Cheese	1	510	30	10	1060	37	2	22
Breakfast Bistro w/ Ham, Egg & Cheese	1	460	24	7	1320	36	2	26
Breakfast Bistro w/ Sausage, Egg & Cheese	1	590	40	13	1000	37	2	23
Breakfast Burrito	jr	330	21	8	790	25	2	13
Breakfast Burrito w/ Bacon, Egg & Cheese	1	450	26	10	1240	38	2	20
Breakfast Burrito w/ Ham, Egg & Cheese	1	440	23	9	1630	37	2	26
Breakfast Burrito w/ Sausage, Egg & Cheese	1	470	30	11	1140	38	2	19
Breakfast Burrito, Super Sonic®	1	550	34	12	1340	47	4	20
Breakfast Toaster® w/ Bacon, Egg & Cheese	1	530	32	10	1440	40	2	20
Breakfast Toaster® w/ Ham, Egg & Cheese	1	490	26	8	1700	40	2	24
Breakfast Toaster® w/ Sausage, Egg & Cheese	1	620	42	13	1380	40	2	20
CroisSonic Breakfast Sandwich w/ Bacon	1	510	36	15	1060	29	0	18
CroisSonic Breakfast Sandwich w/ Sausage	1	600	46	18	1000	29	0	19
French Toast Sticks	4 pcs	500	31	5	490	49	2	7

ITEM DESCRIPTION	Serving Size	Calories	Total Fat (g)	Saturated Fat (g)	Sodium (mg)	Carbohydrates (g)	Fiber (g)	Protein (g)
DESSERTS								
Banana Split	reg	420	9	6	140	80	2	4
Banana Split	jr	180	3.5	2	60	37	1	2
CreamSlush® Treat, Blue Coconut	reg (14 oz)	430	13	8	160	76	0	5
CreamSlush® Treat, Cherry	reg (14 oz)	440	13	8	160	77	0	5
CreamSlush® Treat, Grape	reg (14 oz)	430	13	8	160	76	0	5
CreamSlush® Treat, Lemon	reg (14 oz)	430	13	8	160	77	0	5
CreamSlush® Treat, Lemon-Berry	reg (14 oz)	460	12	7	150	85	1	5
CreamSlush® Treat, Lime	reg (14 oz)	430	13	8	160	77	0	5
CreamSlush® Treat, Orange	reg (14 oz)	430	13	8	160	77	0	5
CreamSlush® Treat, Strawberry	reg (14 oz)	450	12	7	150	84	1	5
CreamSlush® Treat, Watermelon	reg (14 oz)	440	13	8	160	77	0	5
Float, Barq's® Root Beer	reg (14 oz)	300	8	5	110	56	0	3
Float, Coca-Cola®	reg (14 oz)	290	8	5	95	54	0	3
Float, Diet Coke®	reg (14 oz)	220	8	5	100	33	0	3
Float, Diet Dr Pepper®	reg (14 oz)	220	8	5	130	33	0	3
Float, Dr Pepper®	reg (14 oz)	310	8	5	120	58	0	3
Ice Cream, Vanilla Cone	1	180	6	4	80	30	0	2
Ice Cream, Vanilla Dish	1	240	9	5	100	36	0	3
Malt, Banana	reg (14 oz)	490	17	10	200	78	1	7
Malt, Chocolate	reg (14 oz)	550	17	10	280	91	0	7
Malt, Pineapple	reg (14 oz)	510	17	10	210	82	0	7
Malt, Strawberry	reg (14 oz)	520	17	10	210	85	1	7
Malt, Vanilla	reg (14 oz)	480	18	11	210	72	0	7
Shake, Banana	reg (14 oz)	470	16	10	190	76	1	7
Shake, Banana Cream Pie	reg (14 oz)	590	19	11	220	98	1	7
Shake, Chocolate	reg (14 oz)	540	16	10	270	89	0	6
Shake, Chocolate Cream Pie	reg (14 oz)	660	19	11	300	114	0	7
Shake, Coconut Cream Pie	reg (14 oz)	580	20	12	230	93	0	7
Shake, Hot Fudge	reg (14 oz)	570	21	14	240	85	1	6
Shake, Peanut Butter	reg (14 oz)	640	34	13	300	75	0	10
Shake, Peanut Butter Fudge	reg (14 oz)	610	28	14	280	81	1	8
Shake, Pineapple	reg (14 oz)	500	16	10	200	80	0	6
Shake, Strawberry	reg (14 oz)	510	16	10	200	83	1	7

ITEM DESCRIPTION	Serving Size	Calories	Total Fat (g)	Saturated Fat (g)	Sodium (mg)	Carbohydrates (g)	Fiber (g)	Protein (g)
Shake, Strawberry Cream Pie	reg (14 oz)	620	19	11	230	106	1	7
Shake, Vanilla	reg (14 oz)	470	17	11	200	71	0	7
Sonic Blast®, Butterfinger®	reg (14 oz)	580	22	13	240	88	0	8
Sonic Blast®, M&M's®	reg (14 oz)	600	24	15	210	88	1	8
Sonic Blast®, Oreo®	reg (14 oz)	540	21	12	280	80	1	7
Sonic Blast®, Reese's Peanut Butter Cups®	reg (14 oz)	560	19	12	250	89	1	9
Sundae, Banana Fudge	1	440	16	11	170	70	2	4
Sundae, Butterfinger	jr	170	6	3.5	65	26	0	2
Sundae, Chocolate	1	410	13	9	190	67	0	4
Sundae, Hot Fudge	1	440	18	13	170	63	1	4
Sundae, Hot Fudge Cake	1	500	20	12	310	73	2	5
Sundae, M&M	jr	180	7	4.5	55	26	0	2
Sundae, Oreo	jr	150	5	3	90	22	0	2
Sundae, Peanut Butter	1	510	31	12	230	53	0	8
Sundae, Peanut Butter Fudge	1	470	25	13	200	58	1	6
Sundae, Pineapple	1	370	13	9	125	58	0	4
Sundae, Reese's	jr	160	4.5	3	75	27	0	3
Sundae, Strawberry	1	380	13	9	120	61	1	4
DRESSINGS AND SPREADS								
Dressing, Honey Mustard	1 pkg	240	21	3	300	14	0	1
Dressing, Italian, Fat Free	1 pkg	50	0	0	600	13	0	0
Dressing, Ranch	1 pkg	260	28	4.5	490	0	0	0
Dressing, Ranch Light	1 pkg	120	7	1	740	14	0	1
Dressing, Ranch Southwest	1 pkg	120	7	1	770	15	0	1
Dressing, Thousand Island	1 pkg	250	25	4	590	9	0	1
Jam, Strawberry	1	40	0	0	0	9	0	0
Jelly, Grape	1	35	0	0	0	9	0	0
Ketchup	1	10	0	0	110	2	0	0
Mayonnaise	1	80	9	1.5	60	0	0	0
Mustard	1	5	0	0	55	0	0	0
Relish, Sweet	1	10	0	0	65	3	0	0
Sauce, Barbecue	1	45	0	0	390	11	0	0
Sauce, French Fry	1	25	0	0	130	7	1	0

ITEM DESCRIPTION	Serving Size	Calories	Total Fat (g)	Saturated Fat (g)	Sodium (mg)	Carbohydrates (g)	Fiber (g)	Protein (g)
Sauce, Honey Mustard	1	90	7	1	190	7	0	0
Sauce, Marinara	1	15	0	0	270	3	1	0
Sauce, Picante	1	5	0	0	140	1	0	0
Sauce, Ranch	1	150	16	2.5	210	1	0	0
Syrup	1 pkg	80	0	0	0	21	21	0
KIDS MENU								
Burger	jr	310	15	5	610	30	3	15
Cheeseburger	jr	380	20	9	930	31	3	18
Cheeseburger, Double	jr	570	35	16	1290	33	3	30
Cheeseburger, Thousand Island	jr	430	27	10	700	30	3	18
Chicken Strips	2 pcs	200	11	2	470	10	1	14
Corn Dog	1	210	11	3.5	530	23	2	6
Grilled Cheese	1	380	20	8	1010	39	2	12
String Cheese	1	80	5	3	190	0	0	7
MAIN MENU								
Burger w/ Ketchup	1	560	26	9	820	57	5	26
Burger w/ Mayonnaise	1	650	37	10	720	55	5	26
Burger w/ Mustard	1	560	26	9	750	54	5	26
Burger, Dixie	1	660	37	10	810	55	5	26
Burger, Jalapeño	1	550	26	9	610	52	5	25
Burrito	1	370	18	6	480	40	6	10
Burrito Deluxe	1	420	22	7	640	43	6	13
Ched 'R' Bites®	1 serv	280	15	6	740	22	1	13
Ched 'R' Peppers®	1 serv	330	17	6	1110	36	2	8
Cheeseburger w/ Bacon	1	780	48	16	1300	57	5	33
Cheeseburger w/ Ketchup	1	630	31	12	1140	59	5	29
Cheeseburger w/ Mayonnaise	1	720	42	14	1040	56	5	29
Cheeseburger w/ Mustard	1	620	31	12	1070	55	5	29
Cheeseburger, California	1	690	39	13	1060	57	5	29
Cheeseburger, Chili	1	660	35	14	990	56	5	31
Cheeseburger, Dixie	1	720	42	14	1120	56	5	29
Cheeseburger, Green Chili	1	630	31	12	1070	56	5	29
Cheeseburger, Hickory	1	640	31	12	1170	61	5	28
Cheeseburger, Jalapeño	1	610	31	12	930	53	5	28

ITEM DESCRIPTION	Serving Size	Calories	Total Fat (g)	Saturated Fat (g)	Sodium (mg)	Carbohydrates (g)	Fiber (g)	Protein (g)
Cheeseburger, Super Sonic® Jalapeño	1	890	53	22	1600	56	5	46
Cheeseburger, Super Sonic® w/ Ketchup	1	900	53	22	1540	60	5	46
Cheeseburger, Super Sonic® w/ Mayonnaise	1	980	64	24	1430	58	5	46
Cheeseburger, Super Sonic® w/ Mustard	1	890	53	22	1460	57	5	46
Cheeseburger, Thousand Island	1	680	38	13	1130	58	5	29
Chicken Strip Dinner	4 pcs	930	43	8	1610	100	7	36
Chicken, Crispy Bacon Ranch	1	580	30	8	1780	50	4	30
Chicken, Crispy Sandwich	1	560	32	5	780	46	4	23
Chicken, Grilled Bacon Ranch	1	440	17	6	1660	37	3	35
Chicken, Grilled Sandwich	1	420	20	3	670	33	3	29
Chicken®, Jumbo Popcorn	sm	380	22	4	1250	27	3	18
Chicken®, Jumbo Popcorn	lg	560	32	6	1890	41	5	27
Coney, Extra-Long Chili Cheese	1	600	33	11	1700	54	4	24
Corn Dog	1	210	11	3.5	530	23	2	6
French Fries	lg	280	11	2	135	42	3	3
French Fries w/ Cheese	lg	380	19	7	600	44	3	8
French Fries w/ Chili & Cheese	lg	450	25	9	610	48	4	13
Fritos® Chili Pie	1	940	64	18	1540	72	6	25
Hot Dog, Extra-Long Slaw Dog	1	670	38	12	1770	60	4	24
Mozzarella Sticks	1 serv	440	22	9	1050	40	2	19
Onion Rings	lg	640	31	5	300	80	4	9
Salad, Grilled Chicken	1	310	13	6	1070	19	4	29
Salad, Jumbo Popcorn Chicken®	1	480	27	9	1410	39	6	22
Salad, Santa Fe Chicken	1	380	15	7	1180	29	6	30
Sandwich, Bacon Cheeseburger Toaster®	1	670	39	14	1390	52	3	29
Sandwich, Breaded Pork Fritter	1	640	33	6	840	66	7	22
Sandwich, Chicken Club Toaster®	1	740	46	11	1740	55	4	29
Sandwich, Chicken Strip	1	420	22	3.5	710	39	3	18
Sandwich, Fish	1	650	31	5	1160	71	7	22
Tacos	1 serv	340	20	6	360	35	4	8
Tater Tots	lg	370	23	4	790	36	4	3
Tater Tots w/ Cheese	lg	460	31	9	1260	39	4	7
Tater Tots w/ Chili & Cheese	lg	470	31	8	1110	41	5	8

ITEM DESCRIPTION	Serving Size	Calories	Total Fat (g)	Saturated Fat (g)	Sodium (mg)	Carbohydrates (g)	Fiber (g)	Protein (g)
Wrap, Chicken Strip	1	470	20	4.5	1310	54	4	22
Wrap, Fritos® Chili Cheese	1	670	38	13	1360	66	6	22
Wrap, Grilled Chicken	1	380	11	3	1440	44	3	29
TOPPINGS AND EXTRAS								
Bacon	1 serv	70	5	2	260	0	0	4
Cheese	1 serv	60	5	3	310	2	0	3
Chili	1 serv	50	3.5	1.5	160	2	1	3
Cole Slaw	1 serv	45	3	0.5	45	4	1	0
Green Chiles	1 serv	5	0	0	5	1	0	0
Jalapeño	1 serv	5	0	0	280	1	1	0
Nuts	1 serv	20	1.5	0	0	1	0	1
Onions, Grilled	1 serv	25	2	0	200	2	1	0

*Coffee products not currently available in all markets.
Consumer Information Center • 300 Johnny Bench Drive, Suite 400 • Oklahoma City, OK 73104 • 1-866-657-6642 (Toll-free)

SUBWAY

	Serving Size	Calories	Total Fat (g)	Saturated Fat (g)	Sodium (mg)	Carbohydrates (g)	Fiber (g)	Protein (g)
BEVERAGES								
Diet Fountain Soda	21 oz	<10	0	0	<40	0	0	0
Juice Box, Minute Maid®	1	100	0	0	15	24	0	0
Milk, Low Fat***	1	160	3.5	2.5	180	19	0	12
BREAKFAST ITEMS								
Flatbread, Black Forest Ham & Cheese	1	480	22	8	1530	46	3	27
Flatbread, Cheese	1	460	21	7	1170	45	3	23
Flatbread, Double Bacon & Cheese	1	560	28	11	1540	46	3	30
Flatbread, Mega	1	750	48	18	1650	46	3	34
Flatbread, Steak & Cheese	1	521	23	8	1470	48	3	32
Flatbread, Western w/ Cheese	1	490	22	8	1560	47	3	28
Sandwich w/ Cheese	6 in	420	18	7	1060	46	5	22
Sandwich w/ Double Bacon & Cheese	6 in	520	25	11	1440	47	5	29
Sandwich w/ Ham, Black Forest & Cheese	6 in	450	19	7	1450	47	5	27
Sandwich w/ Steak & Cheese	6 in	490	20	8	1400	48	5	31
Sandwich, Mega	6 in	720	45	18	1580	47	5	33
Sandwich, Western w/ Cheese	6 in	450	19	7	1460	48	5	27
DESSERTS								
Cookie, Chocolate Chip	1	210	10	6	150	30	1	2

ITEM DESCRIPTION	Serving Size	Calories	Total Fat (g)	Saturated Fat (g)	Sodium (mg)	Carbohydrates (g)	Fiber (g)	Protein (g)
Cookie, Chocolate Chunk**	1	220	10	5	100	30	<1	2
Cookie, Double Chocolate Chip**	1	210	10	6	170	30	1	2
Cookie, M & M® **	1	210	10	5	100	32	<1	2
Cookie, Oatmeal Raisin	1	200	8	4	170	30	1	3
Cookie, Peanut Butter**	1	220	12	5	190	26	1	4
Cookie, Sugar**	1	220	12	6	140	28	<1	2
Cookie, White Chip Macadamia Nut	1	220	11	5	160	29	<1	2
Pie, Apple**	1	250	10	2	290	37	1	0
DRESSINGS AND SPREADS								
Dressing, Italian, Fat Free	1	35	0	0	720	7	0	1
Dressing, Ranch	1	290	30	4.5	540	3	0	1
Mayonnaise	1 serv	110	12	2	80	0	0	0
Mayonnaise, Light	1 serv	50	5	1	100	<1	0	0
Mustard	2 tsp	5	0	0	115	<1	0	0
Olive Oil Blend	1 tsp	45	5	0	0	0	0	0
Ranch (on Sandwich)	1 serv	110	11	1.5	200	1	0	0
Red Wine Vinaigrette, Fat Free**	1 serv	30	0	0	340	6	0	0
Sauce, Chipotle Southwest	1 serv	100	10	1.5	220	1	0	0
Sauce, Honey Mustard, Fat Free	1 serv	30	0	0	115	7	0	0
Sauce, Sweet Onion, Fat Free	1 serv	40	0	0	85	9	0	0
Vinegar	1 tsp	0	0	0	0	0	0	0
SALADS								
Chicken Breast, Oven Roasted	1	130	2.5	0.5	280	10	4	20
Chicken Teriyaki, Sweet Onion	1	200	3	1	660	25	4	20
Ham	1	110	3	1	850	12	4	12
Roast Beef	1	140	3.5	1	500	10	4	21
Subway Club®	1	140	3.5	1	810	12	4	20
Turkey Breast	1	110	2	0.5	570	12	4	12
Turkey Breast & Ham	1	120	3	0.5	790	12	4	14
Veggie Delite®	1	50	1	0	65	10	4	3
SANDWICHES								
BLT	6 in	360	13	6	990	45	5	17
Cheesesteak, Big Philly	6 in	520	18	9	1710	54	6	39
Chicken & Bacon Ranch	6 in	580	28	10	1330	49	6	35

ITEM DESCRIPTION	Serving Size	Calories	Total Fat (g)	Saturated Fat (g)	Sodium (mg)	Carbohydrates (g)	Fiber (g)	Protein (g)
Chicken Breast, Oven Roasted	6 in	320	5	1.5	880	49	5	23
Chicken Teriyaki, Sweet Onion	6 in	380	4.5	1	1150	60	5	26
Cold Cut Combo	6 in	420	17	6	1590	48	5	21
Double Black Forest Ham	6 in	350	6	2	2120	50	5	27
Double Chicken & Bacon Ranch w/ Cheese	6 in	710	35	12	1720	50	6	55
Double Chicken, Oven Roasted	6 in	410	7	2	1220	53	6	38
Double Cold Cut Combo w/ Cheese	6 in	560	27	10	2420	51	5	31
Double Italian B.M.T. w/ Cheese	6 in	630	34	13	2990	50	6	34
Double Meatball Marinara w/ Cheese	6 in	890	40	15	2570	96	12	38
Double Roast Beef	6 in	400	7	2.5	1410	47	6	44
Double Spicy Italian	6 in	780	50	19	3170	50	6	34
Double Steak & Cheese	6 in	500	14	6	1980	54	6	41
Double Subway Club®	6 in	420	7	2.5	2040	50	5	43
Double Subway Melt® w/ Cheese	6 in	500	17	7	2580	52	5	39
Double Sweet Onion Chicken Teriyaki	6 in	490	7	1.5	1650	66	5	43
Double Turkey Breast	6 in	340	5	1	1550	50	5	27
Double Turkey Breast & Ham	6 in	360	6	1.5	2010	51	5	30
Flatbread, Chicken Breast, Oven Roasted	1	350	8	1.5	960	49	3	24
Flatbread, Ham, Black Forest	1	320	7	1.5	1410	47	3	18
Flatbread, Roast Beef	1	350	8	2	1050	45	3	27
Flatbread, Subway Club®	1	360	8	2	1370	47	3	26
Flatbread, Sweet Onion Chicken Teriyaki	1	410	8	1.5	1220	60	3	26
Flatbread, Turkey Breast	1	320	7	1	1130	47	3	18
Flatbread, Turkey Breast & Black Forest Ham	1	330	7	1.5	1350	47	3	20
Flatbread, Veggie Delite®	1	260	5	1	630	45	3	9
Ham, Black Forest	mini	180	2.5	0.5	670	31	3	10
Ham, Black Forest	6 in	290	4.5	1	1340	48	5	18
Italian B.M.T.®	6 in	450	20	8	1870	48	5	22
Meatball Marinara	6 in	580	23	9	1660	71	9	24
Roast Beef	6 in	320	5	1.5	980	46	5	26
Roast Beef	mini	200	3	1	500	30	4	15
Spicy Italian	6 in	530	28	11	1960	48	6	22

ITEM DESCRIPTION	Serving Size	Calories	Total Fat (g)	Saturated Fat (g)	Sodium (mg)	Carbohydrates (g)	Fiber (g)	Protein (g)
Steak & Cheese	6 in	390	10	4.5	1370	50	6	26
Subway Club®	6 in	330	5	1.5	1300	48	5	26
Subway Melt®	6 in	390	11	5	1670	49	5	25
The Feast w/ Cheese	6 in	550	23	9	2610	51	6	39
Tuna	6 in	540	30	6	1070	46	5	21
Turkey Breast	6 in	290	4	1	1050	48	5	18
Turkey Breast	mini	190	2.5	0.5	610	31	3	12
Turkey Breast & Black Forest Ham	6 in	300	4.5	1	1280	48	5	19
Veggie Delite®	6 in	230	2.5	0.5	550	45	5	9
Veggie Delite®	mini	150	1.5	0	280	30	3	6
SIDES AND SNACKS								
Apple Slices	1 pkg	35	0	0	0	9	2	0
Chips, Baked Lay's®	1 pkg	130	2	0	200	23	2	2
Yogurt, Dannon Light & Fit®	1 pkg	80	0	0	80	16	0	5
SOUPS**								
Broccoli & Cheese	10 oz	180	11	5	990	16	4	5
Chicken & Dumpling	10 oz	170	5	2	810	23	2	8
Chicken & Dumpling w/ Rosemary	10 oz	90	1.5	0.5	810	14	1	6
Chicken & Rice w/ Pork, Spanish Style	10 oz	110	2.5	1	980	16	1	6
Chicken Corn Chowder, Chipotle	10 oz	140	3	1.5	900	22	2	6
Chicken Noodle, Roasted	10 oz	80	2	0.5	950	12	1	6
Chicken Tortilla	10 oz	110	1.5	0.5	440	11	3	6
Chicken w/ Wild Rice	10 oz	230	11	3.5	900	26	1	6
Chili Con Carne	10 oz	340	11	5	950	35	10	20
Clam Chowder, New England Style	10 oz	150	5	1	990	20	4	6
Cream of Potato w/ Bacon	10 oz	240	13	5	870	26	3	5
Minestrone	10 oz	90	1	0	910	17	3	4
Tomato Garden Vegetable w/ Rotini	10 oz	90	0.5	0	820	20	3	3
Tomato Orzo, Fire-Roasted	10 oz	130	1	0.5	410	24	2	6
Vegetable Beef	10 oz	100	2	0.5	960	17	3	5
TOPPINGS AND EXTRAS								
Bacon	2 pcs	45	3.5	1.5	190	0	0	3
Banana Peppers	3 pcs	0	0	0	20	0	0	0
Bread, 9-Grain Wheat	6 in	210	2	0.5	410	41	4	8

ITEM DESCRIPTION	Serving Size	Calories	Total Fat (g)	Saturated Fat (g)	Sodium (mg)	Carbohydrates (g)	Fiber (g)	Protein (g)
Bread, Hearty Italian	6 in	220	2	1	390	41	2	8
Bread, Honey Oat	6 in	260	3	0.5	430	49	5	9
Bread, Italian Herbs & Cheese	6 in	250	5	2	590	41	2	10
Bread, Italian White	6 in	200	2	0.5	390	38	1	7
Bread, Mini Italian	1	130	1.5	0	260	26	1	5
Bread, Mini Wheat	1	140	1.5	0	270	28	3	5
Bread, Monterey Cheddar	6 in	240	5	3	460	39	1	10
Bread, Parmesan Oregano	6 in	220	2.5	1	620	41	2	8
Bread, Roasted Garlic	6 in	230	2.5	0.5	1360	45	2	8
Cheddar**	1 serv	60	5	3	100	0	0	4
Cheese, American, Processed	1 serv	40	3.5	2	200	1	0	2
Cheese, Monterey Cheddar, Shredded	1 serv	50	4.5	3	90	1	0	3
Cheese, Pepperjack**	1 serv	50	4	2.5	140	0	0	3
Cheese, Provolone**	1 serv	50	4	2	125	0	0	4
Cheese, Swiss**	1 serv	50	4.5	2.5	30	0	0	4
Chicken Patty, Roasted	1 serv	90	2.5	0.5	330	4	0	15
Chicken Strips	1 serv	80	1.5	0.5	210	0	0	16
Cucumbers	3 pcs	<5	0	0	0	<1	0	0
Egg Patty**	1 serv	110	8	2	360	3	1	9
Flatbread	1	240	5	1	480	41	2	8
Green Peppers	3 pcs	0	0	0	0	0	0	0
Ham	1 serv	60	2	0.5	790	2	0	9
Jalapeño Peppers	3 pcs	<5	0	0	70	0	0	0
Lettuce	1 serv	<5	0	0	0	0	0	0
Meat, Cold Cut Combo	1 serv	140	11	3.5	830	2	0	10
Meat, Italian BMT®	1 serv	180	14	5	1120	2	0	11
Meat, Subway Club®	1 serv	90	2.5	1	750	2	0	17
Meatballs	1 serv	310	17	6	910	25	4	13
Olives	3 pcs	<5	0	0	25	0	0	0
Onions	1 serv	5	0	0	0	1	0	0
Pickles	3 pcs	0	0	0	115	0	0	0
Pizza w/ Cheese	8 in	680	22	9	1070	96	4	32
Pizza w/ Cheese & Veggies	8 in	740	25	11	2110	100	5	36
Pizza w/ Pepperoni	8 in	790	32	13	1350	96	4	38

ITEM DESCRIPTION	Serving Size	Calories	Total Fat (g)	Saturated Fat (g)	Sodium (mg)	Carbohydrates (g)	Fiber (g)	Protein (g)
Pizza w/ Sausage	8 in	820	34	14	1420	97	4	39
Roast Beef	1 serv	80	2.5	1	430	1	0	18
Seafood Sensation**	1 serv	190	16	2.5	430	7	0	5
Steak, no Cheese	1 serv	112	4	2	560	4	0	15
Tomatoes	3 pcs	5	0	0	0	2	0	0
Tuna	1 serv	260	24	4	310	0	0	10
Turkey Breast	1 serv	50	1	0	500	2	0	9
Veggie Patty**	1 serv	160	5	0.5	520	12	3	15
Wrap**	1	310	8	2.5	610	51	1	8

A Registered Dietitian compiled this nutrition information from the following data: Nutrition analysis from Subway approved food manufacturers, an independent laboratory and the USDA National Nutrient Database for Standard Reference, Release #19. The nutrition information listed here is based on standard recipes and product formulations, however slight variations may occur due to the season of the year, use of an alternate supplier, region of the country, and/or small differences in product assembly.

** Regional and Limited Time Offer subs and menu items are only available in certain regions or at certain times of the year and ingredients and formulas may vary between restaurants. Nutritional information for these sandwiches is based on the most common formulas and ingredients.

† The Exchange Lists are the basis of a meal planning system designed by a committee of the American Diabetes Association and the American Dietetic Association. While designed primarily for people with diabetes and others who must follow special diets, the Exchange Lists are based on principles of good nutrition that apply to everyone.

‡ *** Values differ in California. See nutrition facts on milk container.

TACO BELL

BEVERAGES

ITEM DESCRIPTION	Serving Size	Calories	Total Fat (g)	Saturated Fat (g)	Sodium (mg)	Carbohydrates (g)	Fiber (g)	Protein (g)
Diet Pepsi**	16 oz	0	0	0	50	0	0	0
Dr Pepper**	16 oz	200	0	0	70	54	0	0
Fruit Punch, Tropicana**	16 oz	220	0	0	50	60	0	0
Frutista Freeze®, Mango Strawberry	1	250	0	0	10	62	0	0
Frutista Freeze®, Strawberry	1	230	0	0	55	57	0	0
Iced Tea, Lipton Raspberry**	16 oz	160	0	0	50	42	0	0
Mountain Dew Baja Blast**	16 oz	220	0	0	70	60	0	0
Mountain Dew**	16 oz	220	0	0	70	58	0	0
Pepsi**	16 oz	200	0	0	50	56	0	0
Pink Lemonade, Tropicana**	16 oz	200	0	0	210	54	0	0
Root Beer, Mug**	16 oz	200	0	0	30	52	0	0
Sierra Mist**	16 oz	200	0	0	40	54	0	0

MAIN MENU

ITEM DESCRIPTION	Serving Size	Calories	Total Fat (g)	Saturated Fat (g)	Sodium (mg)	Carbohydrates (g)	Fiber (g)	Protein (g)
Burrito Supreme® w/ Beef	1	410	15	7	1350	51	7	17
Burrito Supreme® w/ Chicken	1	380	12	5	1370	50	6	20
Burrito Supreme® w/ Fresco Chicken	1	330	8	2.5	1360	49	7	18
Burrito Supreme® w/ Fresco Steak	1	330	8	3	1250	48	7	16
Burrito Supreme® w/ Steak	1	380	12	5	1250	49	6	18

ITEM DESCRIPTION	Serving Size	Calories	Total Fat (g)	Saturated Fat (g)	Sodium (mg)	Carbohydrates (g)	Fiber (g)	Protein (g)
Burrito, 7-Layer	1	480	17	6	1350	66	10	17
Burrito, Bean	1	350	9	3.5	1190	54	8	13
Burrito, Beef & Potato †	1/2 lb	520	21	6	1730	67	6	15
Burrito, Beef Combo †	1/2 lb	440	18	7	1630	51	8	21
Burrito, Beef Fiesta	1	370	13	5	1200	49	4	14
Burrito, Cheesy Bean & Rice †	1/2 lb	470	20	6	1400	58	6	13
Burrito, Cheesy Double Beef	1	460	20	7	1620	52	5	18
Burrito, Chicken Fiesta	1	350	10	3.5	1220	47	3	18
Burrito, Chili Cheese	1	370	16	8	1060	40	3	16
Burrito, Fresco Bean	1	330	7	2.5	1200	54	9	12
Burrito, Fresco Fiesta Chicken	1	330	8	2.5	1240	48	3	16
Burrito, Grilled Stuft Beef	1	680	30	10	2120	76	9	27
Burrito, Grilled Stuft Chicken	1	640	23	7	2160	73	7	34
Burrito, Grilled Stuft Steak	1	630	25	8	1930	72	7	30
Burrito, Spicy Chicken	1	400	17	4	1190	48	3	14
Burrito, Steak Fiesta	1	340	11	4	1110	47	3	15
Caramel Apple Empanada	1	290	15	2.5	270	38	2	3
Chalupa Baja, Beef	1	410	27	6	780	30	4	13
Chalupa Baja, Chicken	1	390	23	4	800	29	3	17
Chalupa Baja, Steak	1	390	24	4.5	690	28	3	15
Chalupa Nacho Cheese w/ Beef	1	370	22	4.5	770	32	3	12
Chalupa Nacho Cheese w/ Chicken	1	350	18	3	790	30	2	16
Chalupa Nacho Cheese w/ Steak	1	340	19	3.5	670	30	2	14
Chalupa Supreme w/ Beef	1	370	21	6	630	31	3	14
Chalupa Supreme w/ Chicken	1	350	18	4	650	29	2	17
Chalupa Supreme w/ Steak	1	350	19	4.5	530	29	2	15
Cheese Roll-Up	1	200	10	5	490	19	1	9
Cinnamon Twists	1 serv	170	7	0	200	26	1	1
Crunchwrap Supreme®	1	540	22	7	1430	68	5	17
Crunchwrap Supreme®, Spicy Chicken	1	530	21	6	1370	67	4	19
Enchirito® w/ Beef	1	360	17	8	1420	34	7	18
Enchirito® w/ Chicken	1	340	13	7	1450	33	6	22
Enchirito® w/ Steak	1	330	14	7	1330	33	6	20
Gordita Baja® w/ Beef	1	340	19	5	780	29	4	13

ITEM DESCRIPTION	Serving Size	Calories	Total Fat (g)	Saturated Fat (g)	Sodium (mg)	Carbohydrates (g)	Fiber (g)	Protein (g)
Gordita Baja® w/ Chicken	1	320	16	3.5	800	28	3	17
Gordita Baja® w/ Steak	1	320	17	4	690	27	3	15
Gordita Nacho Cheese w/ Beef	1	300	14	4	770	31	3	12
Gordita Nacho Cheese w/ Chicken	1	280	11	2.5	800	29	2	16
Gordita Nacho Cheese w/ Steak	1	270	12	3	680	29	2	14
Gordita Supreme® w/ Beef	1	300	14	5	630	30	3	14
Gordita Supreme® w/ Chicken	1	280	11	3.5	650	29	2	17
Gordita Supreme® w/ Steak	1	270	11	4	540	28	2	15
MexiMelt®	1	280	14	7	860	22	3	15
Nachos	1 serv	330	21	3.5	530	32	2	4
Nachos BellGrande®	1 serv	760	42	8	1280	77	12	19
Nachos Supreme	1 serv	430	24	6	800	41	7	12
Nachos, Triple Layer	1 serv	340	18	2.5	720	38	6	7
Pizza, Mexican	1	530	30	8	1000	46	6	20
Quesadilla w/ Chicken	1	520	28	12	1420	40	3	28
Quesadilla w/ Steak	1	520	28	13	1300	39	3	26
Quesadilla, Cheese	1	470	26	12	1100	39	2	19
Taco Salad	1	600	31	9	1430	56	14	25
Taco Salad, Chicken Fiesta	1	780	36	7	1830	78	13	37
Taco Salad, Chicken Fiesta w/o Shell	1	420	16	5	1560	38	11	30
Taco Salad, Fiesta	1	840	45	11	1780	80	15	30
Taco Salad, Fiesta w/o Shell	1	460	23	9	1520	41	13	23
Taco Supreme®, Crunchy	1	200	12	5	380	15	3	9
Taco Supreme®, Double Decker®	1	350	15	6	830	40	7	15
Taco Supreme®, Soft Beef	1	240	11	5	650	23	3	11
Taco, Big Taste	1	420	22	6	1030	43	4	14
Taco, Crunchy	1	170	10	3.5	350	13	3	8
Taco, Double Decker®	1	320	13	5	810	38	6	14
Taco, Fresco Crunchy	1	150	8	2.5	370	13	3	7
Taco, Fresco Grilled Steak Soft	1	160	4.5	1.5	550	20	2	10
Taco, Fresco Ranchero Chicken Soft	1	170	4	1.5	730	21	3	12
Taco, Fresco Soft Beef	1	180	7	3	650	21	3	8
Taco, Grilled Steak Soft	1	260	15	4.5	640	20	2	12
Taco, Ranchero Chicken Soft	1	270	14	4	820	21	2	14

ITEM DESCRIPTION	Serving Size	Calories	Total Fat (g)	Saturated Fat (g)	Sodium (mg)	Carbohydrates (g)	Fiber (g)	Protein (g)
Taco, Soft Beef	1	200	9	4	630	21	3	10
Taco, Spicy Chicken Soft	1	170	6	2	580	20	2	10
Taquitos, Chicken, Grilled	1 serv	310	11	4.5	980	37	2	18
Taquitos, Steak, Grilled	1 serv	310	11	5	870	36	2	16
Tostada	1 serv	240	10	3.5	730	27	7	11
SIDES AND SNACKS								
Guacamole	1	70	5	1	180	5	2	1
Pintos 'n Cheese	1 serv	160	6	3	670	19	7	9
Potatoes, Cheesy Fiesta	1 serv	270	15	3	840	30	3	4
Rice, Mexican	1 serv	110	3	0	460	19	1	2
Salsa	1	15	0	0	160	3	0	0
Sour Cream	1	60	4	2.5	40	4	0	1

The Dietary Guidelines for Americans recommend limiting saturated fat to 20 grams and sodium to 2,300 milligrams for a typical adult eating 2,000 calories daily. Recommended limits may be higher or lower depending upon daily calorie consumption.

Product data is based on current U.S. formulations (based on zero grams trans fat canola frying oil) as of the date posted. Product formulations and nutritional values may differ for Taco Bell® Express and "multi-brand" (Kentucky Fried Chicken®/Taco Bell®, Taco Bell®/Pizza Hut®, and Taco Bell®/Long John Silver's®) menu items that may be based on a different type of oil, and for products outside the continental U.S. Although this data is based on standard portion guidelines, variation can be expected due to seasonal influences, minor differences in product assembly per restaurant, and other factors. Substitution of ingredients may alter nutritional values. Menu items and hours of availability may vary by location. Regional Menu items are available only at participating locations. Except for Taco Bell® Express, multi-brand menu items, limited time offerings, and test market menu items, single-brand menu products as of the date posted are included in this Nutrition Guide. For the most current U.S. nutritional information and for Taco Bell® Express, New York City only and multi-brand menu items, see www.tacobell.com. If you have any questions about Taco Bell® and nutrition or are particularly sensitive to specific ingredients or foods, please contact us at 1-800-TACO BELL or visit our Web site at www.tacobell.com.

* "Fresco Style" fat reduction varies per menu item and not all menu items will meet a 25% reduction in fat.

** Nutrition values for fountain beverages do not account for ice. Depending on the sodium content of the water where the beverage is dispensed, the actual sodium content may be higher or lower than the listed values.

† ¼ lb. claim for Beef Combo, Beef & Potato and Cheesy Bean & Rice Burritos is based on average weight. Individual product weights vary.

TIM HORTONS

BAKED ITEMS

Bagel, 12 Grain	1	330	9	1	580	52	6	10
Bagel, Blueberry	1	270	1	0	470	55	2	10
Bagel, Cinnamon Raisin	1	270	1	0.2	350	55	3	10
Bagel, Everything	1	280	2	0.3	460	53	2	10
Bagel, Onion	1	260	1.5	0.2	460	53	3	9
Bagel, Plain	1	260	1.5	0.2	450	52	2	9
Bagel, Poppy Seed	1	270	2	0.3	440	53	3	9
Bagel, Sesame Seed	1	270	2.5	0.4	430	53	3	9
Bagel, Wheat 'N Honey	1	300	3	0.4	600	60	4	10
Biscuit, Plain Tea	1	250	9	2	590	35	1	5
Biscuit, Raisin Tea	1	290	10	2	590	45	2	6
Buns*, Country White	1 serv	240	1	0.3	510	49	2	9

ITEM DESCRIPTION	Serving Size	Calories	Total Fat (g)	Saturated Fat (g)	Sodium (mg)	Carbohydrates (g)	Fiber (g)	Protein (g)
Buns*, Country Whole Wheat	1 serv	230	1	0.3	490	46	4	10
Cinnamon Roll w/ Frosting	1	470	25	12	380	57	2	4
Cinnamon Roll w/ Glaze	1	420	23	11	360	50	2	4
Cookie, Caramel Chocolate Pecan	1	230	11	5	290	32	1	3
Cookie, Chocolate Chunk	1	230	9	6	260	35	1	2
Cookie, Oatmeal Raisin Spice	1	220	8	5	260	35	1	3
Cookie, Peanut Butter	1	280	16	7	260	27	2	6
Cookie, Triple Chocolate	1	250	13	8	220	31	2	3
Cookie, White Chocolate Macadamia Nut	1	240	12	6	270	31	1	3
Croissant, Cheese	1	230	14	8	290	19	1	8
Croissant, Plain	1	200	11	5	210	21	0	5
Danish, Cherry Cheese	1	230	10	4.5	200	27	0	5
Danish, Chocolate	1	340	16	8	180	42	2	6
Danish, Maple Pecan	1	290	12	4.5	190	37	0	5
Donut, Blueberry	1	230	8	3.5	210	36	1	4
Donut, Boston Cream	1	250	8	3.5	260	40	1	4
Donut, Canadian Maple	1	260	8	3.5	260	43	1	4
Donut, Chocolate Dip	1	210	8	3.5	190	32	1	4
Donut, Chocolate Glazed	1	260	10	4.5	300	39	2	4
Donut, Honey Cruller	1	320	19	9	220	37	0	1
Donut, Honey Dip	1	210	8	3.5	190	33	1	4
Donut, Maple Dip	1	210	8	3.5	190	32	1	4
Donut, Old Fashion Glazed	1	320	19	9	230	35	1	3
Donut, Old Fashion Plain	1	260	19	9	230	20	1	3
Donut, Sour Cream Plain	1	270	17	8	230	27	1	3
Donut, Strawberry	1	230	8	3.5	220	36	1	4
Donut, Strawberry Vanilla	1	310	8	3.5	220	55	1	4
Donut, Walnut Crunch	1	360	23	10	320	35	1	4
Dutchie	1	250	10	4.5	210	38	1	4
Fritter, Apple	1	300	11	5	350	49	2	4
Fritter, Blueberry	1	330	10	4.5	340	55	2	6
Muffin, Banana Nut	1	390	17	2	510	56	2	6
Muffin, Blueberry	1	330	11	1.5	580	55	2	4
Muffin, Blueberry Bran	1	300	10	1	770	53	5	6

ITEM DESCRIPTION	Serving Size	Calories	Total Fat (g)	Saturated Fat (g)	Sodium (mg)	Carbohydrates (g)	Fiber (g)	Protein (g)
Muffin, Blueberry, Low Fat	1	290	2.5	0.5	750	62	2	4
Muffin, Chocolate Chip	1	430	16	5	580	69	2	5
Muffin, Cranberry Blueberry Bran	1	290	10	1.5	710	51	5	5
Muffin, Cranberry Fruit	1	350	12	1.5	560	59	2	4
Muffin, Cranberry, Low Fat	1	290	2.5	0.5	750	62	2	4
Muffin, Fruit Explosion	1	360	11	1.5	550	61	2	4
Muffin, Raisin Bran	1	360	10	1.5	790	65	6	6
Muffin, Strawberry Sensation	1	350	11	1.5	580	61	1	4
Muffin, Wheat Carrot	1	400	19	2.5	660	55	4	6
Muffin, Whole Grain Raspberry	1	400	17	4	580	58	5	5
Timbits®, Apple Fritter	1	50	1.5	1	55	9	0	1
Timbits®, Chocolate Glazed	1	70	2.5	1	75	10	0	1
Timbits®, Dutchie	1	50	2	1	40	9	0	1
Timbits®, Honey Dip	1	60	2	1	50	9	0	1
Timbits®, Lemon	1	60	2	1	50	9	0	1
Timbits®, Old Fashion Plain	1	70	5	2.5	60	5	0	1
Timbits®, Raspberry	1	60	2	1	50	10	0	1
Timbits®, Sour Cream Glazed	1	90	4.5	2	65	12	0	1
Timbits®, Strawberry	1	60	2	1	55	10	0	1
Timbits®, Blueberry	1	60	2	1	50	10	0	1
BEVERAGES								
Apple Juice	1 serv	130	0	0	30	32	0	0
Café Mocha	10 oz	180	8	6	170	27	1	1
Cappuccino, English Toffee	10 oz	240	7	6	220	41	2	4
Cappuccino, French Vanilla	10 oz	250	8	7	240	41	1	4
Coffee w/ Cream & Sugar	10 oz	75	3.5	2	15	9	0	1
Coffee, Decaf w/ Cream & Sugar	10 oz	75	3.5	2	15	9	0	1
Flavour Shot	1 serv	4	0	0	0	1	0	0
Hot Chocolate	10 oz	240	6	5	360	45	2	2
Hot Smoothie	10 oz	260	10	9	200	39	2	5
Iced Cappuccino	10 oz	250	11	6	50	33	0	2
Iced Cappuccino w/ Milk	10 oz	150	1.5	1	35	32	0	3
Orange Juice	1 serv	140	0	0	30	35	0	1
Tea w/ Milk and Sugar	10 oz	50	1	0.5	20	10	0	1

ITEM DESCRIPTION	Serving Size	Calories	Total Fat (g)	Saturated Fat (g)	Sodium (mg)	Carbohydrates (g)	Fiber (g)	Protein (g)
BREAKFAST ITEMS*								
Bagel BELT™	1	440	14	6	940	59	3	21
Hashbrown	1	100	5	0.5	210	12	1	1
Sandwich w/ Bacon, Egg, Cheese	1	410	23	14	780	35	1	16
Sandwich w/ Egg & Cheese	1	360	19	13	700	34	1	13
Sandwich w/ Sausage, Egg & Cheese	1	510	33	18	950	35	1	18
DRESSINGS AND SPREADS								
Cream Cheese, Herb & Garlic	1 serv	141	13	8	228	2	0	3
Cream Cheese, Light Plain	1 serv	100	8	5	216	2	0	4
Cream Cheese, Light Strawberry	1 serv	100	6	4	170	8	0	3
Cream Cheese, Plain	1 serv	144	14	9	179	2	0	3
MAIN MENU								
Beans, Baked	1 serv	270	5	1.5	1140	47	12	10
Chili	1 serv	300	19	7	1320	17	4	26
Sandwich, BLT	1	450	18	5	850	53	2	18
Sandwich, Chicken Club, Toasted	1	440	7	2.5	1070	70	2	25
Sandwich, Chicken Salad	1	380	9	1.5	980	54	3	20
Sandwich, Egg Salad	1	390	13	3	780	52	2	17
Sandwich, Ham & Swiss	1	440	12	5	1690	56	3	28
Sandwich, Turkey Bacon Club	1	440	8	2.5	1730	63	2	30
Soup, Beef Noodle	1	130	1.5	0.4	930	23	1	6
Soup, Chicken Noodle	1	120	2	1	820	18	1	5
Soup, Cream of Broccoli	1	160	9	4	820	16	1	6
Soup, Creamy Field Mushroom	1	150	3	2	1080	28	1	3
Soup, Minestrone	1	120	3	0.4	750	24	2	4
Soup, Potato Bacon	1	250	13	6	790	23	1	6
Soup, Split Pea w/ Ham	1	150	2.5	2.5	930	27	5	8
Soup, Turkey & Wild Rice	1	120	1.5	0.2	1000	21	1	3
Soup, Vegetable	1	70	0.4	0.1	930	14	3	4
Soup, Vegetable Beef Barley	1	110	1.5	0.3	930	21	2	4
Yogurt, Creamy Vanilla	1	160	2.5	1.5	45	33	2	4
Yogurt, Strawberry	1	140	2.5	1.5	50	27	2	4

* All nutritional information is based on regular sized sandwiches and standard ingredient servings. Timbits, Tim's Own, and Bagel BELT are all trademarks of The TDL Marks Corporation.

WENDY'S

BEVERAGES

ITEM DESCRIPTION	Serving Size	Calories	Total Fat (g)	Saturated Fat (g)	Sodium (mg)	Carbohydrates (g)	Fiber (g)	Protein (g)
Cherry Coke®	sm	170	0	0	10	45	0	0
Coca-Cola®	sm	160	0	0	0+	45	0	0
Coffee	1	0	0	0	0	0	0	0
Coffee Creamer	1	20	2	1	10	0	0	0
Coke Zero™	sm	0	0	0	10+	0	0	0
Creme Soda, Barq's Red	sm	190	0	0	30+	49	0	0
Diet Coke, Caffeine Free	sm	0	0	0	15+	0	0	0
Diet Coke®	sm	0	0	0	15+	0	0	0
Dr Pepper®	sm	200	0	0	50+	54	0	0
Fanta® Grape	sm	190	0	0	10+	49	0	0
Fanta® Punch	sm	170	0	0	20	45	0	0
Fanta® Strawberry	sm	190	0	0	0+	49	0	0
Fanta® Orange	sm	180	0	0	25+	49	0	0
Frosty™ Float, Vanilla w/ Coca-Cola	1	380	7	4.5	160	75	0	7
Frosty™ Shake, Chocolate Fudge	sm	410	11	7	240	69	1	8
Frosty™ Shake, Strawberry	sm	390	11	7	170	65	0	7
Frosty™ Shake, Vanilla Bean	sm	380	10	6	170	65	0	7
Frosty™, Coffee Toffee Twisted Chocolate	1	550	21	15	240	83	1	9
Frosty™, Coffee Toffee Twisted Vanilla	1	540	20	15	270	83	1	9
Frosty™, Twisted Chocolate w/ M&M's®	1	560	19	12	180	86	1	10
Frosty™, Twisted Chocolate w/ Nestle® Toll House® Cookie Dough	1	480	16	10	220	77	1	10
Frosty™, Twisted Chocolate w/ Oreo®	1	450	14	7	300	72	1	10
Frosty™, Twisted Vanilla w/ M&M's®	1	550	19	12	210	86	1	10
Frosty™, Twisted Vanilla w/ Nestle® Toll House® Cookie Dough	1	480	16	10	240	77	1	9
Frosty™, Twisted Vanilla w/ Oreo®	1	440	14	6	320	72	1	9
Frosty™, Vanilla	1	310	8	5	180	52	0	8
Frosty™, Chocolate	sm	320	8	5	150	52	0	9
Frosty™, Cino	sm	390	10	6	170	62	0	7
Hi-C®, Flashin' Fruit Punch	sm	170	0	0	15+	45	0	0

ITEM DESCRIPTION	Serving Size	Calories	Total Fat (g)	Saturated Fat (g)	Sodium (mg)	Carbohydrates (g)	Fiber (g)	Protein (g)
Hi-C®, Orange Lavaburst	sm	180	0	0	15+	49	0	0
Hi-C®, Poppin' Pink	sm	160	0	0	65+	41	0	0
Iced Tea, Lemon Sweetened Nestea®	sm	120	0	0	15	31	0	0
Iced Tea, Raspberry Nestea®	sm	130	0	0	15	32	0	0
Iced Tea, Sweetened Nestea®	sm	100	0	0	20	28	0	0
Iced Tea, Unsweetened Nestea®	sm	0	0	0	25	0	0	0
Lemonade, Minute Maid®	sm	160	0	0	65+	41	0	0
Lemonade, Minute Maid® Light	sm	10	0	0	15+	2	0	0
Mello Yellow®	sm	180	0	0	10+	45	0	0
Milk, Nesquik® Low Fat	1	100	2.5	1.5	120	12	0	8
Milk, Nesquik® Low Fat Chocolate	1	170	2.5	1.5	160	29	1	8
Pibb Xtra®	sm	160	0	0	25+	45	0	0
Powerade Mountain Blast	sm	100	0	0	90	28	0	0
Powerade® Fruit Punch	sm	100	0	0	90	28	0	0
Root Beer, Barq's®	sm	180	0	0	35+	49	0	0
Root Beer, Caffeine Free Barq's®	sm	180	0	0	35+	49	0	0
Sprite Zero™ Fountain	sm	5	0	0	10	0	0	0
Sprite®	sm	160	0	0	35+	41	0	0
Sugar	1 pkg	15	0	0	0	3	0	0
Sweetener, Non-Nutritive	1	5	0	0	0	1	0	0
Tea	1	0	0	0	0	0	0	0
Tea, Sweet	sm	100	0	0	10	26	0	0
Vault™	sm	180	0	0	15+	45	0	0
DRESSINGS AND SPREADS								
Dressing, Balsamic Vinaigrette**	1 pkg	90	6	1	380	8	0	0
Dressing, Caesar Supreme	1 pkg	120	13	2	200	1	0	1
Dressing, Chunky Blue Cheese**	1 pkg	230	24	5	370	2	0	2
Dressing, French Fat Free**	1 pkg	70	0	0	170	17	1	0
Dressing, Honey Dijon	1 pkg	250	24	3.5	330	9	0	1
Dressing, Honey Dijon Light*	1 pkg	100	5	1	280	13	1	1
Dressing, Italian Vinaigrette**	1 pkg	130	11	1.5	320	8	0	0
Dressing, Oriental Sesame	1 pkg	170	10	1.5	360	19	0	1
Dressing, Ranch	1 pkg	200	20	3	340	3	0	1
Dressing, Ranch Ancho Chipotle	1 pkg	90	8	1.5	240	3	0	1

ITEM DESCRIPTION	Serving Size	Calories	Total Fat (g)	Saturated Fat (g)	Sodium (mg)	Carbohydrates (g)	Fiber (g)	Protein (g)
Dressing, Ranch Light**	1 pkg	90	8	1.5	360	4	0	1
Dressing, Thousand Island**	1 pkg	290	28	4.5	530	9	0	1
Ketchup	1 pkg	10	0	0	115	3	0	0
Mayonnaise	1 serv	40	3.5	0.5	55	1	0	0
Mustard	1 serv	5	0	0	50	0	0	0
Sauce, Barbecue	1 pkg	45	0	0	160	11	0	1
Sauce, Honey Mustard	1 pkg	130	12	2	220	6	0	0
Sauce, Honey Mustard (on Sandwich)	1 serv	40	3.5	0	60	3	0	0
Sauce, Ranch (on Sandwich)	1 serv	35	3.5	0.5	70	1	0	0
Sauce, Ranch Heartland	1 pkg	160	17	2.5	220	1	0	0
Sauce, Sweet & Sour	1 pkg	50	0	0	120	12	0	0
KIDS MENU								
Cheeseburger	kid	260	11	5	700	26	1	15
Chicken Sandwich, Crispy	kid	340	15	3	680	35	2	15
French Fries***	kid	210	10	2	190	27	3	3
Hamburger	kid	220	8	3	490	25	1	12
MAIN MENU								
Burger, Baconator®	1	830	51	23	1880	35	1	56
Burger, Double w/ Everything & Cheese	1	700	40	17	1440	38	2	47
Burger, Single w/ Everything	1	430	20	7	870	38	2	25
Burger, Triple w/ Everything & Cheese	1	970	60	27	2010	39	2	69
Cheeseburger	jr	270	11	5	700	26	1	15
Cheeseburger Deluxe	jr	300	14	6	730	28	2	15
Cheeseburger w/ Bacon	jr	310	16	6	670	25	1	17
Chicken Club Sandwich	1	550	26	8	1290	48	2	34
Chicken Fillet Sandwich, Homestyle	1	440	16	3	1050	47	2	25
Chicken Fillet Sandwich, Spicy	1	440	16	3	1200	49	2	26
Chicken Go Wrap, Grilled	1	250	10	3	730	24	1	17
Chicken Go Wrap, Homestyle	1	310	15	4.5	800	30	1	15
Chicken Go Wrap, Spicy	1	320	15	4	880	30	1	16
Chicken Grill Sandwich, Ultimate	1	320	7	1.5	950	36	2	28
Chicken Nuggets	4 pcs	190	13	3	380	9	0	9
Chicken Nuggets	5 pcs	230	16	3.5	480	11	0	12
Chicken Sandwich, Crispy	1	360	18	3.5	710	36	2	15

ITEM DESCRIPTION	Serving Size	Calories	Total Fat (g)	Saturated Fat (g)	Sodium (mg)	Carbohydrates (g)	Fiber (g)	Protein (g)
Chili	sm	190	6	2.5	830	19	5	14
Chili	lg	280	9	3.5	1240	29	7	21
French Fries***	med	420	20	4	380	55	5	5
Hamburger	jr	230	8	3	490	26	1	13
Hamburger, Double Stack™	1	360	18	8	810	26	1	23
Mandarin Orange	1 cup	80	0	0	15	19	1	1
Potato, Baked	1	270	0	0	25	61	7	7
Potato, Baked w/ Sour Cream & Chives	1	320	3.5	2	50	63	7	8
Salad	side	35	0	0	25	8	2	1
Salad, Caesar	side	70	4	2	170	4	2	6
Salad, Chicken BLT	1	470	27	10	1210	23	3	35
Salad, Chicken Caesar	1	180	4	2	690	8	3	28
Salad, Mandarin Chicken®	1	180	2	0.5	630	16	2	24
Salad, Southwest Taco	1	400	22	11	1140	26	7	27
TOPPINGS AND EXTRAS**								
Almonds, Roasted	1 serv	130	11	1	70	4	2	5
Bacon	1pc	15	1	0	50	0	0	1
Bun, Premium	1	160	2	0	280	31	1	5
Bun, Sandwich	1	120	1.5	0	210	23	1	4
Buttery Best Spread	1 serv	50	5	1	95	0	0	0
Cheese, American	1	70	5	3.5	320	1	0	3
Cheese, American Jr.	1	40	3.5	2	200	0	0	2
Cheese, Shredded Cheddar	1 serv	70	6	3	105	1	0	4
Cheese, Swiss	1	70	6	3.5	85	0	0	5
Chicken Fillet, Homestyle	1	230	11	2	720	14	0	20
Chicken Fillet, Spicy	1	240	10	2	870	16	0	20
Chicken Grill Fillet	1	110	1.5	0	610	1	0	23
Chicken Patty, Crispy	1	210	14	3	460	12	1	11
Crispy Noodles	1 serv	70	2.5	0	190	10	0	1
Croutons, Homestyle Garlic	1 serv	70	2.5	0	125	9	0	2
Hamburger Patty****	1/4 lb	200	14	6	250	0	0	19
Hamburger Patty, Jr.	1	90	6	3	110	0	0	8
Lettuce Leaf	1	0	0	0	0	0	0	0
Onion	4 pcs	5	0	0	0	1	0	0

ITEM DESCRIPTION	Serving Size	Calories	Total Fat (g)	Saturated Fat (g)	Sodium (mg)	Carbohydrates (g)	Fiber (g)	Protein (g)
Pickles, Dill	4 pcs	0	0	0	140	0	0	0
Saltine Crackers	1 serv	25	0.5	0	80	5	0	1
Seasoning, Hot Chili	1 serv	5	0	0	270	1	0	0
Sour Cream, Reduced Fat Acidified	1 serv	45	3.5	2	25	2	0	1
Tomato	1 slice	5	0	0	0	1	0	0
Tortilla	1	130	3	1	320	21	1	3
Tortilla Strips, Seasoned	1 serv	110	5	1	160	13	1	2

* Toppings and Salad Dressings listed separately. ** Not available in all locations. ***Recommended portion sizes. French fries are individually portioned at every restaurant. Variations will exist from restaurant to restaurant.

To determine approximate nutritional information for a Kids' Meal size soft drink, multiply by 0.6; Value soft drink, multiply by 0.8; Medium soft drink, multiply by 1.5; Large soft drink, multiply by 2.0. To determine approximate nutritional information for a Jr. Frosty, multiply the small by 0.5; for a Medium Frosty, multiply the small by 1.3; for a Large Frosty, multiply the small by 1.7.

+ The sodium value will vary based on the level of sodium in your city's water supply.

**** Approximate weight before cooking.

** Note: For your custom sandwich order, add or subtract the nutritional value of any of the following to the totals below.

WHITE CASTLE

BEVERAGES

	Serving Size	Calories	Total Fat (g)	Saturated Fat (g)	Sodium (mg)	Carbohydrates (g)	Fiber (g)	Protein (g)
Apple Juice, Minute Maid***	1	100	0	0	15	23	0	0
Big Red***	sm (21 oz)	270	0	0	60	67	0	0
Cherry Coca-Cola***	sm (21 oz)	230	0	0	10	64	0	0
Coca-Cola Classic***	sm (21 oz)	220	0	0	10	61	0	0
Coffee	med (16 oz)	5	0	0	0	1	0	0
Coke Zero***	sm (21 oz)	0	0	0	10	0	0	0
Crave Cooler Coke***	sm (21 oz)	150	0	0	15	41	0	0
Crave Cooler Fanta Wild Cherry***	sm (21 oz)	150	0	0	10	41	0	0
Cream Soda, Barq's Red***	sm (21 oz)	260	0	0	40	69	0	0
Diet Coke***	sm (21 oz)	0	0	0	20	0	0	0
Diet Coke, Caffeine Free***	sm (21 oz)	0	0	0	20	0	0	0
Fanta Grape Soda***	sm (21 oz)	260	0	0	20	68	0	0
Fanta Orange Soda***	sm (21 oz)	240	0	0	20	64	0	0
Fanta Strawberry Soda***	sm (21 oz)	260	0	0	0	69	0	0
Half & Half	1 serv	15	1.5	0	15	0	0	0
Hi-C, Flashing Fruit Punch***	sm (21 oz)	240	0	0	20	63	0	0
Hi-C, Orange Lavaburst***	sm (21 oz)	250	0	0	0	67	0	0
Hi-C, Poppin' Pink Lemonade Pink***	sm (21 oz)	220	0	0	90	57	0	0

ITEM DESCRIPTION	Serving Size	Calories	Total Fat (g)	Saturated Fat (g)	Sodium (mg)	Carbohydrates (g)	Fiber (g)	Protein (g)
Hot Chocolate	med (16 oz)	300	8	1	410	55	<1	2
Iced Tea, Sweetened w/ Lemon	sm (21 oz)	170	0	0	20	46	0	0
Iced Tea, Unsweetened	sm (21 oz)	0	0	0	30	0	0	0
Lemonade, Raspberry Minute Maid***	sm (21 oz)	290	0	0	5	78	0	0
Orange Juice NTC, Minute Maid***	1	140	0	0	0	33	0	2
Orange Juice, Minute Maid***	1	140	0	0	21	33	0	2
Pibb Xtra***	sm (21 oz)	220	0	0	30	59	0	0
Powerade, Mountain Blast***	sm (21 oz)	140	0	0	119	38	0	0
Root Beer, Barq's***	sm (21 oz)	250	0	0	55	68	0	0
Sprite***	sm (21 oz)	220	0	0	50	59	0	0
Tea, Hot	med (16 oz)	0	0	0	0	0	0	0
Vault***	sm (21 oz)	260	0	0	20	64	0	0
BREAKFAST ITEMS								
Bacon & Cheese Sandwich	1	150	7	3	470	14	<1	7
Bacon & Egg Sandwich	1	210	12	3.5	410	14	<1	12
Bacon Sandwich	1	120	5	2	340	13	<1	5
Bacon, Egg & Cheese Sandwich	1	230	14	5	540	14	<1	13
Bologna & Cheese Sandwich	1	190	11	4	570	15	<1	7
Bologna & Egg Sandwich	1	260	16	5	620	16	<1	12
Bologna, Egg & Cheese Sandwich	1	280	18	6	740	16	<1	14
Egg & Cheese Sandwich	1	190	10	4	350	14	<1	10
Egg Sandwich	1	160	8	2.5	220	14	<1	9
Hamburger w/ Cheese	1	160	8	4	310	14	<1	8
Hamburger w/ Egg	1	240	14	5	360	15	<1	13
Hamburger w/ Egg & Cheese	1	260	16	6	480	15	<1	14
Sausage & Cheese Sandwich	1	250	17	7	590	14	<1	9
Sausage & Egg Sandwich	1	320	23	8	530	14	<1	14
Sausage Sandwich	1	220	15	6	460	13	<1	8
Sausage, Egg & Cheese Sandwich	1	340	25	9	660	14	<1	15
DRESSINGS AND SPREADS								
Butter	1 pkg	30	3.5	2.5	30	0	0	0
Cream Cheese	1 pkg	100	10	6	110	0	0	2
Dipping Sauce, Barbecue	1 pkg	35	0.5	0	390	8	0	0

ITEM DESCRIPTION	Serving Size	Calories	Total Fat (g)	Saturated Fat (g)	Sodium (mg)	Carbohydrates (g)	Fiber (g)	Protein (g)
Dipping Sauce, Cheese	1 pkg	130	10	3.5	560	6	0	3
Dipping Sauce, Honey Mustard, Fat Free	1 pkg	50	0	0	120	13	0	0
Dipping Sauce, Marinara	1 pkg	15	0	0	260	3	0	1
Dipping Sauce, Nacho Cheese	1 pkg	50	4	1	400	3	0	0
Dipping Sauce, Seafood	1 pkg	30	0	0	340	7	0	0
Dipping Sauce, White Castle Zesty Zing	1 pkg	120	11	1.5	190	4	0	0
Dressing, Ranch	1 pkg	150	17	2.5	200	1	0	0
Jam, Strawberry	1 pkg	40	0	0	0	10	0	0
Jelly, Grape	1 pkg	35	0	0	0	9	0	0
Ketchup	1 pkg	10	0	0	100	3	0	0
Lemon Juice	1 pkg	5	0	0	0	1	0	0
Mayonnaise	1 pkg	70	7	1	55	0	0	0
Sauce, Barbecue	1 pkg	15	0	0	130	3	0	0
Sauce, Honey Mustard, Fat Free	1 pkg	20	0	0	50	5	0	0
Sauce, Hot	1 pkg	5	0	0	170	1	<1	0
Sauce, Tartar	1 pkg	25	2.5	0	85	1	0	0
Syrup, Maple	1 pkg	120	0	0	25	31	0	0
MAIN MENU								
Cheeseburger	1	170	9	4	330	15	<1	7
Cheeseburger, Bacon	1	200	11	5	480	15	<1	10
Cheeseburger, Bacon Jalapeño	1	210	12	6	480	15	<1	11
Cheeseburger, Jalapeño	1	180	10	4.5	380	15	<1	8
Chicken Breast Sandwich	1	180	6	1	580	21	1	11
Chicken Breast Sandwich w/ Cheese	1	210	8	2.5	710	21	1	13
Chicken Ring Sandwich	1	180	8	2	380	19	<1	7
Chicken Ring Sandwich w/ Cheese	1	200	10	3	500	19	<1	8
Chicken Supreme	1	230	10	3.5	860	21	1	14
Double Cheeseburger	1	300	17	8	590	23	1	14
Double Cheeseburger, Bacon	1	370	22	10	880	23	1	19
Double Cheeseburger, Jalapeño	1	320	19	9	680	23	1	15
Double Fish w/ Cheese	1	340	15	4.5	790	32	1	18
Double Fish, no Cheese	1	290	11	1.5	540	32	1	16

ITEM DESCRIPTION	Serving Size	Calories	Total Fat (g)	Saturated Fat (g)	Sodium (mg)	Carbohydrates (g)	Fiber (g)	Protein (g)
Double White Castle	1	250	13	5	340	22	1	11
Fish Sandwich	1	160	6	1	300	18	<1	8
Fish Sandwich w/ Cheese	1	190	8	2	430	20	<1	10
Pulled Pork Barbecue Sandwich	1	170	4.5	1.5	490	24	1	9
Surf & Turf w/ Cheese	1	390	22	9	670	28	1	20
Surf & Turf, no Cheese	1	340	18	6	420	28	1	17
Traditional Bun w/ Cheese	1	100	3.5	2	280	13	<1	3
White Castle	1	140	7	2.5	210	14	<1	6
SIDES AND SNACKS								
Chicken Rings	3 pcs	150	10	2	340	8	0	8
Chicken Rings	20 pcs	1020	66	13	2290	56	2	50
Clam Strips	reg	250	22	3.5	620	5	0	8
Fish Nibblers	reg	280	16	3.5	870	24	5	19
French Fries	reg	310	15	3	250	39	4	4
Mozzarella Cheese Sticks	3 pcs	250	14	6	750	22	1	10
Mozzarella Cheese Sticks	5 pcs	420	23	10	1240	37	2	17
Onion Chips	reg	480	23	4	670	62	2	7
Onion Rings	reg	400	21	3.5	460	49	1	4
Onion Rings	reg	200	9	1.5	220	28	1	2
TOPPINGS AND EXTRAS								
Bacon	1 pc	50	4	1.5	190	0	0	3
Bologna	1	80	8	2.5	300	1	0	3
Bun, Golden	1	70	1	0	150	13	<1	2
Bun, Traditional	1	70	1	0	150	13	<1	2
Cheese, American	1 pc	25	2	1.5	125	0	0	1
Cheese, Jalapeño	1 pc	35	3	2	170	0	0	2
Egg	1	90	7	2	70	0	0	6
Hamburger Meat	1	70	6	2.5	15	0	0	4
Hashbrown	1	170	11	4	380	16	2	2
Sausage	1	150	14	5	310	0	0	5

* Sodium values may vary depending on restaurant preparation and on the water used for beverages.
  ** Sandwich weight based on the weight before cooking.
  *** Nutrition based on 1/3 cup of ice for beverages.
  Nutrition Information on all Coca-Cola products provided by the Coca-Cola Company. FDA Rounding Rules used.

NOTES